INTERRUPTIONS IN FAMILY HEALTH DURING PREGNANCY

A Programmed Text

BETTY ANN ANDERSON, R.N., M.A.

Formerly Assistant Professor of Nursing
Long Island University School of Nursing, New York

MERCEDES E. CAMACHO, R.N., M.A.

Director of Hospital Review
Kings County Health Care Review Organization, New York

JEANNE STARK, R.N., Ed.D.

Dean of Instruction
Miami Dade Community College, Miami

VOLUME TWO IN

THE CHILDBEARING FAMILY

SECOND EDITION

McGRAW-HILL BOOK COMPANY

New York St. Louis San Francisco Auckland Bogotá
Düsseldorf Johannesburg London Madrid Mexico Montreal
New Delhi Panama Paris São Paulo Singapore
Sydney Tokyo Toronto

Notice

Medicine is an ever-changing science. As new research and clinical experience broaden our knowledge, changes in treatment and drug therapy are required. The editors and the publisher of this work have made every effort to ensure that the drug dosage schedules herein are accurate and in accord with the standards accepted at the time of publication. Readers are advised, however, to check the product information sheet included in the package of each drug they plan to administer to be certain that changes have not been made in the recommended dose or in the contraindications for administration. This recommendation is of particular importance in regard to new or infrequently used drugs.

Interruptions in Family Health during Pregnancy,
Volume Two in The Childbearing Family

1 2 3 4 5 6 7 8 9 0 D O D O 7 8 3 2 1 0 9 8

Library of Congress Cataloging in Publication Data

Anderson, Betty Ann.
  Interruptions in family health during pregnancy.

  (Her The childbearing family; v. 2)
  Includes bibliographies and index.
      1. Obstetrical nursing—Programmed instruction.
2. Pregnancy, Complications of—Programmed
instruction.   I. Camacho, Mercedes E., joint
author.   II.   Stark, Jeanne, joint author.
III. Title.
RG951.A66   1979   vol. 2   618.2'007'7s   [618.3'007'7]   78–18870
ISBN 0–07–001684–4

This book was set in Times Roman by Offset Composition Services, Inc. The editor was Mary Ann Richter and
the production supervisor was Milton J. Heiberg.
R. R. Donnelley & Sons Company was printer and binder.

CONTENTS

PREFACE

The focus in the second volume is on the critical situation that places a family at high risk and on application of the nursing process in this situation. A chapter has been added on anemias during pregnancy. The second edition of this volume reflects the exciting recent discoveries in perinatology, concerning immunological responses and the new methods of fetal assessment.

This volume continues the innovative approach of the first volume: following pertinent chapters, specific clinical behaviors have been identified and serve as a guide for the clinical competencies. Knowledge gained from the first volume is utilized in this second volume when interruptions of family health status are presented. Together Volumes One and Two provide complete coverage of the childbearing cycle, and family aspects are incorporated throughout. The level of the texts is applicable to any and all nursing students.

Through the use of a programmed text the learner actively participates in acquisition of the subject matter. The unique aspect of these texts lies in the use of two methods of programming—linear and branching (scatter)—to provide reinforcement of learning throughout. Students are able to self-pace their learning. The linear method enhances the acquisition of specific information and theory. The branching, or scatter, method provides for applications of learned theory to realistic situations.

The comprehensive body of knowledge concerning the interruptions of family health during the childbearing process has been delineated by specific objectives that guide students' learning. At the beginning of the chapters there is a glossary of new terms to prepare the student. A pretest serves as a further guide to important aspects of the new material and will enable students, when reviewing, to evaluate recall of the material. Tests after chapters and units enable students to recognize their difficulties as they encounter them; the program then directs them back to review specific material. The student also gains experience in the skill of test taking.

The text also assists the student in developing a personal philosophy with positive attitudes toward family nursing.

ACKNOWLEDGMENTS

We are indebted to all those who gave us support and encouragement during the writing of this text. Our special thanks go to David Aurell for assistance with the cover design and to Iris Vaughan for typing the manuscript. Our personal thanks to Jeanne, Hugh, and Larry.

We wish to add a special dedication in tribute to Mary Ann Richter, our late editor, whose vivaciousness and enthusiasm aided us in the task of rewriting the manuscript for this edition. Her sudden death before the fruits of her labor appeared has left us with a profound sense of personal and professional loss.

Betty Ann Anderson
Mercedes E. Camacho
Jeanne Stark

TO THE STUDENT

Volume Two has been developed to assist you in the study of the various interruptions in the family health status during the childbearing cycle. Major emphasis will be on identifying the dynamics of the different interruptions, the family's adaptations, and the role of the nurse in meeting identifiable needs.

Mastery of the content presented in the first volume is a prerequisite to the study of the material presented in this volume. Some chapters are preceded by pretests. The objective of the pretests is to acquaint you with content covered in the chapters and to allow you to identify areas to be learned.

The core chapters are not preceded by pretests because we consider this material fundamental to your complete understanding of the program. We suggest that you study these chapters thoroughly.

Throughout this program, two different types of programming are used:

1. *Linear*, in which the answers are on the same page on which the material is presented. These answers are to be covered as you study the material and uncovered to check your learning. The mask enclosed in your book should be used to conceal the answers while you read. An arrow appears in the upper right-hand corner on pages where the mask should be used. As you study, you may write your answers in the spaces provided in the text.

2. *Branching*, or *scatter*, in which you are directed to turn to other pages to reinforce your learning.

Achievement tests follow each chapter and each unit so that you can check your comprehension of the completed material. Remember that when you answer the evaluation questions, you are not competing with anyone else for a grade. Rather, you are evaluating your own understanding to see if there are any sections of the material that you did not comprehend. Directions following the questions will help you decide how much of the material you will need to review.

At the ends of pertinent chapters you will find modules of behavioral objectives that have been developed to describe significant behaviors in the clinical area. These objectives provide examples of how theoretical knowledge is applied in the clinical portion of a program.

In order to meet the needs of programs having different emphases, a wide range of behavioral objectives is presented. This range should be wide enough to provide close similarity to those clinical competencies measured in your individual program.

These objectives are to help you become familiar with the application of theory in a clinical setting. Your ability is then measured by your performance: Are you able to meet this objective, and if so, how well? These behavioral objectives should serve as a guide in the critical task of self-evaluation of your clinical ability. The grade that appears on the left side of each objective indicates the suggested ranking of the behavioral objectives. An asterisk indicates minimal passing behavior. The B and A indicate that additional knowledge and skill are required for the objective. Your own program may alter this ranking to be consistent with your curriculum.

TO THE INSTRUCTOR

The purpose of this volume is to provide nursing students with a comprehensive body of knowledge concerning the various interruptions in the family health status during the childbearing cycle. The programmed approach of this book will enable students to learn at their own pace with immediate reinforcement. In the second volume the material presented in the first volume is used as a basis to enable the students to assess the alterations that occur if an interruption in health is present. The volumes may be used in combination to provide any desired sequence of topics; for example, the unit on normal labor in Volume One can be followed by the unit on interruptions of labor in Volume Two.

To assist the student in exploring topics in greater depth, pertinent reading lists are provided at the ends of most chapters. Pretests precede most chapters to enable the student to review knowledge already acquired and identify areas for further study. Achievement tests follow each chapter and each unit. This double testing is intended to further reinforce the knowledge assimilated in the program and to direct the learner to portions of the chapter or the unit which may need reviewing.

This program can be used by the instructor as a basis for seminars, role-playing exercises, and teaching in the classroom or clinical laboratory. Family models introduced in the text can be used to engage the students in realistic situations requiring them to apply their understanding of the concepts learned in the various units.

At the ends of pertinent chapters you will find modules of behavioral objectives. These objectives have been tested in a clinical setting, and we feel that they describe a broad spectrum of behaviors to be achieved by students in the clinical setting. You may wish to use these behaviors for your clinical competencies, either adding or deleting behaviors to be consistent with your own curriculum.

The behavioral objectives allow the student to be familiar with the expected behaviors that are measured in the clinical setting. The clinical setting can be simulated in a laboratory or classroom. The grade indicated on the left side of each objective is an example of the suggested ranking of the behavioral objectives. An asterisk indicates minimal passing behavior. The B and A indicate that additional knowledge and skill are required for the objective. You may wish to alter this ranking to be consistent with your program.

UNIT I

INTERRUPTIONS IN HEALTH STATES

CHAPTER ONE

INTERRUPTIONS IN HEALTH

OBJECTIVES *Identify the concept of interruptions in health.*

Identify the six features characterizing interruptions in health.

Identify the characteristics of a crisis state.

Apply these concepts to specific situations.

Define "high-risk."

A state of health exists whenever there is harmony within the homeodynamic systems; when this harmony is interrupted, then a nonhealth state ensues. Nonhealth states have in the past been vaguely defined by other terms such as "illness," "disease," "sickness," etc. In examining the definitions of these terms, you will find that they are as vague and as general as the original words being defined. For instance, Webster refers to "illness" as being "an unhealthy condition of body or mind," yet what is meant by "unhealthy" is not clearly understood since when once again the same reference is consulted, it is found that the state of being "unhealthy" is defined in terms of "diseased, not evidencing health, not conducive to health, unwholesome," etc.

It becomes apparent, therefore, that the concept "illness" is as difficult to define as the concept "health" and that, in fact, in itself the word "illness" has little or no meaning unless its basic components are identified.

In her book *Behavior and Illness*,[1] Ruth Woo has extensively examined and analyzed the historical meaning and nature of the term "illness" and how this concept has been variously interpreted and utilized throughout the past. To primitive people, according to Woo, illness came about as the result of malignant forces acting upon them, overwhelming and destroying them. In this context, illness was given supernatural powers that human beings could not control. With the passage of time, as the scientific approach to the study of disease grew with human knowledge, changes in definition and thus in the conceptual frame of reference came about. Illness began to be viewed as resulting directly from aberrations of anatomical structures, and disease was seen as merely a process brought about by specific organic occurrences and changes based on cause-and-effect relationships of physiological nature.

Dissatisfied with this somewhat limiting view and definition, scientists then approached the concept of illness from the standpoint that disease processes came about as a result of disturbances in the interactions of the host-agent-environment triad. These interactions are dependent on the strength of the host (human being); the action of the agent (any number of unfavorable circumstances, be they chemical, biological, thermal, social, or psychological in nature); and the positive or negative influences of the environment.

It became apparent that these interactions are never static, but rather are constantly in a state of change. Whenever an alteration occurs in any one of the components (either in the host, the agent, or the environment), it brings about reciprocally some type of action by the other components. Thus a dynamic state of equilibrium is achieved and maintained among these three elements.

We have previously stated that preexisting or emergent disruptive conditions will prevent the restoration and/or maintenance of a dynamic state of equilibrium within the health continuum. Whenever such an imbalance occurs, a nonhealth state ensues.

Interruptions in health, or nonhealth states, may be defined as those situations in which individuals are unable to call forth successful and effective adaptive mechanisms that would enable them to modify or overcome the strength of a stressor.[2]

The severity of the interruption is dependent upon the operations of external and internal variables acting on homeodynamic systems. *Internal variables* are elements related to the individual's physiological and psychological makeup; examples of internal variables that will determine the degree of nonhealth are the nature of the physiological and/or psychological system being affected, the health status of other supporting systems, and the individual's own energy resources and potential to overcome and/or modify the stressor.

External variables are elements outside the individual, such as environmental, social, biological, and physiological stressors, that act to bring about an interruption in health. It must be added that the severity of the interruption is also dictated by whether there is a single stressor or multiple interacting stressors and by the duration and strength of the stressor(s).

An interruption in health occurs _____

_____

_____.

    when the individual is unable to modify or reduce the strength of the stressor

The internal factors that determine the degree of the interruption are _____,

_____

_____, and _____

_____.

    the system that is affected; the health state of the other systems; the resources of the individual

The external factors that are operating to determine the degree of the interruption are _____, _____,

_____, and _____.

    environmental; social; biological; physiological

The appearance of a nonhealth state and thus the emergence of a serious interruption in health is not necessarily due to the action of a single, powerful, clearly identifiable stressor; rather interruptions may arise as a result of the simultaneous interaction of many apparently insignificant stressors to which the individual would have been able to adapt had they emerged singly or in a less powerful combination. Moreover, the effects of previous stressors may have so depleted the indi-

vidual's available resources that subsequent adaptation to other im-
pinging forces may become impossible. Previous demands made upon
the human system may have been so great that an interruption in the
homeodynamic balance at this time may become the triggering element
in eliciting a serious nonhealth state and may even produce a crisis
situation.

Generally, interruptions of health are characterized by one or a
combination of the following factors:

1. Resources, structures, or functions may be inadequate.
    Reserves are so affected that the organism is unable to
    maintain a homeodynamic balance.

2. Adaptive responses may be inadequate, excessive, inap-
    propriate, or injurious to the organism so that the present
    interruption may be further complicated by the response
    to the disturbance.

3. Loss of equilibrium in one area may lead to disturbances
    of function, structure, and resources in another area or
    system.

4. Although the adaptation may be successful in some re-
    spects, it may prove unsuccessful in others; that is to say,
    at one point the organism is unable to respond adequately
    to the stressor whereas it may have been successful in
    doing so previously.

5. Disturbances of the internal or external environments may
    be of such intensity that they lie outside the organism's
    ability to respond to them or to effect successful adaptation.

6. The operation of one stressor for a short period of time
    may not affect the system, but if the stress is prolonged,
    failure to maintain the homeodynamic balance results.

When an interruption in health occurs, the individual may have
limited _____, the response of the individual may be   resources;
_____, or the interruption in one system may lead to   inappropriate;
_____   an interruption in another
_____.   system

If the stressor originally was mild in strength and then increased,
then _____.   a nonhealth state may ensue

A stressor may be of such magnitude and force that the organism
_____.   is unable to respond or adapt

The length of time during which a stressor is operating affects the organism's ability to respond, especially if the stressor is _____.

prolonged

It is well documented that mothers from lower socioeconomic backgrounds are often under great stress in their daily lives. During pregnancy these mothers may know the kinds of foods that are recommended but be unable to afford them. Also, these mothers may understand that rest is important, but with crowded living quarters and no help with the children, they may find it impossible to rest more. These are only some of the stressors operating to limit maternal adaptation. It follows that the fetus must adapt within these limits which interrupt the homeodynamic balance of mother and child, so the baby is often born prematurely because of disturbances of function and lack of supporting resources.

In the following situation, identify the system that is under stress and factors that may produce an interruption in health. A twenty-three-year-old woman has hypertension, but by following a medical regimen, she maintains an adequate homeodynamic balance. She becomes pregnant and during the second trimester, her blood volume increases at a rapid rate. When she next visits the doctor, the concern will be about what system? _____.

vascular system

The factors that are operating are _____

the increased

_____

volume and the sustained

_____,which may produce an interruption in health.

period of time

We have identified that health and nonhealth exist on a continuum. At the extreme nonhealth end, there may be interruptions of health which occur to such an extent that the organism or system involved is unable to solve this state. This means that the adaptive mechanism of the organism is unable to reduce or avert the strength of the stressor or stressors. This state of nonhealth is referred to as a "crisis." In a *crisis* state, outside intervention is needed to effect successful adaptation toward a homeodynamic balance. If there is no outside intervention, the crisis state may progress to the point of permanent loss of function or death of the system or organism. A crisis state may be precipitated initially by a physical stressor such as loss of an arm; the psychological aspect quickly becomes an integral component and may in fact act as an additional stressor. It also is possible that the initial stressor is psychological in nature, for example, fear of the labor process; this may interfere to such an extent that the progress of labor is slowed and outside intervention, often in the form of medication, is necessary to assist the process. Once the initial stressor begins operating, it becomes difficult to clearly isolate physiological and psychological stressors. A crisis state exists in degree: there is no one absolute level of a crisis state, but rather the degree of crisis is related to the interactions of the stressors and the resources of the person. Stressors that produce a crisis for one individual may not create the same degree of disruption for another individual.

A crisis state exists when _____

_____

_____

_____.

> the individual
> is unable to effect adequate
> adaptation, and outside
> intervention is necessary

A mother who was 18 weeks pregnant was driving home and sustained minor injuries, such as bruises and a few small lacerations, when her car collided with a delivery truck. The mother became terrified that her baby had been harmed, and she could not stop shaking. She was taken to the hospital and was thoroughly examined by the physician, who assured her that there were no broken bones, the baby's heart rate was good, and there was no problem. She then stopped trembling.

The crisis for this mother was the fear that her child had sustained injury and that she was unable to do anything about it. Only after the doctor examined her and ascertained that the baby was without harm could she begin to relax.

The term "high-risk" is usually applied to those situations in which potential, emergent, or previously existing interruptions of health threaten the viability of the pregnancy.

Complicating conditions such as interruptions associated with the pregnancy (toxemias as an example) or previous interruptions antecedent to the pregnancy will seriously jeopardize maternal and fetal health. In general, the presence of any factor that will decrease the opportunity for a normal, healthy delivery will represent a high-risk situation.

Interruptions in health antecedent to or coincidental with the pregnancy are usually classified as _____

since these are _____ conditions that will seriously

_____ maternal and infant health.

Any factor that _____ the expectancy of a normal, healthy delivery therefore will represent a _____ situation.

> high-risk;
> complicating;
> jeopardize
> decreases;
> high-risk

POST-TEST Indicate whether each statement is true or false by circling the appropriate letter. Then turn to page 10 and see how well you have done.

1. When a health state is interrupted, this means that there is no harmony in any of the homeodynamic systems. T F

2. If the homeodynamic system has utilized its limited resources and a stressor is introduced, this situation can produce an interruption in the health state. T F

3. The environment in no way can become so stressful as to alter the homeodynamic system's balance and produce a nonhealth state. T F

4. If one system is unable to maintain adequate function, then other systems are affected. T F

5. When the degree of stress an organism is exposed to is maintained for a long period of time, the organism may no longer be able to adapt successfully. T F

6. If the adaptive mechanism of the homeodynamic system is unable to reduce the strength of the stressor, a state of nonhealth may ensue. T F

7. In a crisis state, the individual is able to avert the strength of the stressor. T F

8. A crisis state can exist at different levels. T F

9. Particular stressors may be able to produce a crisis state for one individual but not for another. T F

10. The term "high-risk" applies only to those complicating conditions arising during the pregnancy. T F

11. High-risk situations usually threaten only the health of the pregnant mother. T F

12. High-risk conditions have the potential for eliciting serious crisis states. T F

In the specific areas with which you had difficulty, return to the material and review.

REFERENCES   1.   Ruth Woo: *Behavior and Illness*, Prentice-Hall, Inc., Englewood Cliffs, N.J., 1973, pp. 5–24.

2.   Betty Ann Anderson, Mercedes E. Camacho, and Jeanne Stark: *Pregnancy and Family Health*, Vol. I in *The Childbearing Family*, 2d ed., McGraw-Hill Book Co., New York, 1979, p. 12.

BIBLIOGRAPHY   Bloom, Bernard L., "Definitional Aspects of the Crisis Concept," in Howard J. Parad (ed.), *Crisis Intervention*, Family Service Association of America, New York, 1972, pp. 303–311.

Matheney, Ruth and Mary Topalis: *Psychiatric Nursing*, 5th ed., C. V. Mosby Co., St. Louis, 1970, pp. 321–322.

Rapoport, Lydia, "The State of Crisis: Some Theoretical Considerations," in Howard J. Parad (ed.), *Crisis Intervention*, Family Service Association of America, New York, 1972, pp. 22–31.

Woo, Ruth: *Behavior and Illness*, Prentice-Hall, Inc., Englewood Cliffs, N.J., 1973, pp. 5–24.

**POST-TEST
ANSWERS**   1. F   2. T   3. F   4. T   5. T   6. T   7. F   8. T   9. T
10. F   11. F   12. T

CHAPTER TWO

RESPONSES TO A LOSS

Identify the five stages of the grieving process in response to a loss.

Identify nursing intervention measures that must be instituted when families have suffered a loss.

During pregnancy, potential or preexisting nonhealth states become serious stressors affecting either the mother or the baby. These states may lead to serious interruptions of the homeodynamic systems, causing the death of either the fetus, the mother, or both.

Typically, the obstetrical unit of any hospital is perceived as being the "happiest" area of the institution: assisting with the emergence of a new life is its objective and birth, not death, the purpose of its existence. Nevertheless, death of the baby or of the mother does at times take place within such settings. When this occurs, not only the family but also the staff receive the full impact of the loss.

The psychological reaction of the grief process as a result of a loss can be measured in relationship to the meaning of the loss object to those undergoing the experience and to the investment they have made in the loss object. Therefore, a miscarriage or abortion in early pregnancy will have a different impact than a stillborn birth.

According to Dr. Elisabeth Kübler-Ross, the threat or impact of a loss brings about a sequence of psychological responses to which the individual must successfully adapt so as to restore a positive homeodynamic balance. The five stages that Dr. Kübler-Ross has identified are denial, anger, bargaining, depression, and acceptance.[1] It is important that the nurse recognize these various stages and be able to identify when a family member is at a specific stage. As the person works through these stages, he or she may fluctuate back and forth, and may not always move continuously in the direction of the final stage. Also, different family members pass through the stages at varying rates.

Generally, the first reaction to a loss is one of *denial*: the thought or possibility that a loss through death may occur is expressed in statements such as "It can happen to someone else but not to me." Such denial may also become apparent in behavioral expressions of evasiveness, such as changing the topic of conversation or negating the significance of the event.

The second reaction coming about as a result of a loss is *anger*. Behaviorally, this feeling is expressed through physical or verbal outbursts of resentment. Often, mothers when approached by the nursing personnel attempt to deal with their loss by crying, "How can you know what I feel; you've never gone through this!"

The third phase of the grieving process is that of *bargaining*. It is at this point that the individual, although recognizing the seriousness of the situation, begins to seek ways and means to diminish or obliterate the threat of the loss or to reverse the event.

Bargaining phases are expressed in compromises or in promises made to a higher force or to persons who are perceived as possessing the controls that will serve to prevent the loss; as a rule, bargaining behavior is tempered by socioeconomic backgrounds or by psychological reactions taking place during this time. Sometimes it is seen when family members offer to assist the staff with some of their tasks, such as answering the phone or doing paperwork.

The fourth phase in the grieving process is that of *depression*. When the latest activity (that of bargaining) has been unsuccessful in stopping or reversing the loss, the individual moves into a state of despair. Behavioral expressions of this phase may be withdrawal, non-participation, and the experience of an overwhelming sense of alone-ness: the mother may reject the father and other family members and may seek expression of feelings of depression by making statements such as "What's the use of going home?" or "I had some plans and now there is nothing."

The depression may come about as a result of the woman and family's perception of the event as being due to something they may have done in the past; as such, the loss is perceived as a punishment and the prevailing underlying feeling is one of guilt. This in turn can add to the feelings of worthlessness, despair, and rejection. The depres-sion can also be in anticipation of an impending loss. This phase is the crucial one for the individual since, depending upon the amount of support and understanding given at this time, the woman (or the family) may be successful in adapting to these feelings and be able to go on to the next phase, that of acceptance of the loss.

When appropriate intervention measures in the form of interper-sonal activities and therapeutic responses and reactions are instituted, the individual or the family unit is assisted toward the achievement of *acceptance*. It is during this phase that the individual becomes able to adapt to the stresses brought about by the loss and, within the limitation imposed by the situation, able to achieve a positive homeodynamic balance. The nursing approach to mothers and families who have ex-perienced the loss of their baby should definitely include specific op-portunities for the nurse to spend time with the family unit so as to allow their expression of feelings. Requests such as that of wanting to see the baby's body should be fulfilled, for these activities aid the family in accepting the reality of the death.

When a person attempts to prevent or postpone a loss or death by some special activity, then he or she is in the stage of _____.　　bargaining

When a person withdraws from activities, this is typical of the stage of _____.　　depression

When a person refuses to accept the possibility of a loss, this is indication of the stage of _____.　　denial

When a person blames other persons for not assisting him properly and meeting his needs, this is a sign of the stage of _____.　　anger

When a person has come to terms with the reality of the loss, he or she is in the stage of _____.

acceptance

When the mother who has lost her baby is on the postpartum floor, it is important not to isolate her completely from other people. It is at this time that personal contact with the staff and family members is very important as the mother and family begin to work through the stages of grief. Since the staff also must deal with the loss, it is important for them to identify their feelings and assist each other to accomplish the tasks of the different stages. At times it is necessary to bring in professionals from another area, such as a clinical nurse specialist in psychiatry, or the clergy, who are able to provide the needed support to the staff. Before the staff can successfully interact with and provide support to the family, they must have identified and dealt with their feelings.

Nursing intervention is geared to providing the needed support to the mother and family so that they are able to work through the stages of grief. If the family is unable to deal with the loss, then many psychological problems usually ensue.

During the phase of denial, the nurse must recognize that the mother or family member is at this stage. Attempts to push the person through to another stage, such as acceptance of reality, are not helpful. Responses that are helpful at this time are supportive of the person's feelings and allow the person to verbalize the feeling that the situation is too impossible to happen to him or her. Usually after expressing these feelings and finding acceptance, the person can progress to the next stage.

The stage of anger can be quite frightening to the staff member who is unprepared, since often the staff may take the brunt of the angry feelings. Effective intervention at this time is a response to the effect that, "Yes, I would be very angry too in your situation." In this way, you are accepting the person's anger as a valid feeling; you are not rejecting him or her, and you are indicating that the feelings are not overwhelming you but rather are normal responses. When possible, allowing the person to control certain routines is helpful and can alleviate some of the anger.

As the person works through and enters the stage of bargaining, it is important to recognize what the person's behavior is indicating and when possible, to allow him or her to attempt to control the situation. Thus, you will not negate the person's attempts to alter what seems to be an impossible situation.

When the mother or family member is in the stage of depression, often he or she does not wish to eat and does not participate in any activity but rather withdraws and stays in bed all the time. At this time, intervention is important to maintain personal contact and to allow the person to express the feelings of hopelessness. It is by this activity that the mother or family member is able to move through into the final stage, that of acceptance.

In the stage of acceptance the person is not happy but rather has reached a kind of peace and then becomes able to participate again in the responsibilities and activities of life.

In the following situation, identify the appropriate nursing assessment and intervention. A mother came in in labor, Stage One, relaxation phase, and during the labor fetal distress developed. A cesarean section was performed (emergency intervention). This was unsuccessful in saving the baby; it was a stillborn. You are the nurse on the postpartum floor the following day. When you go into the room and introduce yourself, the mother asks you why, if the doctors know so much, they didn't do something better and save the baby.

Which of the following choices indicates the stage of grieving the mother is in and is the best response?

A.   The mother is in the denial stage and is not accepting reality. Your response to the mother's question is, "Things are difficult now but they will work out later."   Go to page 16.

B.   The mother is in the bargaining stage now, and your best response is to agree with her that the doctors should have done something else and the baby would have been saved   Go to page 17

C.   The mother is in the stage of anger and, since the doctors are supposed to save lives, she is angry at them for letting her down. Your best response is, "It is a very normal feeling to be angry when you have lost your baby and especially when doctors and nurses are supposed to save people's lives. It is a very difficult time now; maybe there is something I can do to help."   Go to page 18.

Your choice, response *A*, that the mother is in the denial stage, is incorrect. Reread the situation and identify exactly what the mother is saying: Is she saying that everything is all right? The response of false reassurance is not helpful to the mother who is attempting to work through her feelings of loss.

Return to page 12. Review the material and choose another response from page 15.

Your choice of response *B* is wrong. Is the mother promising to do something special so that she will not lose the baby? Your agreement to the doctors' wrongdoing is inappropriate and certainly not therapeutic for the mother.

Return to page 12. Review the material and choose another response from page 15.

Good. Your choice of response *C* indicates that you were able to identify the stage of grieving that the mother was in as that of anger. You were able to sort out that the mother was angry that this event should have happened to her and that when she relied on experts to take care of her, they let her down. "They should make everything all right" is a normal feeling. Your support of her feelings as valid and your staying with her are important at this time; also, offering to assist her provides her with the needed support.

Advance to page 19 and take the post-test.

POST-TEST Indicate whether each statement is true or false by circling the appropriate letter. Then turn to page 20 and see how well you have done.

1. People respond to death differently according to their past experiences. T F

2. The staff does not go through the same emotional process as the person suffering the loss. T F

3. The person who is going through the grieving process always goes directly from the beginning to the end stages. T F

4. Denial is the first stage of the grieving process. T F

5. Acceptance is the stage in which there is happiness. T F

6. Anger is one of the easiest stages for the nurse to accept. T F

7. Bargaining is not a worthwhile activity for the person to engage in since it does not change things. T F

8. When the person is in the depression stage, it is important to encourage him or her to look at the bright side of things and stop being unhappy. T F

In the specific areas with which you had difficulty, return to the material and review.

REFERENCES   1.   Elisabeth Kübler-Ross: *On Death and Dying*, The Macmillan Co., New York, 1969, pp. 34–121.

BIBLIOGRAPHY   Baird, S. F., "Crisis Intervention Theory in Maternal-Infant Nursing. Emotional Crisis and Maternal Child Nursing," *JOGN Nurs.*, pp. 30–39, Jan.–Feb. 1976.

Chiota, B. J., et al., "Effects of Separation from Spouse on Pregnancy, Labor and Delivery, and the Post-Partum Period," *JOGN Nurs.*, pp. 21–24, Jan.–Feb. 1976.

Halstead, L., "The Use of Crisis Intervention in Obstetric Nursing," *Nursing Clinics of North America*, pp. 69–76, 1974.

Kübler-Ross, Elisabeth: *On Death and Dying*, The Macmillan Co., New York, 1969.

Lindemann, Eric, "Symptomatology and Management of Acute Grief," in Howard J. Parad (ed.), *Crisis Intervention*, Family Service Association of America, New York, 1972, pp. 7–21.

Schoenberg, Bernard, et al.: *Loss and Grief—Psychological Management in Medical Practice*, Columbia University Press, New York, 1971.

Yates, Susan A., "Stillbirth—What A Staff Can Do," in Murray H. Browning and Edith P. Lewis (eds.), *Maternal and Newborn Care, Nursing Interventions*, The American Journal of Nursing Co., New York, 1973, p. 103.

POST-TEST ANSWERS   1. T   2. F   3. F   4. T   5. F   6. F   7. F   8. F

CHAPTER THREE

INTERVENTION DURING INTERRUPTIONS IN HEALTH STATES

OBJECTIVES *Identify areas of prevention during interruptions in health.*

Identify areas of promotion during interruptions in health.

Identify areas of restoration during interruptions in health.

Apply these concepts to specific situations.

We have mentioned the fact that the sustained presence of any given stressor over a prolonged period of time reduces the individual's ability to effect adaptive responses because energies and reserves often become depleted or exhausted to such a degree that the organism cannot by itself maintain a homeodynamic balance. During interruptions in health, the preventive and promotive aspects of health care function on the one hand to avoid disabilities and/or interruptions in the homeodynamic systems not directly affected by the stressor, while on the other hand they aid in maintaining the functioning capacity of the system being affected. Therefore, preventive and promotive measures enhance the individual's ability to cope with the stressor in such a way that the strength of the stressor may be averted, diminished, or redirected. For example, when an individual has suffered a cardiovascular accident, three levels of rehabilitative measures are immediately instituted: (1) to prevent further disabilities such as deterioration of muscle tone and death of other nerves and cells; (2) to promote the function of other systems, such as bladder and bowel; and (3) to restore the individual's ability and potential to function to optimum capacity, in spite of apparent limitations imposed by the existing disability. Thus, it becomes essential that preventive and promotive measures be immediately instituted so that further degeneration and failure of the affected system or systems and/or involvement or interruptions of any other interacting systems are avoided.

It is difficult to identify at what point preventive and promotive measures become restorative measures, i.e., measures that serve to restore the individual's ability to adapt to the adverse effects of the stressor. Preventive, promotive, and restorative goals often can be accomplished by instituting the same activity. For example, in the above situation, when establishing range-of-motion exercises, the nurse is preventing loss of muscle tone and development of edema and is promoting circulatory function. At the same time, these exercises restore the individual's ability to maintain function in the affected part by encouraging motion of that part within the limitations imposed by the disability. Achievement of a homeodynamic balance is dependent also upon the individual's ability to adjust to the disability imposed by the negative stressor; psychological factors have an important role in restoring a positive homeodynamic balance. The essential characteristic of "restoration" can be summarized as follows: *Restoration* is any process tending to assist the individual in effecting adaptation to a stressor so that harmony in the homeodynamic balance can be achieved.

To summarize, let us consider the measures taken to reinstate homeodynamics in the case of a bone fracture. A fracture of the ulna is aligned, and the limb is supported by a cast. The use of the cast is a *preventive* measure because it prevents the bones from changing position and causing further complications. A sling is used around the cast to distribute the weight and support the arm in a position that *promotes* good circulation through the affected area. These preventive and promotive measures, once initiated, allow for the *restoration* of the system, i.e., the actual healing of the fractures to take place. Once the fracture has healed, the cast is removed and restorative measures are initiated in the form of physical therapy, which aids the muscle function to achieve good tone.

Restorative measures, therefore, are usually goal-directed toward a specific system and geared to lessening the effects of the stressor by increasing or replenishing the adaptive resources of the individual. It is not possible to restore a system to a previous state of health, but rather the system is helped to achieve a new state of health.

Preventive and promotive measures are usually directed to more than one system.

When activities are carried out toward a specific goal of assisting a system toward adaptation, these are _____ measures.

restorative

Activities that are carried out to arrest the development of other complications are _____ measures.

preventive

Support of systems not involved directly in coping with a particular stressor is a _____ measure.

promotive

The following example will indicate stressors that produce interruption within the health status of the mother and, ultimately, of the fetus during pregnancy, labor, and delivery.

During pregnancy a mother's cervix may begin to dilate around the fourth month as the products of conception grow and have more weight. With further growth there may be more dilatation, and the pregnancy is lost because of the incompetent cervix. The physical stressor, the inability of the cervix to function adequately, disturbs the environment of the developing fetus and produces an interruption in the homeodynamic balance to a point where there is a loss of the pregnancy. This pattern of interruption, once identified, can be altered, for if the dilatation of the cervix is diagnosed, sutures can be placed within the cervical os, securing the closure of the cervix until term. Successful intervention is able to alter the pattern of stress adaptation by restoring function to the cervix, thus preventing the loss of the pregnancy and promoting the health status of both the mother and the baby.

POST-TEST   Indicate whether each statement is true or false by circling the appropriate letter. Then turn to page 25 and see how well you have done.

1. When a nonhealth state exists, then there is no need for preventive measures.   T   F

2. "Restoration" means that, following a stressful situation, a homeodynamic system can return to a previous state and be the same as before.   T   F

3. Preventive and promotive measures often are in combination when intervention occurs.   T   F

4. Restoration assists the individual in effective adaptation to a disruptive stressor.   T   F

5. Restorative measures are not goal-directed.   T   F

In the specific areas with which you had difficulty, return to the material and review.

BIBLIOGRAPHY   Beland, Irene L.: *Clinical Nursing—Pathophysiological and Psychological Approaches*, The Macmillan Co., New York, 1970.
Dubos, René: *The Mirage of Health*, Harper and Row, New York, 1959.
Kintzel, Kay Corman: *Advanced Concepts in Clinical Nursing*, J. B. Lippincott Co., Philadelphia, 1971.

POST-TEST ANSWERS   1. F   2. F   3. T   4. T   5. F

CHAPTER FOUR

THE FAMILY SYSTEM AND INTERRUPTIONS IN HEALTH

OBJECTIVES *Identify the types of interruptions in the family system.*

Identify the states of disorganization, crisis, and termination of the family system.

Identify the nursing intervention when the family is in a nonhealth state.

PRETEST   In the spaces provided, fill in the word or words that best complete(s) the
statements. Then turn to page 36 and check your answers.

   1.   Interruptions in health of the family system are due to _____

_____

_____.

   2.   If the resources of the family system are limited so that outside assistance
is necessary, the family is considered to be in _____.

   3.   The first indication of a nonhealth state of the family system is

_____.

   4.   If the functional roles are not shared by the family members, but rather are
occupied primarily by one member, this situation often produces

_____.

The family system, functioning as a unit, adapts to achieve a homeo-dynamic balance as the members interact within the system and outside of the system. Stressors affecting the family system may be in the form of alterations of organization or of mode of functioning of the system. For example, if one member acts as a dissonant force within the family system or is subject to a strong stressor from the outside, the family system's balance may be altered to such a degree that a nonhealth state of the family ensues.

The normal process of childbearing produces stress within the family system and causes the family members to utilize their various resources in the process of adaptation. At this time, when interruptions of physical, psychological, or social impact are introduced into the system, the ability of the family to respond may not be adequate to achieve harmony of the homeodynamic system. What then ensues is an interrupted state of health of the system.

The strength of the stressor may be sufficient to negate the re-sources of the system; should this situation occur, a crisis state is produced. When there is a crisis state, the family system is so vulnerable that if no outside assistance introduces resources to modify and/or lessen the impact of the stressors, a progressive disruption of the ho-meodynamics of the family system will occur.

It is important to recognize that the same stressor introduced in or affecting one family system will have a different effect in another family system. Family systems are unique and have varied resources, so adaptive processes vary from time to time and system to system. Thus the breadwinner's loss of a job may produce a crisis for one family whereas for another family the interruption may be minimal and last for a short time.

A family state of nonhealth also can occur if the functional roles of the family members are not shared but rather are occupied primarily by one member. When this happens, that individual's resources often are depleted, and, as the stressors persist or new ones are introduced, the family's adaptive processes are limited, and further interruptions are created within the system. The first indication of the nonhealth process is *disorganization of the family system*. The nonhealth state can be resolved at this point or can progress to further disruption where the resources are so limited that a state of *crisis* evolves.

The absence of a vital family member from the family system, such as occurs during the hospitalization of the mother, produces stress within the system. Often if there is a long period of absence, another family member must assume all the responsibility and roles; this sit-uation causes disorganization of the family system and can lead to a crisis state. The process may be seen most readily in single-parent families.

Often cultural differences among family members produce conflict due to members' various expectations about the other members' behavior and role: for example, the parents' different expectations of their roles often are a source of difficulty and can produce disruptions of the family system's organization and mode of functioning. If the result of the differences means that one member must assume all the responsibility, then often the same disruptive situation as described above occurs.

Interruptions in the health of one member may have similar effects, depending on the length of time the interruptions last. For example, if the mother has a cardiac problem during pregnancy, she may be on bed rest for many months and further disruptions within the family system may be created.

It also is possible for the family system to *terminate* or, in essence, die. This condition occurs in instances where there is only one surviving member left in the family system, following the death of the other members or after legal termination of the relationship, such as the giving up of a child for adoption or the ending of a relationship between the members. When the single parent gives up a child for adoption, this termination of the family system usually follows the exhaustion of available resources, indicating that even with outside support the family is incapable of reducing or altering the stressors.

Successful nursing intervention is geared to the whole family system. Basic to the nursing process is the assessment of the family membership and the dynamics of the family system. It is essential to identify the stressors that the family perceives. It often is easier to identify stressors that are familiar to you from your background rather than the actual stressors that are affecting the family. Once you determine the stressors (and there usually is no one isolated stressor but rather many stressors interwoven), it is important to recognize the positive strength and the available resources of the family system as you determine the ways in which the family members have approached the situation.

If the family is in a state of disorganization, often by your help in identifying the stressors and the possible adaptations the family system then is able to adapt successfully. Sometimes, if this adaptation is not possible and the family system is becoming more disruptive, then the nursing intervention is to provide support either directly or by referral. For example, in a family where the mother is placed on bed rest and the father becomes increasingly unable to cope with all the responsibility, the help or support in this situation may be a homemaker service. Thus the mother may share responsibility by making schedules and lists, thereby not abdicating all functional roles, the father may not be so tired and overwhelmed, and they will be able to share interests and relax together.

It also is important for the nurse to be supportive in the situation of the termination of the family system. This situation often can be encountered when a single mother who has had a child is in the process of deciding to give the child up for adoption. Before beginning nursing intervention, it is important to identify your feelings so that as you approach this mother you will be nonjudgmental; otherwise, it is desirable to have another person give care to this mother. Your nursing intervention is geared to allowing the mother to express her feelings and, once she has made her decision, giving her support. Often the stressors in the environment are so great that the mother recognizes her limitations and decides to give the baby up. Then the mother must go through a period of grieving over her loss. It is extremely important for the nurse to help the mother so that sometime in the future, when she wants children, she may be able to establish a satisfactory parental relationship.

In the following situation, you are the nurse with the Soyre family. Nancy and Joe Soyre have two girls at home, two and four years of age, respectively, and a premature baby boy who is still in the hospital because he weighs only 3½ pounds. Nancy was discharged two and a half weeks ago after an uncomplicated postpartum stay. The Soyres live an hour and a half away from the hospital, and Joe is employed as a full-time accountant in a department store. Nancy has been getting up early to take the children to a neighbor's before coming to the hospital to feed the baby. She arrives a little before the 9 A.M. feeding and stays through until after the 3 P.M. feeding. The baby's condition has stabilized, and he is gaining weight. You talk with Nancy and find out that by the time she gets home in the evening she feels too tired to cook, so Joe has been opening cans for their evening meal. During dinner Nancy tells the family how the baby was during the day and how much of the feedings he took, and after dinner Joe gets the two youngsters off to bed. Your assessment of the family situation is which of the following choices?

A.   The family has adapted successfully following the crisis state that occurred with the birth of the premature son. Everyone is participating and sharing the responsibility.

Go to page 31 top.

B.   Nancy seems to be able to adapt effectively and has begun her mothering role with her new son, but Joe seems to have a problem since he does not come in to visit or participate in the care.

Go to page 32 top.

C.   The family roles and responsibilities are not shared but rather rest primarily on Joe's shoulders, and Nancy has abdicated much of her family responsibility since she is at the hospital so much.

Go to page 33.

If you chose *A*, you did not clearly identify the dynamics of the interaction within the family and the kinds of adaptations that are occurring.

Reread this chapter before making another selection. Return to page 30 and choose another response.

In choosing *C*, you have decided for the family that having the children leave the house will solve the problem. Remember, it is important to have the family involved with the decision. Does it mean that the responsibilities are shared when the children are no longer physically present?

Return to page 28. Review the situation and choose another response from page 33.

Your choice of *B* indicates that you have isolated one aspect of the family dynamics, but that the family as a system with all the various interactions has been ignored.

Review the material in this chapter before making another selection. Return to page 30 and choose another response.

_____

You chose *A*, indicating that you felt that the outside help of a homemaker would assist the family with successful adaptations. Your action is not based on a good understanding of the needs of the family.

Return to page 33. Review the situation and choose another response.

Excellent! Your selection of *C* demonstrates your ability to assess the dynamics of the family system and to identify factors that indicate that there is a crisis within the family. You identified that Joe is the one member who is presently occupying most of the functional roles within the family and has most of the responsibility for meeting the needs of the family. The nursing intervention that is most appropriate in this situation is which of the following?

A. Referring the family to the homemaker service so that someone will come into the home and look after the children and prepare all the meals. Go to page 32 bottom.

B. Helping Nancy identify her feelings about the baby and then helping her plan a schedule so that she is able to spend more time with the girls, visit the hospital every other day, yet keep in touch by phone. Go to page 34.

C. Suggesting that the children stay with their grandparents for several weeks so that Joe can pick Nancy up at the hospital and then they can go out to dinner. In this way, Joe will not have to worry about the girls or make the dinner. Go to page 31 bottom.

Your choice of *B* indicates a very good understanding of effective intervention with this family. You allowed Nancy to identify the problem and then gave support as she determined suitable means to meet the needs of the family. Nancy is now assuming some of the functional roles of the family, and the responsibility no longer rests with Joe alone. In this way, the adaptation to this crisis state has decreased the force of the stressor, and the family is functioning as a unit.

Advance to page 35 and take the post-test.

POST-TEST Indicate whether each statement is true or false by circling the appropriate letter. Then turn to page 36 and see how well you have done.

1. A state of nonhealth is present when the family system is not able to achieve harmony of the homeodynamic systems. T F

2. In a crisis state, the family does not need outside resources. T F

3. The first sign of the family system's disruption is disorganization. T F

4. In a crisis state, it is important that you as the nurse inform the family about which stressors are producing this crisis. T F

5. The nurse cannot function in the supportive role when the family system is in the process of termination. T F

6. It is important to find out how the family members have attempted to deal with the stressor. T F

7. If a stressor is capable of producing a crisis state in one family, it will have the same effect in all the other family systems. T F

In the specific areas with which you had difficulty, return to the material and review.

BIBLIOGRAPHY   Halstead, L., "The Use of Crisis Intervention in Obstetric Nursing," *Nursing Clinics of North America*, pp. 69–76, 1974.

Liberman, Samuel: *Stress Situations*, J. B. Lippincott Co., Philadelphia, 1955.

Menniger, Karl: *The Vital Balance*, The Viking Press, New York, 1965.

Minuchin, Salvador, et al.: *Families of the Slums*, Basic Books Inc., New York, 1967.

Parad, Howard J. (ed.): *Crisis Intervention*, Family Service Association of America, New York, 1972.

**PRETEST
ANSWERS**
1. Stressors producing a disruption of the harmony of the system's homeodynamics   2.   Crisis
3. Disorganization   4.   A nonhealth state

**POST-TEST
ANSWERS**
1. T   2.   F   3.   T   4.   F   5.   F   6.   T   7.   F

CHAPTER FIVE

EMERGENCY OBSTETRICS

OBJECTIVES   *Identify the information pregnant women should have concerning their obstetrical status.*

Identify the equipment pregnant women should have at home in case of an emergency.

Identify the role of the professional nurse during a disaster.

Identify how the nurse could manage the four stages of labor during a disaster.

PRETEST In the spaces provided, fill in the word or words that best complete(s) the statements. Then turn to page 45 and check your answers.

1. The pregnant woman should be informed about her obstetrical _____.

2. Pregnant women should be prepared for a home delivery and should have

    _____, _____, _____,

    _____, _____, and _____ on hand.

3. During a disaster, the expectant mother feels more isolated than if she were
    in a hospital during normal times because she probably _____

    _____

    _____.

4. The nurse should recognize the need to utilize other women and men to help
    and to give _____

    _____.

5. After the delivery the umbilical cord can be cut if the nurse has a

    _____.

6. To ensure proper identification, the mother and baby must be _____

    _____.

The sudden occurrence of a major catastrophe gives rise to high-risk situations that endanger the viability of the fetus and the life of the mother. Whether man-made or natural in origin, major disaster situations may disrupt ecological, social, and human systems to such an extent that the life of entire groups of people and communities is seriously threatened and the existence of generations of families extinguished. Under such circumstances, it is the responsibility of those who are members of the health care professions to provide swift, necessary, appropriate, and competent emergency services. Therefore, it is essential that professional nurses recognize and accept the importance of being prepared to assume a leadership role in providing care during emergency situations.

A disaster can completely isolate areas: water, electricity, telephone, radio, television, and other means of communication may not be functioning. Roads may be blocked and medical help unavailable. It is estimated that at any given moment, 2 percent of the total population is pregnant, and in a catastrophe, as many as 25 percent of all pregnant women in the area may deliver or abort.

It is essential that every pregnant woman be informed by her physician as to the status of her health and whether or not she is expected to be able to have a normal vaginal delivery. It also is essential that the pregnant woman know if any special facilities will be necessary in order for her to deliver a healthy child. If the triage of care is being utilized during a disaster, this information is vital.

In a disaster, pregnant women will be exposed to all of the problems faced by the general population. In addition, they will have the problem of pregnancy and, possibly, imminent labor.

Ideally, every pregnant woman should be informed about the equipment that it is advisable for her to have readily available in case of an emergency. This equipment should include:

1. Clean linen such as a sheet, towels, and a washcloth; soap

2. Baby equipment such as blanket, clothing, nipple, and bottle

3. Pair of blunt scissors and two pieces of binding tape 6 inches long and $\frac{1}{4}$ inch wide, wrapped separately from the other items, to tie and cut the cord

4. Container of drinkable water and powdered milk

In order for the nurse to care effectively for a mother in labor during a disaster, the mother must inform the nurse of her expected

type of delivery

The mother should have an emergency bundle that contains

several types of equipment. The equipment for general use is
_____, _____, _____, and
_____.

    For the baby she should have _____, _____,
and _____.

    She should be told also to have for herself some _____
_____.

sheet; soap; towel;

washcloth

clothes; bottle;

nipple

powdered

milk

    If the mother is separated from her family and is unsure of their whereabouts or safety, her needs will be even greater. Her concern for their safety and that of herself and the unborn baby will greatly increase the stress with which she has to contend.

    It is essential that the nurse be cognizant of these needs and do her utmost to exude confidence and provide a feeling of acceptance.

    During emergencies, it will be most helpful for you, as a nurse, to seek and utilize the aid of other women and/or men available to assist you. Try to determine quickly which men or women in the community have had some training or experience. If any of these persons are available, they can help you with some rapid on-the-job training for other people whom you might be able to utilize. If there are no trained persons available, you must be able to select from among the persons available those who seem able to function in adverse situations and inform them of the ways in which they can best assist you.

    For your women in labor, if possible, clear an area away from rubble and crowds. During the early stages of labor, these women can be watched and supported by other people, thus freeing you for the care of those in greater need or for the preparation of an area and equipment for deliveries.

    During the first stage of labor, the mother's physical and emotional strength must be maintained. She must be kept informed of her progress and encouraged to relax and rest when possible. Remember that the equipment available to you may be makeshift. Most people do not carry around a fetascope, sphygmomanometer, or stethoscope. You will not have sterile gloves or drapes, yet asepsis must be maintained. You will have to use all other observation techniques to determine the progress of labor.

    Separation from husband and children will cause the pregnant mother to have _____.

increased stress

    In addition to her fears for them, she will be increasingly anxious about _____ and _____.

herself; the baby

    The nurse must appear to be _____.

confident

The nurse is unable to do everything herself; therefore, it might be wise if she _____.

utilizes other people

The nurse may have to prepare these helpers by immediate _____.

on-the-job training

Children should be kept away from the area in which you expect to have a delivery. In addition, this area should be away from _____ and _____.

rubble; crowds

The mother must be kept well informed about her _____ and helped to _____ and _____.

progress;
relax; rest

To determine progress, you must be aware of the observations to be made. During the first stage, you will be able to check changes in contractions as labor progresses from the effacement to the dilatation phase. These changes will be in _____, _____, and _____.

intensity;
duration; frequency

As transition approaches, you will be able to see physical as well as emotional changes. The mother's demeanor will become more _____.

angry

Some of the physical changes will be _____, _____, and _____ of the legs.

nausea;
vomiting; trembling

In addition, the labia will _____, the rectum will _____, and there may be an increase in _____ _____.

separate;
dilate; bloody
show

Remember that it is important to have the mother frequently empty her _____.

bladder

During the second stage of labor, it is essential to try to provide an area with some privacy. The mother needs special care and encouragement as well as continuous explanation about what is occurring. Exhaustion and dehydration must be prevented.

When caput is observed, the mother must be taught to push in order to help you. When crowning occurs, the perineum must be supported with a clean towel and the head slowly guided as it begins to emerge. If the membranes are present around the baby's head, they should be removed immediately. If the cord is around the baby's neck, remove it by slipping it over the baby's head as soon as this can be done easily. Wipe the mucus from the baby's mouth, and use a finger to clear the mouth. If external rotation does not take place spontaneously, gently turn the head in the direction in which it will go most easily, thus presenting the shoulders to the pubic arch. Deliver the shoulders slowly by first applying traction upward to free the posterior shoulder, then reversing the traction downward, delivering the anterior shoulder.

To prevent perineal lacerations, the perineum must be _____.

supported

The head should be guided and delivered _____.

slowly

If present, membranes immediately should be _____.

removed

The cord must be felt for and if necessary _____.

unlooped

The mouth should be cleared of _____ as soon as possible.

mucus

Restitution can be affected by the nurse by _____ _____ _____.

turning the

head in the direction it will

go most easily

The shoulders should be delivered _____ and by the use of upward and downward _____.

slowly;

traction

The baby should be wrapped in a warm, clean towel, blanket, or cloth and placed in Trendelenburg position on the mother's abdomen. This will facilitate drainage of mucus from the nasopharynx.

When the cord stops pulsating, it can be tied in two places with the binding tape. The first tie is placed about 2 inches from the umbilicus, the next tie about 2 inches closer to the maternal end of the cord. If a pair of sterile scissors is available, the cord may be cut between these two ties. However, if no pair of sterile scissors or aseptic tapes are available, *do not* cut or tie the cord.

Carefully observe the mother for signs of placental separation; when this occurs, have the mother bear down again to help expel the placenta. If the cord has not been cut, wrap the placenta with the baby. If it has been cut, wrap it in newspaper and discard it, after examining to be sure it is intact.

The mother and baby should be identified and kept together as one unit. The mother should be made comfortable and given fluids. When the baby's color is good and respirations clear, the baby should be put to breast to help keep the uterus contracted.

As always, the mother should be observed carefully for bleeding during the fourth stage. Again, other people can be utilized to check on the fundus and massage it if indicated, and to report any changes to you.

After the delivery, the baby should be kept warm. Clearing the nasopharynx of mucus may be facilitated if the baby is placed on the mother's abdomen with its head _____.

down

The binding tape is used to tie the cord in two places after it stops _____.

pulsating

The cord can be cut between the two ties if there is an available

_____.

pair of sterile scissors

The mother and baby should be _____ and

_____.

identified;
kept together

If the baby is breathing well and its color is good, it may

_____.

be breast-fed

During the fourth stage, other people may be utilized to observe the mother for _____.

bleeding

It is the responsibility of all nurses, whether employed or not, to be aware of the emergency facilities in their own communities. They can be helpful also in teaching classes in first aid, nurses' aides, and emergency procedures. This is an obligation of every citizen and especially of those who are prepared in these areas.

POST-TEST Indicate whether each statement is true or false by circling the appropriate letter. Then turn to page 45 and see how well you have done.

1. It is important that the pregnant woman be knowledgeable about her health status and the type of delivery expected.   T   F

2. The pregnant mother should not be advised to prepare equipment for use during delivery in an emergency because she will become frightened.   T   F

3. During an emergency situation in an isolated area, you as the nurse will often be responsible for the medical care of the women in labor.   T   F

4. Other people can assist in the care of the women in labor during an emergency.   T   F

5. In a disaster situation, the progress of labor is determined by the amount of cervical dilatation.   T   F

6. Once the newborn's respirations and color are good, it is helpful to put the baby to breast so that the uterus will contract firmly.   T   F

7. It is the nurse's responsibility to be aware of the emergency facilities in the community.   T   F

In the specific areas with which you had difficulty, return to the material and review.

BIBLIOGRAPHY Brown, Janet, et al.: *Two Births*, Random House, New York, 1972.
Pritchard, Jack and Paul MacDonald: *Williams Obstetrics*, 15th ed., Appleton-Century-Crofts, New York, 1976.
Reeder, Sharon R., et al.: *Maternity Nursing*, J. B. Lippincott Co., Philadelphia, 1976.

PRETEST ANSWERS 1. Status   2. Clean linens; soap; baby clothes; bottle; nipple   3. Does not know where members of her family are   4. On-the-job training (on-the-spot teaching)   5. Sterile scissors   6. Kept together as a unit

POST-TEST ANSWERS 1. T   2. F   3. T   4. T   5. F   6. T   7. T

**UNIT I
EXAMINATION** The following multiple-choice examination will test your comprehension of the material covered in the first unit of this program. Remember, you are not competing with anyone but yourself. Therefore, do not guess in order to answer the questions; if you are unsure, this means that you have not learned the content. Return to the areas that give you difficulty and review them before going on with the examination.

Circle the letter of the best response to each question. After completing the unit examination, check your answers on page 541 and review those areas of difficulty before proceeding to the next unit.

1. An interruption in health occurs when the individual:
   a. Adapts successfully to a stressor
   b. Is unable to modify the strength of the stressor
   c. Is able to maintain his homeodynamic balance in the presence of a stressor
   d. Maintains an equilibrium while a stressor is operating

2. The internal factor of the individual which determines the degree of the interruption is:
   a. The length of time during which the stressor is operating
   b. The environment in which the stressor is operating
   c. The health state of the other systems
   d. The fact that the stressor is operating in combination with another stressor

3. When an individual's adaptive mechanism is inappropriate, this means that:
   a. There is no problem incurred
   b. The health state of the individual is not altered
   c. The individual will respond to all stressors in this manner
   d. The response of the individual further disrupts the equilibrium of the individual

4. The nonhealth state that ensues following a strong stressor:
   a. Might not have occurred if the stressor had been operating at a lower level of intensity
   b. Is only a transitory state, and the individual returns readily to a health state
   c. Is perceived only by the individual
   d. Is always a learned response to this specific stressor

5. A crisis state exists when the individual:
   a. Is able to modify the strength of the stressor
   b. Is aware that the strength of the stressor can be reduced by his or her own actions
   c. Is unable to adapt effectively without outside intervention
   d. Has sufficient resources to adapt successfully

6. In response to the death of the baby, the parents go through stages of grief in the following order:
    a. Depression, denial, bargaining, anger, and acceptance
    b. Bargaining, anger, denial, depression, and acceptance
    c. Anger, denial, depression, bargaining, and acceptance
    d. Denial, anger, bargaining, depression, and acceptance

7. Parents who are in the bargaining stage may display:
    a. Anger at the staff for not assisting them
    b. Signs of sadness and of being overwhelmed
    c. Activities to gain the favor of God
    d. Signs of isolation and withdrawal from daily activities

8. Nursing activities with a family who have just lost their newborn infant should be geared to:
    a. Helping the family to get through the stages of grief as soon as possible
    b. Accepting the response of each member even if the members are at different stages
    c. Sitting down and telling them that they must accomplish these various stages
    d. Providing reassurance to the parents that if they get through the first two steps in the hospital, they can do the rest at home

9. Areas of prevention, promotion, and restoration:
    a. Operate separately depending on the nonhealth state
    b. Follow a specific pattern, with preventive measures first, promotive measures next, and restorative measures last
    c. Operate together in only health states
    d. Often are found in combination as the organism adapts toward a state of homeodynamic balance

10. Restorative measures usually are:
    a. Nonspecific in nature
    b. Directed toward a specific system
    c. Of value only if used for a short period of time
    d. Kept constant once identified

11. The degrees of nonhealth states that can exist within a family system include:
    a. Interruptions, disorganization, and crisis
    b. Reorganization and readaptation
    c. Restoration and resolution
    d. Disorganization and reorganization

12. Disorganization of the family system can result from:
    a. Successful adaptation to a new member
    b. Ineffective adaptation to a new member
    c. Ability to reorganize the system when a new member joins
    d. Ongoing adaptation to the presence of a new member

13. A crisis state occurs within the family system when:
    a. The family is unable to adapt to the stressor without outside intervention
    b. The family is able to adapt successfully when the members discuss the difficulty
    c. The family is able to modify the stressor and maintain a homeodynamic balance after a period of disorganization
    d. The family is adapting to a stressor and reducing the strength as the members continue the adaptation

14. When the family is in a state of disorganization, the nurse can intervene effectively by:
    a. Identifying for them the specific stressors that seem to be causing the difficulty
    b. Assisting the family to develop their positive strengths and adapt to the stressor
    c. Separating the family members so that they can individually try to modify the stressor
    d. Encouraging the family to accept the disorganization since it could be worse

15. When the family system terminates, the nurse can effectively intervene by:
    a. Providing reassurance that everything happens for the best
    b. Attempting to help the person identify what went wrong
    c. Taking the place of the lost members
    d. Providing support for the persons' feelings and allowing them to go through the grieving process

16. The pregnant woman should be aware of her health status and the type of delivery she is expected to have:
    a. Since this will serve to prevent any complications
    b. So that in case of an emergency she will get proper care
    c. Since it is important for the hospital to keep good records
    d. So that the baby may be born on the due date

17. In a church basement, during a disaster situation, you are responsible for giving care to five women in labor. You would:
    a. Keep the whole family together as a unit
    b. Keep only the children with their mothers
    c. Clear the area and have present only other people who are assisting
    d. Clear the area of all lay persons and have only professionals to help

18. In an emergency situation, your assessment of the mother's progress during labor is dependent upon:
    a. The mother's cervical dilatation
    b. The amount of discomfort the mother is experiencing
    c. The type of breathing the mother is using
    d. The changes in the contractions and the physical signs such as trembling and nausea

19. To ensure the expulsion of the placenta after an emergency delivery, uterine contractions may be stimulated by:

    a. Administering an oxytocic intravenously
    b. Massaging the fundus
    c. Pulling on the umbilical cord
    d. Putting the baby to breast

UNIT II

INTERRUPTIONS IN HEALTH SYSTEMS DURING FETAL GROWTH AND DEVELOPMENT

CHAPTER ONE

FACTORS AFFECTING FETAL GROWTH

OBJECTIVES   *Identify how the genetic factors affect fetal growth.*

Identify how the environmental factors affect fetal growth.

Identify the methods of assessment of the fetus.

Identify the nursing intervention.

GLOSSARY   *Fetology:* The study of fetal growth and development
Gamete: The germ cell—spermatozoon or ovum
Gametogenesis: The development of mature gametes
Dominant trait: The characteristic that is expressed in the offspring
Recessive trait: The characteristic that is not expressed in the offspring if one trait of the pair is dominant but which will be evidenced if both traits are recessive
Autosome: Any chromosome excluding the sex chromosomes
Infant mortality rate: The number of infant deaths during the first year after birth as a ratio per 1,000 live births
Maternal morbidity: Interruptions in the health state of the mother occurring during the antepartum, intrapartum, or postpartum period
Amniocentesis: The procedure in which some amniotic fluid is removed transabdominally
Sonography: The use of ultrasonic waves to detect various tissues and the relaying of this information on a graph
Amnioscopy: The visualization of the amniotic sac and fluid using an endoscope
Lecithin: A phospholipoid found in the fetal lungs and amniotic fluid
Sphingomyelin: A phospholipoid found in the fetal lungs and amniotic fluid

PRETEST   In the spaces provided, fill in the word or words that best complete(s) the statements. Then turn to page 67 and check your answers.

1. The factors affecting the fetal pattern of growth are from two sources: _____ and _____.

2. A genetic error in the gamete can occur at the time of _____ _____.

3. Abnormal chromosomes can carry traits that are _____.

4. Poor nutrition of the mother may affect the fetal development _____.

5. Fetal growth and development are dependent on the mother's psychological well-being and her use of _____.

6. Rubella can be prevented by the use of _____.

7. Amniocentesis is _____ _____.

8. The L/S ratio determines the _____ _____.

9. Amnioscopy is _____ _____.

10. If the amniotic fluid is dark green, it contains _____.

11. An ultrasonic scanner can be used to determine _____ _____.

There is much study in the field of fetology concerning the factors that can alter and/or change the pattern of fetal growth and development. These factors are from two sources: they are either *genetic* (from each parent) or *environmental* (from the maternal source).

The basic genetic factors are established at the time of *fertilization*. During normal gametogenesis and meiosis, the 46 chromosomes divide so that each gamete contains 23 complete chromosomes. If there is an error in this process and the gamete contains other than the normal number of chromosomes or any fragmented chromosomes, at the time of fertilization this error will become part of the new life and act as a stressor, causing abnormal growth and development. If the genetic error is very great, often the result is incompatible with life at this time and results in a spontaneous abortion. Some of the genetic abnormalities arise from parents who are carriers of an abnormal trait, often recessive in the parents but becoming expressed with certain parental combination so that the abnormality is present, as, for example, in cystic fibrosis. Genetic counseling will be discussed in the next chapter.

Currently much research is being done to determine the extent of the alterations of the genes and chromosomes in the gametes as a result of the effects of drugs, those taken in therapeutic dosages and in abusive dosages, and of radiation. The types of sequelae that may follow the exposure to these agents are being studied.

Factors from two sources may affect the development of the fetus; these sources are _____ and _____.

genetic; environmental

Genetic errors can occur randomly during the processes of _____ and _____.

meiosis; gametogenesis

Some genetic abnormalities are inheritable because the parents are _____.

carriers of the trait

Chromosomal aberrations in the gametes may follow the exposure to _____ and _____.

drugs; radiation

After fertilization, the maternal body is the environment for the developing fetus, with direct influence on the patterns of growth. There are various stressors arising from this source which can alter and change the patterns of growth, producing a nonhealth state in the fetus since the effects of the stressor often are magnified because of the small size of the fetus.

Maternal nutrition has a direct effect on the number of cells within the body of the developing fetus. Studies have found that the children of severely malnourished women have a smaller number of brain cells. Although these extremes are rarely seen in this country, the amount and quality of the nutrients are thought to have a direct bearing on the well-being of the fetus.

Fetal malnutrition can also occur in instances where the mother is receiving adequate nutrients. There are maternal interruptions in health that limit blood supply so that the transfer of nutrients at the placenta is reduced, as seen with cardiac problems, hypertension, or renal problems. There are also instances in which the mother is receiving adequate nutrition yet there seems to be an interference within her system which makes the nutrients unavailable to the infant. Studies being carried out with mothers who smoke cigarettes seem to indicate that indeed this may be the case since maternal smoking seems related to reduced fetal growth. Out of these studies also comes a correlation of fetal nutritional well-being with the status of the maternal leukocytes.

Since fetal malnutrition is closely related to perinatal mortality and to problems of the central nervous system, including retardation, much attention is being directed toward identifying malnutrition and the actual dynamics occurring in utero.

A method to determine the rate of fetal growth in utero involves the use of the *ultrasonic B-mode scanner*. This method uses ultrasound waves that bounce back from soft tissues and form a pattern on an oscilloscope from which a photograph can be taken. This picture can then be used to measure the biparietal diameter of the fetal head. Since growth occurs at a specific rate, norms have been established. If the growth rate is less than 1 millimeter per week in the last trimester, then there is arrested or minimal growth.[1]

The biparietal diameter of the fetus is an indication of

_____.

     fetal growth in utero

This measurement is made by using _____

     an ultrasonic

_____.

     B-mode scanner

The mother's emotional status has a direct effect on the levels of various hormones circulating in the blood, and the fetus, in turn, will be affected by these hormones. Studies have indicated that if the mother is under much emotional stress without adequate support from family members, the effects of her body chemistry alter the pattern of growth and, in many cases, there is an increased incidence of prematurity. It therefore is important for the nurse to assess the emotional status of the mother and the family dynamics so that intervention can be at the appropriate time and of the appropriate kind.

Often associated with the mother's emotional status is her use of chemicals: drugs, alcohol, and nicotine. Drugs taken during the first three months of gestation often interfere with the organ development of the fetus. Later, ingestion or administration of drugs can interfere

USE TH
TO CONCEAL
ON THOSE
WITH AN A[
AT THE T[

Interruptions in
Family Health
during
Pregnancy

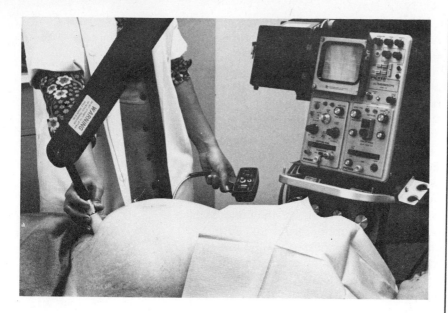

B-mode sonography. (*From Williams Obstetrics, 15th ed., by Jack Pritchard and Paul MacDonald. Copyright © 1976 by Appleton-Century-Crofts. Used with permission of Appleton-Century-Crofts*).

with the body physiology to such an extent that such problems as hyperbilirubinemia (high levels of bilirubin in the blood), goiter, and early fetal death occur as a result. The use of alcohol has been associated with bone and other changes in the fetus, while following delivery the infant may go through withdrawal symptoms. The nurse must advise caution in the use of any chemicals in women of childbearing age since often in early pregnancy the woman is unaware that she is pregnant. Pregnant women should always consult with their physicians before taking any medication. If the mother tells you that she already has used drugs or is a heavy smoker, it is important not to raise her level of anxiety about the outcome of the pregnancy and to be as supportive as possible.

Maternal nutrition affects the _____ _____.

well-being (growth)

of the fetus

The mother's emotional status has a direct _____ _____.

effect on fetal

growth and development

Drugs taken by the mother affect the _____ _____.

physiology

of the fetus

Alcohol produces changes in _____.

fetal bones

It is important for women of childbearing age _____ _____.

to use

drugs with caution

Certain drugs and radiation are capable of producing chromosomal breaks in the developing fetus not thought to be present at the time of fertilization. The extent of these aberrations and the possible sequelae are not well known. There may be permanent genetic changes that will be passed on to the next generation, or there may be higher incidence of problems such as leukemia occurring later. There is known to be a certain amount of fetal loss since these radiation and chemical stressors can be overwhelming to the developing fetus.

Viruses are able to cross the placental barrier, and, during the first three months of development, these stressors are capable of producing severe adverse effects within the fetus. The effects of viruses are dramatically illustrated when the mother has rubella during the first trimester and the fetal development is interrupted so that the children are often blind, deaf, retarded, and/or have cardiac problems. In the instance of rubella, the nurse can be effective by promoting the use of vaccines among school-age children to prevent spread to their mothers and by cautioning the pregnant women to avoid contact with persons who have viral infections.

Many *infectious agents* are able to cross the placental barrier. In the case of many of these agents, if the mother has been exposed previously then her antibodies will effectively remove the agents as antigens, as seen with polio, variola, and rubella, whereas if the mother has had no previous exposure to any or all of the agents, both mother and fetus will be affected.

Bacterial infections early in pregnancy may result in abortions; such infections later in pregnancy may result in stillbirths, as seen with syphilis. In cases of less severe infection the infant may survive but have the symptoms, e.g., congenital syphilis. Studies of the amniotic fluid reveal that there is a bacteriostatic action present. Infections can occur, however, even when the amniotic membrane is intact. Bacteriostatic action is especially important at the end of pregnancy, as the cervix begins to dilate slightly. If the mother has a poor nutritional status, as seen more prominently in the developing countries, then the amniotic fluid does not have the necessary bacteriostatic action and there is a high premature and stillbirth rate.

The maternal antibodies provide protection for the developing fetus and passive immunity for the infant. The infant's own immunological system begins to develop at the eighth week of gestation and functions at about the sixteenth to twentieth week, but normally the uterine environment is protective and there is limited exposure to antigens. Maternal antibodies circulating in the infant after birth provide passive immunity and protection against such agents as diphtheria, providing that the mother has been immunized. Problems arise when the maternal antibodies produce reactions in the developing fetus. This is frequently seen when the mother has Rh negative blood and the fetus is Rh positive. The mother's antibodies cross the placental barrier and destroy the red blood cells of the fetus. (This situation is discussed further in the chapter entitled "Hemolytic Incompatibilities.")

Studies have indicated that in low socioeconomic groups there is a higher incidence of prematurity, infant mortality, and maternal morbidity than there is in higher socioeconomic groups. Teen-age mothers who are unwed also have a high incidence of these events. No one cause of these events has been identified, but higher levels of stress present, such as those associated with poor living conditions and poor nutrition, seem to contribute.

Viruses and drugs are capable of _____ _____ and _____ _____.

changing chromosomal structure; altering growth patterns

Maternal antibodies are able to cross _____ _____.

the placental barrier

In low socioeconomic groups, mothers have a higher incidence of _____, _____, and _____ than do mothers in higher socioeconomic groups.

prematurity; infant mortality; maternal morbidity

Now that you are cognizant of the factors that affect fetal growth and the kinds of stress these factors produce, let us look at the methods of assessment of the fetal status. This is a relatively new area and is in the process of expanding as new techniques are learned and developed.

Characteristics of the fetus and problems related to its growth and development can be determined by various studies that are carried out using samples of amniotic fluid obtained by amniocentesis. *Amniocentesis* is the procedure by which a sample of amniotic fluid is removed, usually by means of a needle inserted into the uterine cavity transabdominally. Studies of the amniotic fluid and the fetal cells contained in it can determine genetic information, such as chromosomal abnormalities, as in Turner's syndrome, and the possible presence of sex-linked problems such as hemophilia, a disorder of the blood-clotting mechanism. Certain enzyme deficiencies associated with disorders such as Tay-Sachs disease and Hurler's syndrome can be identified. Other problems that can be identified during fetal life are erythroblastosis (associated with hemolytic disorders) and postmaturity. Amniocentesis is considered to be a relatively safe procedure, although problems do occur in a very small number of instances. A problem that may be encountered during the procedure is the needle hitting the fetal parts, with the possibility of fetal death occurring as a result of hemorrhage.

There is also a chance of introducing an amniotic fluid embolism into the maternal bloodstream.

As the nurse, you are involved in clarifying the explanation of the procedure and the reasons for its being performed to the mother and the family. Once the results have been interpreted, further clarification of the implications is necessary. At the time of the procedure, which usually is done on an outpatient basis, the mother empties her bladder, she may receive an analgesic, and the fetal position is checked. Before the procedure, the placenta often is localized by *sonography*, the use of ultrasonic waves that are reflected by tissue to create a picture on a graph. At the time of the amniocentesis, an explanation of the ongoing procedure helps to reduce the level of the mother's anxiety about it. The skin area is anesthetized before the insertion of the needle, and sterile technique is extremely important. Following the procedure the nurse observes the status of the mother and fetus in order to assess if there is any change. The parents often are very anxiously awaiting the outcome of the results of the tests; they need acceptance of their feelings and fears.

Examination of the amniotic fluid can reveal _____ _____.

> information about the status of the fetus

The cells in the amniotic fluid carry _____ information.

> genetic

During the procedure it is important that you prepare the mother and _____ _____.

> explain what is happening during the procedure

Following the procedure it is important to _____ _____.

> check the fetal and maternal status

Another method of assessment of the fetus is *amnioscopy*, which is the visualization of the amniotic fluid through the intact membranes. This procedure, done in late pregnancy, involves inserting an endoscope (a plastic cone or stainless steel tube with a light) through the slightly dilated cervix. The amniotic fluid normally is clear. If meconium is present, indicating that there is fetal anoxia and that the fetus is compromised, the amniotic fluid appears dark green. Amnioscopy is easier to do and has fewer side effects than amniocentesis. However, some of the problems that may occur as a result of this procedure are infection, rupture of membranes, and, if the placenta is implanted low, bleeding. Often if there is heavy meconium, indicating that the fetus is in jeopardy, labor is artificially stimulated. Since the majority of mothers who undergo this procedure have a diagnosed problem, they are aware of the possibility of an untoward outcome of the pregnancy. These mothers need much support from the nurse. The nurse must provide sufficient time and a comfortable atmosphere enabling families to express their fears and anxieties. The nurse must give careful and complete explanation before, during, and after the procedure, obtaining feedback in order to validate the family's understanding.

Amnioscopy is done _____ in pregnancy.

By amnioscopy one is able to _____

_____.

late

visualize the

amniotic fluid

If the amniotic fluid appears dark green, this means that _____ is present, indicating _____.

If the fetus is in jeopardy, often labor is _____

_____.

meconium; fetal anoxia

artificially

stimulated

These methods of fetal assessment enable determination of the maturity of the fetus. Since the EDC (expected date of confinement) is an approximate date and there may be a slight amount of bleeding in the first months of pregnancy around the time of the menstrual period, often it is difficult to determine the gestational age of the fetus. If for some medical reason based on the maternal or fetal health status, it is deemed advisable to intervene and to terminate the pregnancy, it is important to know the maturity of the baby, which provides some indication of the baby's ability to survive outside the uterine environment. There is no accurate way of determining when the fetus is at term or the degree of postmaturity. Tests available indicate only immaturity or relative maturity of some of the systems, or fetal distress.

One of the most significant tests of fetal maturity reflects the development of the lungs. The phospholipoids lecithin and sphingomyelin make up the surfactant that lines the alveoli of the lungs. These must attain a certain ratio in order to decrease the surface tension of the lungs. A test is performed to determine the *lecithin, sphingomyelin (L/S) ratio* using amniotic fluid. The L/S ratio should be 2:0 or above to indicate adequate lung maturity and thus a decreased risk of idiopathetic respiratory distress syndrome, which has a high mortality rate.

This test is 95 to 99 percent accurate when the mother has no interruption in health. Problems occur when the mother has preeclampsia, chronic hypertension, diabetes, or sickle cell anemia: reliability drops to 81 to 83 percent.[2] This is in contrast to the "nile blue" test of fat cells, which maintains its accuracy even during interruptions in maternal health.

A quick estimate of the L/S ratio is done by taking amniotic fluid and adding 95 percent ethanol and isotonic saline in a test tube, shaking it, and measuring the amount of foam that remains on top 15 minutes later.

The L/S ratio is an indication of _____ _____. A ratio of _____ or above indicates that the lungs are mature enough. A difficulty with the L/S ratio occurs when the mother has _____ _____.

fetal lung maturity; 2.0;

interruptions in health

The L/S ratio is used in combination with other tests to determine the status of the fetus. Currently there is investigation of the relationship between the percentage of fat cells and increase in lecithin.

Estriol levels are another determinant of fetoplacental well-being. Estriol is produced by a complex method whereby the fetal adrenals produce dehydroepiandrosterone, which is hydroxylated in the liver of the fetus and then converted by the placenta to estriol. During the end of pregnancy the estriol levels increase, and these levels can be assessed from the maternal urine or blood. A 24-hour urine specimen is necessary. This may be awkward for the mother to obtain. Assessment of blood estriol levels is accurate, and the specimen is more easily obtained than a 24-hour urine collection. Blood levels are examined for both free and conjugated estriol. If these levels drop appreciably then the fetus is assumed to be in danger. It is important to be sure the mother is not taking medication or changing her activity greatly, since both these factors can alter the level of estriol and give false results. There are also difficulties in interpreting the test if the mother has renal disease.

Estriol levels must be assessed serially, since one test is not significant by itself. Values for urinary estriol above 12 milligrams per 24 hours are acceptable; values between 12 and 4 milligrams indicate problems; and values below 4 milligrams mean severe fetal jeopardy.

Tests are also being done on the levels of placental lactogen. Low levels (below 4 micrograms) have been correlated, in some studies, with fetal jeopardy, especially if the mother is hypertensive.

Estriol levels indicate _____ _____. Normally at the end of pregnancy estriol levels _____. These levels can be altered by the mother's _____ _____. Urinary levels of

fetoplacental well-being;

rise;

taking medication or changing activity;

estriol that indicate severe fetal jeopardy are _____

_____.

> below 4
> milligrams

Other studies utilize amniotic fluid obtained by amniocentesis to assess fetal status. Fat cells of the fetus contained in the amniotic fluid react with a dye called "nile blue" and turn an orange color. If there are a large number of fat cells, in excess of 30 percent after 36 weeks, this indicates that the fetus is close to term since the integumentary system has matured.

The amniotic fluid also can be tested for the ratio of bilirubin to creatinine. At term, the bilirubin level lowers as the liver matures, and the creatinine level rises as the kidney matures.

An indication of the maturity of the integumentary system is the

_____

_____.

> number of fat cells in the
> amniotic fluid
> goes down;
> liver

At term the level of bilirubin _____,

indicating maturity of the _____.

The *oxytocin challenge test* is used to determine whether the fetoplacental unit can withstand the stress that would occur during the contractions of labor. This test is not used as the only parameter but rather as part of the battery of tests utilized to determine the well-being of the fetus in utero. Oxytocin is administered to the mother to induce contractions, and the fetus is monitored to determine the response to this simulated labor.

The procedure is as follows. The mother comes into the clinical unit, and after emptying her bladder, she assumes a semi-Fowler's position or lies on her left side so that there is less of a problem of maternal hypotension due to compression of the inferior vena cava. Blood pressure is assessed, and then the fetal heart tones are located and an external monitor is used. The ultrasonic transducer is placed over the area where the fetal heart was heard. Then the pressure transducer is placed above the umbilicus, where contractions of the fundus are best felt. A tracing is done to determine if the mother is having any spontaneous contractions and to also determine a baseline for the fetal heart rate. Then an intravenous infusion of oxytocin is started. It is given very slowly, often with a pump such as an Ivac that delivers a prescribed dosage very slowly. The dosage of oxytocin is increased to the point where the mother is having at least three contractions in a ten-minute period which last for 30 to 60 seconds. If there are persistent late decelerations of the fetal heart rate, indicating fetal jeopardy, the test is considered positive. Late deceleration means that following or at the peak of the contraction, the fetal heart rate drops and then slowly recovers. If there are no persistent decelerations then it is felt that the fetus is safe in utero for another week, when the test is repeated. If there is fetal jeopardy, it is confirmed by other tests, such as estriol levels; then an elective cesarean section is usually performed.

The oxytocin challenge test may take three hours or more of the parents' time, so they should be prepared for this. During the procedure they need complete explanations of what is occurring. The fetal heart tones are audible with the monitor, and the parents are relieved when they hear a steady heartbeat. If the fetus is in jeopardy, the parents can comprehend the concern of the staff and are better able to make choices about intervention.

The oxytocin challenge test is used to determine _____ _____.

The test is considered positive if there are _____ _____, which indicate that _____, _____. During the test the mother should be positioned in a way that prevents _____ _____. During the test the parents should be provided with _____.

the

fetal response to labor;

persistent

late decelerations; the fetus

is in jeopardy;

hypotension

from developing;

complete explanations

Studies are being done to watch the fetal heart rate for accelerations during the time that the oxytocin test is being performed. These increases in the fetal heart rate are considered evidence of fetal well-being. The increases may occur as the baseline of the tracing is being done, with fetal movement, or during a contraction. The accelerations have been classified. Minimal acceleration is an increase of less than 10 beats per minute; average acceleration is 10 to 20 beats per minute; and marked acceleration is 20 to 50 beats per minute. If the oxytocin challenge test is suspicious, that is, if there are occasional late decelerations, then the presence of average to marked acceleration is evidence that the fetus is responding adequately to the stress. But if there is only minimal acceleration, then often the oxytocin challenge test converts to a positive test subsequently.

Average to marked accelerations are indicative of _____ _____. Average acceleration is _____ beats per minute.

fetal

well-being;

10–20

POST-TEST Indicate whether each statement is true or false by circling the appropriate letter. Then turn to page 67 and see how well you have done.

1. Once the gametes are formed, there is no chance of a genetic error occurring.   T   F

2. Only dominant genetic traits will be seen in the offspring.   T   F

3. The quality of nutrition of the mother is important for the developing fetus.   T   F

4. If the mother is under the effects of many emotional stressors, the well-being of the fetus can be affected.   T   F

5. Viral infections in the mother do not affect the fetal growth and development.   T   F

6. Amniocentesis always is performed after the cervix has begun to dilate.   T   F

7. Cells from the amniotic fluid can be cultured to give genetic information.   T   F

8. It is possible to determine the relative maturity of the pulmonary system by the L/S ratio.   T   F

9. It is possible to visualize the amniotic fluid by using an endoscope and to determine if fetal distress has occurred.   T   F

10. The number of fat cells in the amniotic fluid will help to determine the maturity of the fetus.   T   F

11. Sonography can be used to determine where the placenta is located.   T   F

In the specific areas with which you had difficulty, return to the material and review.

REFERENCES   1. Warren M. Crosby et al., "Fetal Malnutrition: An Appraisal of Correlated Factors," *American Journal of Obstetrics and Gynecology*, Vol. 128, No. 1, p. 29, May 1, 1977.
2. J. C. Morrison et al., "Amniotic Fluid Tests for Fetal Maturity in Normal and Abnormal Pregnancies," *Obstetrics and Gynecology*, Vol. 49, No. 1, p. 23, Jan. 1977.

BIBLIOGRAPHY   Arias, Fernando, "The Diagnosis and Management of Intrauterine Growth Retardation," *Obstetrics and Gynecology*, Vol. 49, No. 3, pp. 293–297, March 1977.

Crosby, Warren, et al., "Fetal Malnutrition: An Appraisal of Correlated Factors," *American Journal of Obstetrics and Gynecology*, Vol. 128, No. 1, pp. 22–29, May 1, 1977.

Doran, T. A., et al., "Amniotic Fluid Tests for Fetal Maturity in Normal and Abnormal Pregnancies," *American Journal of Obstetrics and Gynecology*, Vol. 125, No. 5, pp. 591–592, July 1, 1976.

Evans, Hugh E., et al., "Effect of Amniotic Fluid on Bacterial Growth," *Obstetrics and Gynecology*, Vol. 49, No. 1, pp. 35–37, Jan. 1977.

Farahani, Gholamali and Arnold Fenton, "Fetal Heart Rate Acceleration in Relation to the Oxytocin Challenge Test," *Obstetrics and Gynecology*, Vol. 49, No. 2, pp. 163–165, Feb. 1977.

Galloway, Karen G., "Placental Evaluation Studies: The Procedures, Their Purposes, and the Nursing Care Involved," *Maternal Child Nursing*, Vol. 1, No. 5, pp. 300–306, Sept./Oct. 1976.

Gewolb, I. H., et al., "Amniotic Fluid Cortisol as an Index of Fetal Lung Maturity," *Obstetrics and Gynecology*, Vol. 49, No. 4, p. 462, April 1977.

Hudson, Elizabeth A. and Janice Gauntlett, "Amniotic Fluid Cells and the Lecithin/Sphingomyelin Ratio," *Obstetrics and Gynecology*, Vol. 49, No. 3, pp. 280ff., March 1977.

Larsen, Bryan and Rudolph P. Galask, "Protection of the Fetus Against Infection," *Seminars in Perinatology*, Vol. 1, No. 2, pp. 183–193, April 1977.

Miller, Carol, et al., "Maternal Serum Unconjugated Estriol and Urine Estriol Concentrations in Normal and High-Risk Pregnancy," *Obstetrics and Gynecology*, Vol. 49, No. 3, pp. 289–291, March 1977.

Miller, Herbert C., "Fetal Growth Retardation in Relation to Maternal Smoking and Weight Gain in Pregnancy," *American Journal of Obstetrics and Gynecology*, Vol. 125, No. 1, p. 55, May 1, 1976.

Morrison, J. C., et al., "Amniotic Fluid Tests for Fetal Maturity in Normal and Abnormal Pregnancies," *Obstetrics and Gynecology*, Vol. 49, No. 1, pp. 20–24, Jan. 1977.

Mukherjee, Trisht Kumar, et al., "Significance of Amniotic Fluid Corticosteroid Levels in Human Pregnancies," *Obstetrics and Gynecology*, Vol. 49, No. 2, pp. 145–147, Feb. 1977.

Naeye, Richard, et al., "Amniotic Fluid Infections in an African City," *Journal of Pediatrics*, Vol. 90, No. 6, pp. 967–969, June 1977.

Ott, William J., et al., "Analysis of Variables Affecting Perinatal Mortality," *Obstetrics and Gynecology*, Vol. 49, No. 4, pp. 481–485, April 1977.

Pierong, Sophie, et al., "Withdrawal Symptoms in Infants with the Fetal Alcohol Syndrome," *Journal of Pediatrics*, Vol. 90, No. 4, pp. 630–633, April 1977.

Pritchard, Jack and Paul MacDonald: *Williams Obstetrics*, 15th ed., Appleton-Century-Crofts, New York, 1976.

Trieweiler, Michael W., "Baseline Fetal Heart Rate Characteristics as an Indicator of Fetal Status During Antepartum Period," *American Journal of Obstetrics and Gynecology*, Vol. 125, No. 5, p. 622, July 1, 1976.

PRETEST ANSWERS
1. Genes; environment (maternal body)   2. Gametogenesis or meiosis   3. Inheritable
4. Adversely   5. Drugs or chemicals   6. Immunization   7. The removal of amniotic fluid, usually intra-abdominally   8. Lung maturity by the ratio of lecithin to sphingomyelin   9. The visualization of the amniotic sac and fluid through the cervix   10. Meconium
11. The biparietal diameter of the fetal head

POST-TEST ANSWERS
1. F   2. F   3. T   4. T   5. F   6. F   7. T   8. T   9. T
10. T   11. T

CHAPTER TWO

GENETIC COUNSELING

OBJECTIVES   *Identify the need for genetic counseling.*

Identify the steps used in providing genetic counseling to families.

Identify the nurse's role.

GLOSSARY   *Chromosomes:* Material carrying genetic information
Autosomes: The 22 pairs of chromosomes, excluding X and Y, that have no sexual
characteristics

PRETEST In the spaces provided, fill in the word or words that best complete(s) the statements. Then turn to page 76 and check your answers.

1. The total number of human chromosomes is _____.

2. There are 22 pairs of autosomes and _____

   _____.

3. The material that makes up the genes is _____.

4. The functions of genes are _____

   _____

   _____.

5. When a chromosomal aberration occurs, then often there is seen

   _____.

6. Genetic counseling is available to _____

   _____.

7. Those persons who are considered to be in a high-risk group are

   _____

   _____, _____ _____

   _____, and _____

   _____.

8. Genetic counseling is _____

   _____

   _____.

9. The first step in genetic counseling is to _____

   _____.

10. After the tests are complete, then the information is provided to the families
    so that _____

    _____.

The field of genetic counseling has developed as the knowledge of genetics has grown in recent years through the discovery of the structure of the genes. The total number of human chromosomes is 46, and the chromosomes are paired, making a full complement of 23 pairs of chromosomes. Twenty-two of these pairs are the autosomes and one pair is the sex chromosomes. Each chromosome is made up of genes, molecular structures of DNA (deoxyribonucleic acid) material, which are responsible for protein, enzyme, and hormone synthesis.

The total number of human chromosomes is _____.

46

There are 22 pairs of autosomes and _____

_____.

one pair

of sex chromosomes

The molecular structure of the genes is made up of _____.

DNA

When the chromosomes are paired, there are matching genes on each pair of chromosomes responsible for a specific aspect of growth and development. For example, if a person has two matching recessive genes bb, for blue eyes, then the person will have blue eyes, but if the person has one gene b and the other B, for brown eyes, the person will have brown eyes, since the B is dominant. In some instances, there are multiple genes that are responsible for a particular characteristic; height is such a characteristic.

Specific aspects of growth and development are governed by

_____.

genes

	B	b
b	**Bb** brown eyes	**bb** blue eyes
b	**Bb** brown eyes	**bb** blue eyes

Bb - Heterozygous brown eyes

bb - Homozygous blue eyes

An example of the Mendelian law of independent assortment.

When a recessive gene or trait is expressed, this means that

_____

_____.

> there is a matching recessive gene

When chromosomal aberrations arise, the defect of development which follows is dependent on the gene or genes involved and on what segment of development they are responsible for.

Should a child with a genetic disorder be born to a family, this event often produces a state of disruption and disorganization, and in some families it produces a state of crisis.

Should a chromosomal aberration occur, the result often is seen

_____.

> in a defect of development

Genetic counseling is the provision of information about the chromosomal structure and functioning of genes with the prediction of the potential effect parental genes will have on the offspring or the prediction of genetic disorders of the developing fetus. This information is made available to families so that they are better able to decide about future plans to have more children or the desirability of continuing the present pregnancy.

Genetic counseling of families has become more easily available as research in the field of genetics has developed rapidly. Now families who have had one child with a genetic problem and who wish to know what the chances are of having a normal child are usually able to obtain answers. Genetic counseling presently is available only to families who are a high-risk group: this group is made up of families who have one child with a chromosomal defect, families in which the mother is over forty, and families whose family history presents a high probability of transmitting a genetic disorder such as hemophilia.

Genetic counseling is available to _____

_____

_____.

> members of
> families who are in a high-risk
> group

Genetic counseling provides information about _____

_____

_____ so that it is possible to

_____

_____.

> the
> structure and functioning
> of one's genes;
> predict the effect on one's
> offspring

The first step involved in providing genetic counseling is to determine that the family is in a high-risk group. This is done on the basis of the family history of the parents, the diagnosis of the specific genetic disorder in a child, or the age of the mother. A detailed family history is taken, determining the age of death and cause of death of the members of the extended family and any genetic disorder—such as muscular dystrophy (fascioscapulchumeral type), which appears in the school-age child—that has appeared during the lifetime of the various members of the family.

The second step is to do a chromosomal study of the parents; this is called karyotyping. If the counseling is being done before the mother becomes pregnant, a blood sample usually is used for the study. If the mother is pregnant at the time, amniocentesis is performed and cells are cultured to determine the genetic makeup. If the genetic disorder cannot be seen on genes, as is the case with cystic fibrosis, then studies of the various enzymes in the amniotic fluid can be done and values established determining the probability that the disorder exists.

The third step is to assemble all the facts from the family history, physical findings, and chromosomal studies. This information then is analyzed according to the probability of the occurrence of a recessive trait or a dominant trait in future pregnancies. If the trait is sex-linked, as in the case of hemophilia, in which 50 percent of males inherit the problem, this information can assist the families in making their decisions.

The beginning step in genetic counseling is _____ _____ _____.

identifying that the family is in the high-risk group

It is important to do a thorough family history determining the _____ _____.

cause of death and presence of any genetic disorder

Karyotyping is the _____.

study of the chromosomes

The last step in genetic counseling is to _____ _____ _____ _____.

determine the probability of a genetic disorder occurring in future pregnancy or being present in the developing fetus

Nursing intervention may begin by referral of the family for genetic counseling. When the nurse is with the family at the time of the birth of a child with a genetic problem, the nurse must give much support to the family members. Often the mother feels very guilty or another member may be blamed for causing the problem. Following the birth, it is important for the family members to express their fears and anxieties so that the nurse can clarify information. The family may have many questions about the genetic makeup, and, since the culturing of the cells usually takes several weeks, waiting may be difficult for them. Once the family is informed of the findings, it is important to obtain feedback to clarify the facts and enhance the family's understanding. Often difficulties arise when the chances or percentages are given, e.g., the families often misinterpret the probability to mean one out of four of their children rather than one out of four chances with each pregnancy.

Once the diagnosis of a child born with a genetic problem is established, the parents may have many questions and concerns about what difficulties may arise and how they will handle them. Referral to various agencies, especially to a parents' association, can provide much needed support and realistic approaches to problems. The child's health often is followed by specialists, and the family may need referral for assistance with medical expenses.

If the genetic counseling is being done when the mother is pregnant, and she decides to terminate the pregnancy once the results indicate that there is a high chance that the fetus is affected, then the mother needs to be able to verbalize her feelings of loss. If this is the first pregnancy, the parents may feel that there is something wrong with them.

If the parents have just had a child born with a genetic problem, then the nursing intervention is to _____.

| allow them to express and work through their feelings and refer them for counseling |

When the family is going for genetic counseling, the nurse can provide _____.

| information about the procedure for genetic testing |

Once the results have been determined, it is helpful to get _____ from the family.

| feedback |

Referral to various agencies for help with the child may include _____ and _____.

| parents' associations; official agencies for care and financial aid |

If the family or mother decides to terminate the pregnancy, then
nursing intervention is to _____
_____
_____.

$\Downarrow$

be supportive and

allow for feelings to be

expressed

POST-TEST Indicate whether each statement is true or false by circling the appropriate letter. Then turn to page 76 and see how well you have done.

1. There are 46 chromosomes in human beings.   T   F

2. There are two pairs of sex chromosomes.   T   F

3. Genes control the growth and development.   T   F

4. Genetic counseling is available to people who have family histories of genetic problems.   T   F

5. It is possible to be certain that the next child will develop a genetic disorder.   T   F

6. Genetic disorders may not show up in early childhood.   T   F

7. Karyotyping refers to the culturing and studying of the chromosomes.   T   F

8. Some genetic disorders are sex-linked and show up only in males.   T   F

9. Genetic counseling can be done only after the birth of the baby.   T   F

10. It is important for the nurse to obtain feedback from the family after they have been given the results.   T   F

In the specific areas with which you had difficulty, return to the material and review.

BIBLIOGRAPHY   Howell, Rodney R., "Prenatal Diagnosis in Prevention of Handicapping Disorders," *Pediatric Clinics of North America*, Vol. 20, No. 1, pp. 141–149, Feb. 1973.

Moore, Mary Lou: *The Newborn and the Nurse*, W. B. Saunders Co., Philadelphia, 1972.

Nadler, Henry L., "Prenatal Diagnosis of Inborn Defects: A Status Report," *Nursing Digest*, pp. 63–67, Fall 1976.

Pritchard, Jack and Paul MacDonald: *Williams Obstetrics*, 15th ed., Appleton-Century-Crofts, New York, 1976.

Romney, Seymour L., et al.: *Gynecology and Obstetrics: The Health Care of Women*, McGraw-Hill, New York, 1975.

Sly, William S., "What Is Genetic Counseling?" *Birth Defects: Original Article Series*, Vol. IX, No. 4, The National Foundation of the March of Dimes, New York, April 1973.

Vaughan, C. and R. James McKay: *Nelson Textbook of Pediatrics*, 10th ed., W. B. Saunders Co., Philadelphia, 1975.

PRETEST ANSWERS   1. 46   2. One pair of sex chromosomes   3. DNA   4. To control growth and development by controlling protein, enzyme, and hormone synthesis   5. A defect in development   6. Families or persons in a high-risk group   7. Families who have a child with a genetic problem, families with a history of genetic problems, and families in which the mother is over forty   8. The provision of information about the effect of one's genes on the growth and development of one's offspring   9. Take a complete family history   10. They can make decisions about having children or continuing the present pregnancy

POST-TEST ANSWERS   1. T   2. F   3. T   4. T   5. F   6. T   7. T   8. T   9. F   10. T

CHAPTER THREE

HEMOLYTIC INCOMPATIBILITIES

OBJECTIVES   *Identify the factors that produce Rh incompatibility.*

Identify the effects of Rh incompatibility on the fetus.

Identify the types of treatment instituted with Rh problems.

Identify the factors producing ABO incompatibility.

Identify the nursing intervention with families who have Rh and ABO hemolytic incompatibilities.

GLOSSARY   *Kernicterus:* A condition in the fetus or neonate occurring when bilirubin, because of its elevated level, crosses the barrier and affects the central nervous system, especially the brain

Hydrops fetalis: A condition of the fetus which indicates severe involvement with extreme anemia, producing generalized edema often followed shortly by circulatory collapse

Coomb's test: A measurement of antibody levels against the Rh factor

Rh: A factor found in the blood of a portion of the population. When the Rh factor is introduced into the system of a person who normally does not have this factor, an antigen-antibody response occurs

PRETEST   In the spaces provided, fill in the word or words that best complete(s) the statements. Then turn to page 87 and check your answers.

1. The Rh negative mother forms antibodies when _____
   _____ .

2. During pregnancy the maternal anti-Rh antibodies _____
   _____ , and if the fetus has Rh positive blood,·
   _____ .

3. In erythroblastosis, the fetus has _____
   levels and _____ .

4. Neurological damage in the fetus can result from _____
   _____ .

5. Hydrops fetalis is the condition in which _____
   _____
   _____ .

6. If the father also is Rh negative, _____
   _____
   _____ .

7. A Coomb's test indicates _____
   _____ .

8. Intrauterine transfusions are performed when _____
   _____
   _____
   _____ .

9. After delivery, if the bilirubin levels of the neonate are extremely high, the
   treatment is _____ .

10. Bilirubin lights are used _____
    _____ .

11. ABO incompatibility results when the mother is _____ and
    the fetus is _____ .

12. Treatment during pregnancy if there is an ABO problem is _____
    _____.

13. RhoGam consists of _____
    and is given to the _____

    _____

    _____.

The maternal-fetal immunological interaction is a complex phenomenon that is currently under much investigation. The mechanism during pregnancy which suppresses the maternal immunological response to the fetus is not well understood. One theory is that a factor is present in the maternal plasma which inhibits the response to the placental antigen.[1] Thus in most pregnancies no difficulty arises; yet there are certain instances in which the maternal-fetal immunological interaction creates problems, such as hemolytic incompatibilities. The most prevalent and potentially devastating problem occurs when the mother has Rh negative blood and antibodies against the fetal Rh positive cells.

The Rh factor, when present, is found only in one site, the erythrocyte. *Rh negative* means that there is no Rh factor present. For example, if this factor is introduced into the Rh negative woman before any pregnancy, as in the case of a transfusion of Rh positive cells, then her body responds to the Rh positive antigen by producing immunoglobin G (IgG) antibodies. The most common Rh factor that causes problems in the neonate is D; the antibodies formed are specific anti-D. These IgG anti-D antibodies are of low molecular weight and therefore are able to cross the placental barrier and enter the fetal system. The possible ways that the woman can be sensitized, that is, have exposure to and develop antibodies against the Rh factor, are a transfusion of poorly cross-matched blood; an abortion, either spontaneous or induced; a ruptured ectopic pregnancy; amniocentesis, if the needle traverses the placenta; antepartum bleeding, placenta abruptio, or placenta previa; and delivery of an immature, premature, or full-term infant.

In the situation in which the mother has Rh antibodies and the fetus is Rh positive, as these antibodies cross the placenta they destroy the fetal erythrocytes. This condition is known as *erythroblastosis fetalis*.

The Rh factor is found on the _____. When a person is Rh negative, this means that _____ _____.

The most common Rh factor is _____.

If the Rh D factor is introduced into a Rh negative person, there is production of _____. Once the mother has been exposed to Rh positive blood, during the next pregnancy _____ _____ _____.

erythrocytes;

he or she has no

Rh factor on the erythrocytes

D

IgG anti-D antibodies

antibodies will cross

over, and, if the fetus is Rh

positive, destruction of the

fetal cells will occur

   The effects on the fetus are dependent on the degree of the force
of the stressor, i.e., the antibody level of the mother. The greater the
antibody level, usually the greater the force; a crisis situation for the
fetus and even death in utero or shortly after birth may be produced.
The amount of red blood cell destruction produces various degrees of
anemia and high bilirubin levels. The bilirubin level may be so high as
to produce central nervous system problems such as kernicterus, which
causes lasting neurological damage. The anemia may be severe enough
to produce *hydrops fetalis*, in which there is edema of the whole body,
then often circulatory collapse occurs and death ensues.

   The maternal antibodies as they cross over into the fetal
circulation _____
and produce _____ and _____
_____.

    destroy red blood cells;
anemia; high bilirubin
levels

   If hydrops fetalis develops, often _____.

    death ensues

   During the antepartum care, the mother who has a blood type Rh
negative will be asked to bring the father of the baby in to have his
blood typed. If the father also is Rh negative, there is no problem, but
should he be Rh positive, antibody levels of the maternal blood are
determined by a Coomb's test. If the Coomb's test is positive, this
indicates that the mother has antibodies against the Rh factor. Often
the mother has her blood tested for these antibody levels throughout
pregnancy. If the titer level should rise in pregnancy, then often an
amniocentesis is more reliable in determining the amount of fetal blood
destruction than is a Coomb's test. The amniotic fluid is tested for
bilirubin levels; if these are high and if it is early in the pregnancy, then
the physician may consider an intrauterine blood transfusion if hydrops
fetalis is not present. This is done by administering 100 cubic centimeters of Rh negative, type O blood into the abdomen of the fetus. A
needle is inserted through the abdominal and uterine walls after the
fetal position has been located by fluoroscopy. This blood is absorbed
into the fetal circulatory system and alleviates some of the problems
of anemia since these erythrocytes are not destroyed by the antibodies.
It is possible to repeat this procedure every two weeks. Delivery is
effected as soon as the fetus has attained sufficient maturity to survive
outside, since remaining in utero increases the risk to which the fetus
is subject.

   If the mother's Coomb's test is positive, this means that
_____
_____.

    she has antibodies against
the Rh factor

If the mother's titer level should rise high in early pregnancy, the treatment that may be instituted is _____ _____ .

Delivery of the baby is _____ _____ .

⟱
intrauterine
transfusion
effected as soon
as the fetus can survive

After delivery, if the baby has much cell destruction, the bilirubin levels will be very high. The treatment is to do a complete exchange transfusion, replacing the baby's blood with Rh negative, type O blood. This procedure may have to be repeated if the bilirubin levels stay high. During this time, the baby is in a crisis state, but with the new blood often adaptation is successful.

If, after the delivery, the baby's bilirubin levels are elevated but not over 14 grams per cent, often the treatment is to place the infant under the bilirubin lights. These are special lights that emit light from the blue spectrum, which breaks down the bilirubin so that it can be excreted, thus lessening the risk of neurological problems.

After delivery, if the baby has extremely high levels of bilirubin, then the treatment is _____ .

exchange transfusions

If the baby's bilirubin levels are high but not over 14 grams per cent, then often the baby is _____ _____ .

placed under the
bilirubin lights

Nursing intervention is geared to helping the family understand what is happening. If the mother is having titers done every two weeks, then it is very important that she understand why she is having all the blood drawn. As the physician informs the family of the prognosis, it is very important that the nurse obtain feedback before explaining the specific tests and possible developments. If the mother is scheduled for an intrauterine transfusion, she needs much support during the procedure since she is awake and must participate by keeping still during the transfusion. Helping the family to explore their feelings and concerns about the outcome of the pregnancy is very necessary. If the baby dies in utero or shortly after birth, then the emotional impact is great and it is important to help the family deal with the grief, guilt, depression, and often anger that may be present.

If there are exchange transfusions after delivery, it is important that the parents be kept informed of the baby's status. They should understand the purposes of the various pieces of equipment and the treatments, such as the bilirubin lights and the fact that the baby has its eyes covered with patches to protect them from the lights. Often the parents fear that there is something wrong with the baby's eyes.

Before the nurse gives information to the family after the doctor has told them about the prognosis, it is important for her to
_____ .

⬇

obtain feedback

During the intrauterine transfusion, the mother needs much support since _____
_____ .

she is awake and often anxious

After delivery, it is important to inform the parents of
_____ and _____
_____ .

the baby's status; the equipment being used

Often during a first pregnancy when the mother is Rh negative and the fetus is Rh positive, there has been no previous exchange of cells and the mother has not produced any antibodies against the Rh factor. The fetal cells normally enter the maternal circulation at the time of delivery, when the placenta separates. At this time the fetal cells enter the bloodstream of the mother. Normally about 10 to 30 milliliters of fetal blood are absorbed. This amount increases when there is any operative intervention and especially if there is manual removal of the placenta. Once the positive cells enter the maternal system, after a few days these antigens stimulate the maternal system to produce antibodies. This interaction can now be interrupted by administering Rh anti-D antibodies to the mother in the form of *RhoGam*. The antibodies then coat the fetal cells that have entered the maternal system, and thus the erythrocytes of the fetus no longer have the Rh sites exposed and the maternal system does not have any antigen to stimulate a response. RhoGam is administered when the mother does not have a high antibody level and the fetus has the Rh D factor. The mother's blood is cross-matched with RhoGam before administration.

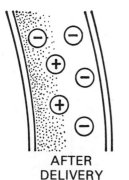

AFTER
DELIVERY

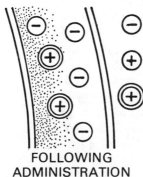

FOLLOWING
ADMINISTRATION
OF RhoGam

⊖ Maternal red blood cells

⊕ Fetal red blood cells

⊕ RhoGam combined with fetal cell, which is no longer an antigen

MOTHER'S CIRCULATION

RhoGam.

To be effective the RhoGam must be administered within 72 hours of delivery. This regime is not 100 percent effective in preventing maternal antibody formation, so currently it is recommended that when the father is Rh positive, RhoGam be given following all abortions and ectopic pregnancies. If there is a bloody amniocentesis or antenatal bleeding, RhoGam should also be given to the mother. The RhoGam should be given at each possible exposure, since it is only effective at that time. Cost is a factor that also must be considered, and the parents should be informed of the benefits of receiving the preparation.

Normally the mother is exposed to the fetal cells at _____ _____. The amount of fetal blood that enters the maternal circulation is increased if _____ _____.

delivery, when the placenta separates; operative intervention occurs

Antibody formation in the mother can be inhibited by _____, which is _____. It serves to _____ _____. To be effective RhoGam must be given within _____ _____.

administering RhoGam; anti-D Rh antibody; coat the fetal cells and remove their antigenic quality; 72 hours of delivery

If the Rh negative mother has an abortion, it is important to _____ if _____ _____.

administer RhoGam; the father is Rh positive

ABO incompatibility is different from Rh incompatibility since the A and B factors are found as antigens in other tissues besides the erythrocytes. In mothers who have type A or type B blood, the antibody they form against the foreign antigen, B or A, respectively, is IgM. This is a very large molecule, and therefore it does not cross the placental barrier. When the mother has type O blood IgG is also formed against A and B, often before any pregnancy, since these antigens are present in other tissues besides the red blood cells. During pregnancy if the mother has type O blood and the fetus has type A, for example, the antibodies that cross into the fetal system will become attached to other tissues besides the erythrocytes; therefore, anemia and high bilirubinemia are not found as frequently as with the Rh problem. Although it is possible that fetal death may occur as a result of incompatibility of the ABO systems, this is rare and so early termination of the pregnancy is not recommended. After delivery the newborn may need exchange transfusions or treatment under the bilirubin lights, but generally there is less of a problem.

The A and B factors are different from the Rh factor because they are found on _____ and _____ _____. If the mother has type A blood, she may form _____. The mother with type O blood will also form _____ _____ that can cross over the placental barrier.

erythrocytes, other
tissues;

IgM anti-B antibodies;

IgG anti-A and

anti-B antibodies

POST-TEST Indicate whether each statement is true or false by circling the appropriate letter. Then turn to page 87 and see how well you have done.

1. Antibodies against the Rh factor are formed by the Rh positive mother.   T   F

2. Fetal cells cross the placental barrier during pregnancy and set up the antigen-antibody response.   T   F

3. Erythroblastosis fetalis occurs when the maternal antibodies cross over and destroy the fetal blood cells.   T   F

4. Kernicterus is caused by severe anemia.   T   F

5. Hydrops fetalis occurs when there is severe involvement of the fetus.   T   F

6. The Coomb's titer indicates the level of antibodies against the Rh factor.   T   F

7. During an intrauterine transfusion, the blood is injected into the abdomen of the fetus.   T   F

8. The blood used for exchange transfusion is Rh negative.   T   F

9. The baby's eyes are patched if it is under the bilirubin lights.   T   F

10. ABO incompatibilities are not as severe problems as is Rh incompatibility.   T   F

11. RhoGam always is given to the Rh negative mother.   T   F

12. RhoGam coats the fetal cells so that the mother does not form antibodies of her own.   T   F

In the specific areas with which you had difficulty, return to the material and review.

REFERENCE 1. Stanley A. Gall, "Maternal Immune System During Human Gestation," *Seminars in Perinatology*, Vol. 1, No. 2, p. 129, April 1977.

BIBLIOGRAPHY Goplerud, Clifford P., "Remaining Problems in the Prevention of Rh_0 Isoimmunization," *Seminars in Perinatology*, Vol. 1, No. 2, pp. 177–181, April 1977.

Scott, James R., et al., "Pathogenesis of Rh Immunization in Primigravidas," *Obstetrics and Gynecology*, Vol. 49, No. 1, pp. 9–14, Jan. 1977.

Zlantik, Frank J., "Non-Rh_0(D) Hemolytic Disease of the Newborn: An Obstetric Point of View," *Seminars in Perinatology*, Vol. 1, No. 2, pp. 169–175, April 1977.

PRETEST ANSWERS 1. The Rh factor is introduced in her blood   2. Cross the placental barrier; the fetal cells are destroyed   3. High bilirubin; anemia   4. High bilirubin levels, as seen in kernicterus   5. There is generalized edema of the fetus and circulatory collapse is imminent   6. The fetus will be Rh negative and there will be no problem   7. The antibody level for the Rh factor, determined by a titer   8. The antibody levels of the mother are high and the fetus has a high bilirubin level early in pregnancy   9. Exchange transfusion   10. To break down the bilirubin so that it can be excreted   11. Type O; types A, B, or AB   12. Not possible   13. Anti-Rh D antibodies; Rh negative mother after delivery of a positive fetus when her antibody level is low or absent

POST-TEST ANSWERS 1. F   2. F   3. T   4. F   5. T   6. T   7. T   8. T   9. T   10. T   11. F   12. T

The following multiple-choice examination will test your comprehension of the material covered in the second unit of this program. Remember, you are not competing with anyone but yourself. Therefore, do not guess in order to answer the questions; if you are unsure, this means that you have not learned the content. Return to the areas that give you difficulty and review them before going on with the examination.

Circle the letter of the best response to each question. After completing the unit examination, check your answers on page 541 and review those areas of difficulty before proceeding to the next unit.

1. Factors that alter the growth of the fetus:
    a. Are easily controlled by the mother
    b. Occur by random chance and can be dependent on the mother's activity
    c. Are a result of only the father's health status
    d. Operate only after fertilization takes place

2. A fetal chromosome that has been fragmented:
    a. May act as a stressor during fetal growth
    b. Always has no effect on the fetal development
    c. Can produce changes in the mother
    d. May cause the pregnancy to advance

3. If the mother has poor quality and quantity of nutrients during pregnancy, then:
    a. The growth of the fetus will not be altered
    b. The fetal development is speeded up
    c. The fetal pattern of growth can be slowed
    d. The fetal growth continues at a constant rate

4. During pregnancy it is important to assess the factors that affect fetal growth and development. These include:
    a. The time of year conception took place
    b. The mother's awareness of the process of fertilization
    c. The emotional status of the mother
    d. The father's attendance at the clinic

5. The effect of congenital rubella interrupts the development of certain major systems. These include the:
    a. Respiratory system
    b. Urinary system
    c. Gastrointestinal system
    d. Cardiac system

6. Amniocentesis can be done in pregnancy to determine:
    a. The health status of the mother
    b. The relative maturity of the fetus
    c. The advisability of adding nutrients to increase the fetal well-being
    d. The number of fetuses in utero

7. The ratio of lecithin to sphingomyelin indicates the maturity of the:
   a. Lungs
   b. Kidneys
   c. Liver
   d. Brain

8. Upon analysis of amniotic fluid during pregnancy, if meconium is found, this indicates that:
   a. The baby is in breech presentation
   b. The fetus has been in jeopardy and has suffered a period of anoxia
   c. The fetus has an imperforate anus
   d. The fetus is immature and should stay in utero another three weeks

9. Genetic counseling is a service that provides:
   a. Cures for genetic problems
   b. Information for the parents as to what to do when there is a genetic abnormality
   c. Identification of carriers of a disorder and explanation of the chances of the disorder repeating
   d. Suggestions of the need to terminate the pregnancy if there is a chance the child will develop the genetic problem

10. When a recessive gene is expressed, this means that it:
    a. Has become a dominant gene
    b. Has produced the disorder singly without a similar gene
    c. Has produced the disorder in combination with another similar gene
    d. Has been lost during cell division

11. Karyotyping is the process of:
    a. Removing the genes from the chromosomes
    b. Studying a cell culture of the chromosomes
    c. Destroying the abnormal genes
    d. Adding karo to the genes and correcting any imbalances

12. Often when the parents have a child born with a genetic disorder, they express feelings of guilt. The nurse at this time may:
    a. Help the parents identify who was responsible for transmitting the disorder
    b. Explain to the parents that they are lucky since the child could be worse off
    c. Explain to the parents that they should not consider having any more children
    d. Explain that many people have genetic errors and that they are not to blame; it was just a chance occurrence

13. Parents often are overwhelmed by the thought of caring for a child with a genetic disorder. The nurse may:
    a. Explain that if they are organized, then the care will not seem to be so difficult

b. Introduce them to other parents who have encountered the same problem
c. Inform them that problem-solving activities directed at specific areas would be helpful for them to do
d. Inform the parents that it takes professional people to give the adequate care

14. An Rh incompatibility means that:
  a. The mother is Rh positive and the baby is Rh negative
  b. The mother is Rh negative and the baby is Rh negative
  c. The mother is Rh negative and the baby is Rh positive
  d. The mother is Rh positive and the father is Rh negative

15. If the mother's Coomb's titer is increasing during pregnancy, this indicates that:
  a. The baby's cells are crossing over into the maternal circulation
  b. The baby's antibodies are crossing over into the maternal circulation
  c. The mother's red blood cells are crossing over and affecting the fetus
  d. The mother has been immunized and is developing antibodies that can cross over and affect the fetus

16. ABO incompatibility occurs when:
  a. The mother is group A and the baby is group O
  b. The mother is group AB and the baby is group B
  c. The mother is group O and the baby is group A
  d. The mother is group B and the baby is group O

17. After delivery, if the baby develops high bilirubin levels due to incompatibility, then:
  a. The baby is given medication to reduce the amount of bilirubin
  b. The baby is given Rh positive blood by exchange transfusion
  c. The baby is placed under specialized blue lights
  d. The baby is sedated so that the bilirubin levels will not increase

UNIT III

INTERRUPTIONS IN HEALTH IN EARLY PREGNANCY

CHAPTER ONE
ABORTION

OBJECTIVES *Define the term "abortion."*

Identify two classifications of abortions.

Identify stressors that are known to be associated with spontaneous abortions.

Identify the characteristics of the four types of spontaneous abortions.

Identify the three types of medical abortions.

Identify possible family reactions and response to abortions.

Identify the nursing intervention with the families.

Identify nurses' feelings and responsibilities during medically induced abortions.

GLOSSARY *Abortion*: The termination of pregnancy before viability of the fetus
Spontaneous abortion: A termination of pregnancy as a result of natural causes

PRETEST   In the spaces provided, fill in the word or words that best complete(s) the statements. Then turn to page 110 and check your answers.

1. "Abortion" means_____

    _____.

2. A spontaneous abortion occurs as a result of _____

    _____

    _____.

3. An induced abortion occurs as a result of _____

    _____.

4. Fetal stressors causing a spontaneous abortion are _____

    _____.

5. Stressors from the maternal source producing abortions are _____

    _____ , _____ ,

    _____ , _____ , _____

    _____ , and _____.

6. A "miscarriage" is _____

    _____.

7. A "threatened abortion" is _____

    _____

    _____.

8. An "inevitable abortion" is _____

    _____.

9. A complete abortion usually occurs _____

    _____.

10. In an incomplete abortion the tissue that is often retained is the

    _____.

11. A mother is an habitual aborter if _____

    _____.

12. The type of medical abortion done within the first twelve weeks is

    _____ , _____

    _____ , or _____.

13. A saline abortion is _____
   _____
   _____
   _____.

14. Side effects from saline administration are _____
   _____, _____, and _____
   _____.

15. Another hypertonic solution being used to induce the termination of a
   pregnancy is _____ and the hormones used are
   _____.

16. Side effects from prostaglandin administration are _____,
   _____, and _____.

Abortion is the termination of the pregnancy before viability of the fetus is reached. "Viability" means that _____

_____.

the fetus

can survive outside the uterus

Specialized supportive care has enabled 500-gram babies to survive so that when "viability" is used in the definition of abortion, it is synonymous with the fetus reaching 500 grams.

"Abortion" is _____

_____

_____ or weighs _____.

the termination of

pregnancy before the fetus

reaches viability; 500 grams

There are two classifications of abortions: spontaneous and induced. *Spontaneous abortions* occur as a result of stressors within the homeodynamic systems, while *induced abortions* occur directly as a result of mechanical or medicinal agents. Induced abortions can either be medical, under legal jurisdiction, or criminal, outside the legal realm.

The two classifications of abortions are _____ and _____.

spontaneous;

induced

"Spontaneous abortions" are _____

_____

_____.

a result of stressors

within the homeodynamic

systems

"Induced abortions" occur following the use of

_____.

mechanical or medicinal agents

There are two categories of induced abortions: _____ and _____.

legal;

criminal

SPONTANEOUS ABORTIONS

The stressors that result in the termination of the pregnancy are found within either the fetal or maternal homeodynamic systems or are caused by disharmony between the two systems. Those stressors that are of fetal origin are abnormalities of the ovum and/or the placenta. The structural abnormalities resulting from alterations of the chromosomal structure interfere with development to such a degree that the fetus often succumbs.

The stressors within the homeodynamic systems are either of _____ or of _____ origin.

fetal; maternal

There may be disharmony _____ ⟱
_____.   between the two

Stressors that are of fetal origin are defects in the _____   systems
and/or _____.   ovum;
                                                         placenta

The known stressors found within the maternal system arise from interruptions in production of the hormones such as thyroxin and progesterone; ingestion of heavy metals; conditions such as pneumonia, typhoid fever, pyelonephritis, and severe malnutrition. Trauma rarely is the stressor that produces an abortion.

Stressors within the maternal system are _____   interruptions
_____,   of hormone production;
_____,   ingestion of heavy metals;
_____, and _____   severe malnutrition; specific
_____.   conditions of infection
Trauma is not considered to _____   often cause
_____.   abortion

The layman, when referring to a spontaneous abortion, uses the term ''miscarriage.'' Spontaneous abortions are further divided according to the clinical signs and symptoms. A *threatened abortion* presents as any bloody vaginal discharge or vaginal bleeding that occurs during the first 20 weeks of pregnancy. The mother may experience mild uterine cramping or backache, but there is no cervical dilatation or rupture of membranes, and the mother may or may not lose the pregnancy. A threatened abortion is a frequent occurrence. One out of five pregnant women may experience these signs and symptoms, and of this number one-half carry the pregnancy to term.

It is important for you to know that certain occurrences of vaginal bleeding early in pregnancy do not signify a possible termination of the pregnancy. Some pregnant women have mild vaginal bleeding about one month after the last prepregnant menses or if there are cervical or endometrial lesions or polyps. This bleeding stops spontaneously and needs no intervention other than advising abstinence for a period of two weeks following the bleeding.

When the mother has a threatened abortion, she will have
_____ or   bloody vaginal discharge;
_____ and she may feel   vaginal bleeding;
_____ and _____.   mild cramps; backache

A mother who has vaginal bleeding becomes alarmed, and, since she has no way of stopping this bleeding, she is frightened by it. She fears losing her own life and is concerned over possible loss of the pregnancy. The medical treatment for a threatened abortion is for the mother to remain in bed, often on sedation. It is felt that possibly the rest will allow the body to adapt successfully to the pregnancy and to the inherent stressors that have caused this bleeding. Two urine samples are taken and tested for the presence of chorionic gonadotrophins. If these tests are consecutively negative, then it is assumed that the pregnancy will terminate since the test results indicate that there is no placental function.

Medical treatment for a mother who has a threatened abortion consists of _____ and _____.   bed rest; sedation

Urine samples are tested for the presence of _____   chorionic

_____, which are produced by the   gonadotrophins;

_____.   placenta

Nursing intervention is geared to assisting the family to understand the diagnosis and the reasons for treatment when the mother is hospitalized. By providing information about the vital signs and any tests that you are taking, you allay heightened anxiety. As you assess the amount of blood loss by a perineal pad count and other physical responses, color, skin temperature, and respirations, you may be able to help the mother and also the father express their fears and concerns. Reassurance should be given about the facts that definitely occur, but you cannot guarantee that the mother will carry the pregnancy to term. You should not leave alone the mother who is continually losing blood, since her anxieties and fears may become overwhelming and her physical status may change quickly. The mother's status may change to a crisis state in which the cervix becomes dilated and the membranes rupture; this event is classified as an *inevitable abortion*.

Another mother may present herself initially to the clinic or physician with all the signs of an inevitable abortion: vaginal bleeding, cervical dilatation, and ruptured membranes. The pregnancy will terminate in an abortion; it is thought that the fetus has been dead for several weeks before most abortions take place. If the abortion occurs before the tenth week, then it is usually a *complete abortion*, that is, all the products of conception are passed together. Should the abortion occur later than the tenth week, part of the products of conception may be retained and usually all or part of the placenta is retained; this condition is termed an *incomplete abortion*.

The signs of an inevitable abortion are _____

_____ , _____ ,

and _____ .

vaginal

bleeding; ruptured membranes;

cervical dilatation

A complete abortion occurs when _____

_____

_____ .

all the

products of conception are

passed at the same time

A spontaneous abortion in which tissue is retained is an

_____ ; it usually occurs

after the _____ .

incomplete abortion;

tenth week

At the time of an inevitable abortion, the mother is very vulnerable to other stressors, such as hemorrhage, shock, and infection. Nursing intervention is geared to the prevention of the emergence of these stressors. The amount of bleeding is observed, and a count of the number of perineal pads that are saturated within a specified time helps to estimate the amount of blood loss. Any tissue that is passed vaginally is saved for analysis to determine how much of the products of conception has been expelled. The vital signs are monitored, the mother is observed for signs of shock, and a type and cross match of the mother's blood is done. Strict aseptic technique is very important since, with the blood loss, the mother's resistance to infections is low. If the mother has an incomplete abortion, then she will need to have a dilatation and curettage (D and C) to remove the remaining parts of the products of conception in order for the uterus to contract effectively and bleeding to stop.

As you are making the physical observations, you should assess the fears and anxieties of the family. They may be experiencing fear of dying, helplessness at not being able to control the events, guilt that they have done something wrong to cause this, and the feeling of loss. The woman often may feel failure and a loss of femininity, since at this time she is unable to be a mother. Allowing the family to verbalize and explaining all the facts as they happen help to limit the family's fantasies and help them to deal with the reality of the situation, i.e., that they did not do something wrong which caused this abortion. Promises of future success in other pregnancies are not helpful at this time because the family must go through the grieving period for this loss. It is important to spend time with the family after the abortion has occurred so that they are able to work through their feelings within a comfortable environment before they go home and begin interactions with their friends and neighbors.

Physiologic stressors to which the mother is more vulnerable at

this time are _____ , _____ , and
_____ .

    A method of assessing the amount of blood loss is _____
_____ .

    It is important to save tissue passed in order to _____
_____
_____ .

    Aseptic technique is important _____
_____ .

    The fears and anxieties of the family concern _____ ,
_____ , _____ , and _____ .

hemorrhage; shock;

infection

counting

perineal pads

assess

how much of the products

of conception is retained

to reduce the

possibility of infection

death;

helplessness; guilt; loss

    Habitual abortion occurs when a mother has three consecutive spontaneous abortions. The increase in frequency of abortions is related directly to the decrease in ability to carry the pregnancy to term. The physical care of the mother having habitual abortions is similar to that offered in other spontaneous abortion situations, but the psychological problems tend to be manifold.

    Although the definitive causes of habitual abortion are unknown, they are thought to include an incompetent cervical os; that is, for some reason the cervix dilates prior to term. The McDonald or the Sherodkar surgical procedure is sometimes employed to suture the cervix closed. Either of these procedures may be done after pregnancy has been confirmed.

    Missed abortions are discussed in Unit IV, Chapter 5.

INDUCED ABORTIONS

In 1973 the U.S. Supreme Court agreed that termination of pregnancy was a woman's right. This decision caused many moral issues to be raised and created personal conflicts in members of health teams. Women's rights organizations spearheaded the fight for this decision. Studies have indicated that women elect to terminate a pregnancy for various reasons including marital status, socioeconomic factors, relationship with the father, professional and educational aspirations, health, and family size.

    Because of the continuing controversy and the increased cost of federally assisted medical care, in 1977 the Supreme Court passed another decision, stating that federal funds will not be used to subsidize terminations of pregnancy. This decision primarily affects women of lower socioeconomic groups, those who proponents of equal rights state need this prerogative most. It is obvious that the issue will continue to exist. Nurses must be aware of federal and local legislation that affects termination of pregnancy. Medical abortions also are performed when the mother's health is in jeopardy or if the fetus has a genetic disorder, when the family agrees.

There are three methods of surgical intervention: D and C, abdominal hysterotomy, dilation and suction. Except for hysterotomy the procedures are done on a short-stay basis. The mother comes into the hospital in the morning, goes to the operating room, returns to a recovery area, and is discharged from the hospital later that same day. Prior to this admission, the mother has a pregnancy test, blood work, and a general physical examination. RhoGam is given to Rh negative mothers following the abortion. The D and C and dilation and suction procedures are usually done only up to the twelfth week of pregnancy because of the problems of uterine perforation after this time.

At this time in pregnancy, the reality of the pregnancy itself is often vague and there is no sense of a baby. Thus, the mother has to deal with the feelings of loss of the state of pregnancy rather than loss of a baby. Depending on the stressors that caused the mother to decide to terminate the pregnancy, the mother may be able to adapt more effectively to those stressors now that the crisis state of the pregnancy is over.

Complications that may occur during or after these procedures are perforation of the uterus; hemorrhage; infection; retained clots (so that the procedure must be repeated); and an incompletely closing or contracting cervix, leading to possible incompetent cervical os with spontaneous abortion or prematurity as a result.

Nursing intervention is aimed at assisting the mother, and father when present, to adapt successfully and preventing the emergence of additional stressors.

Dilatation and suction can be used to abort the pregnancy until the _____ week. After this time the danger of perforation is too great.

twelfth

After the abortion the mother must deal with _____ _____.

the loss
of the pregnancy

Complications that may arise following this procedure are: _____, _____,

perforation; hemorrhage;

_____, _____

infection; retained clots;

and _____.

incompetent cervix

A mother who is ambivalent about or wishes to deny her pregnancy often delays going to a doctor until the second trimester, and this means that she will have a medically induced abortion. Medically induced abortions can be done late in the first trimester with prostaglandins being administered either orally, parenterally, in the form of vaginal suppository, or extravulvarly. When prostaglandins or hypertonic solutions of saline or urea are administered intra-amniotically, this necessitates an adequate intrauterine space and is done after the fourteenth week of pregnancy. Exactly how these chemical agents work has not been clearly delineated; however, the fetus usually dies in utero, uterine contractions occur, and the products of conception are passed vaginally. All these chemical agents are usually used in conjunction with intravenous drips of oxytocin to speed the process. Often prostaglandins are used in combination with urea and oxytocin.

During the administration of the saline, the mother is awake and may be very fearful and responsive to the feelings of those who are caring for her. The physician withdraws 50 to 250 cubic centimeters of amniotic fluid and then slowly begins to administer the 20 percent saline solution. Up to 250 cubic centimeters of the solution is given. As the saline is given, the mother is watched closely for signs of intravascular injection, such as dryness of the mouth, heat sensation, tinnitus, severe headache, and tachycardia. Should any of these signs develop, intravenous dextrose and water are given, as are oral fluids to restore fluid and electrolyte balance. Sometimes with the contractions the saline will leak out of the amniotic sac in the place where the needle was inserted and spill into the peritoneal cavity, and the mother will experience severe abdominal pain and tachycardia; fluids are rapidly administered. Occasionally the bladder is accidentally entered and saline injected; the mother will feel backache, burning, and urgency almost immediately after injection. Immediate treatment is irrigation of the bladder with normal saline. Amniotic fluid embolism may occur, but this is rare. (See page 340.)

The time from the administration of the saline to the expulsion of the products of conception is usually from 32 to 48 hours. Signs of water intoxication, such as drowsiness, confusion, edema, headache, and decreased urinary output may occur because of the oxytocins. Ringer's lactate frequently is used to reverse these effects.

During the time that the mother is in the hospital for a termination of pregnancy, she does not like to be left alone. She usually finds it helpful to talk about her decision and about her future plans in an accepting atmosphere.

Sometimes the placenta or parts of it are retained after a saline abortion so that surgical intervention (D and C) is necessary to stop hemorrhaging and to prevent infection. It is important to assess the amount of bleeding the mother has and to maintain asepsis.

A saline abortion can be done between the _____ and _____ weeks.

When the saline is being administered, it is important for the nurse to observe the mother for signs of _____ _____, _____, and later _____.

If the mother complains of a dry mouth and severe headache, you would suspect _____ and give _____ _____.

Since large amounts of oxytocins are used, the nurse must watch for signs of _____.

It is important to assess how much bleeding there is and if any of the products of conception are _____, since if this occurs the uterus _____ _____.

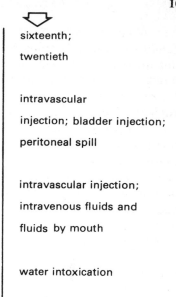

sixteenth;

twentieth

intravascular injection; bladder injection; peritoneal spill

intravascular injection; intravenous fluids and fluids by mouth

water intoxication

retained; will not contract tightly

Prostaglandins E_2 and F_{2a} produce the side effects of nausea, vomiting, and/or diarrhea. The added use of urea and oxytocin in combination helps to decrease the time to when the fetus is aborted. Often Laminaria tent is injected into the cervical canal to promote cervical dilation and prevent cervical rupture. An occasional complication of prostaglandin injection is retention of products of conception, necessitating a D and C.

Thirty to 40 percent urea in a 5 percent dextrose and water solution has also been used to terminate pregnancy through intra-amniotic instillation.

The morning-after pill or injection is a high-dosage synthetic estrogen that must be administered within 72 hours after coitus. When a woman of childbearing age has intercourse without the use of contraceptives or feels she is in danger of having conceived, this chemical therapy may be medically administered. It should be made clear that this treatment is an emergency measure and should not be considered a form of birth control. Side effects such as severe nausea and vomiting often accompany the use of this treatment.

Further studies are being carried out on using different and more effective means to abort the pregnancy. There is the menses extractor, which can be used if the woman misses her period. She goes to the physician's office, and the endometrium is removed by suction whether or not the mother is pregnant and as early as five weeks from her last menstrual period. The suctioning of the uterine contents requires no cervical dilation or administration of anesthesia, but some problems of retained tissue and bleeding occur.

In many clinics and hospital centers, nurses are involved in giving preabortion and postabortion counseling. In these sessions, which may be carried out in groups or on an individual basis, the nurse helps the mother to clarify her thinking and reasoning so that her decision about the abortion is as rational as possible. The nurse helps the mother to be fully aware of what she is doing so that after the abortion she will have fewer regrets about her decision. Often in the group the mothers are able to share some of their feelings and concerns about the procedure they will undergo. During the follow-up sessions, the nurse helps the mothers to gain a positive attitude about themselves after working through their feelings of loss. Guidance is given about the uses of family planning methods, and suggested follow-up is arranged.

The number of criminal abortions has decreased as a result of liberalized abortion laws. Previously various chemical and mechanical devices often were used to induce abortions illegally. The side effects and maternal mortality rate with these methods were very high.

Let us look at the following situation. Jane and Harry Stone visited the obstetrician one week ago. At that time the physician performed a pregnancy test, and the results were positive. Jane was considered to be eight weeks pregnant at the time. This morning Jane had vaginal bleeding, backache, and cramps. She called the doctor, who advised her to go to the hospital, where he could examine her. Upon examination, he found the cervix to be 4 centimeters dilated and the membranes to be intact. Jane was admitted to the hospital, and Harry accompanied her.

You would expect which of the following diagnoses, and the most appropriate nursing intervention with Jane and Harry would be which of the following?

A. This is a threatened abortion. Your response is to reassure them by telling them everything is going to be all right, they have nothing to worry about. Go to page 105.

B. This is an inevitable abortion; most likely it will be a complete abortion. You explain your activities of assessment and provide information about current treatment measures. Go to page 106.

C. This is an inevitable abortion; most likely it will be an incomplete abortion. You explain that Jane will lose the pregnancy and need follow-up surgery. Go to page 107.

Your choice is *A*. This is incorrect. Remember the criteria for the various spontaneous abortions. Your reassurance to the couple is very empty because you cannot assure them that there will be no problems.

Review the material on abortions on pages 96–100. Return to page 104 and choose another response.

Your choice of *B* is excellent. You identified that once the cervix started to dilate this would be an inevitable abortion. You also recognized that before ten weeks most abortions are complete. Your response to the couple provided reassurance that measures were being taken to assess her condition and provide the proper treatment. It helped them to understand what was occurring so that they could adapt more easily to this crisis situation.

Advance to page 108 and take the post-test.

You chose *C*, which is wrong. Although you were right about this being an inevitable abortion, did you consider how many weeks pregnant Jane was? Look at your response: It sounds awesome and very frightening. How might you help the family to adapt?

Return to page 96. Review the material and choose another response from page 104.

POST-TEST Indicate whether each statement is true or false by circling the appropriate letter. Then turn to page 110 and see how well you have done.

1. The fetus is considered viable at 500 grams.   T   F

2. A spontaneous abortion occurs as a result of natural causes.   T   F

3. Trauma will always cause an abortion.   T   F

4. A criminal abortion is an induced abortion.   T   F

5. In a threatened abortion there is no cervical dilatation.   T   F

6. About half the number of women who experience bleeding and cramps will eventually lose the pregnancy in an abortion.   T   F

7. If the mother's cervix has started to dilate, the membranes rupture, and she has vaginal bleeding, this is an inevitable abortion.   T   F

8. An incomplete abortion usually occurs before the tenth week.   T   F

9. Complications associated with spontaneous abortions are hemorrhage, shock, and infection.   T   F

10. During an abortion the mother may feel helpless and afraid that she may die.   T   F

11. Following the abortion, it is important that the family members have a chance to work through their feelings of loss.   T   F

12. A habitual abortion always occurs at the same time in the pregnancy as the previous abortion occurred.   T   F

13. Medical abortions can be performed legally if the mother's health is in danger or if the fetus is adversely affected.   T   F

14. Complications following the dilatation and curettage are hemorrhage, infection, and retention of clots.   T   F

15. A saline abortion can be performed between the fourteenth and twentieth weeks of pregnancy.   T   F

16. Should intravascular injection of saline occur, it is important to stop the intravenous fluids immediately.   T   F

17. Water intoxication may occur as a side effect of oxytocin.   T   F

18. It is important to spend as much time as possible with the mother while she is undergoing an abortion, allowing her to verbalize her feelings.   T   F

19. Criminal abortions have high maternal morbidity and mortality rates.   T   F

In the specific areas with which you had difficulty, return to the material and review.

BIBLIOGRAPHY Beck, Paul and Max Lilling, "Induction of Labor with Intravenous Prostaglandins," *American Journal of Obstetrics and Gynecology*, Vol. 125, No. 5, p. 648, July 1, 1976.

Clark, Ann and Dyanne D. Alfonso: *Childbearing: A Nursing Perspective*, F. A. Davis Co., Philadelphia, 1976, pp. 823–829.

Donovan, Cornelia, Rhoda Greenspan, and Fay Mittleman, "Postabortion Psychiatric Illness," *Nursing Digest*, pp. 12–17, Sept.–Oct. 1975.

Eastbrook, Bonnie and Beth Rust, "Abortion Counseling," *Canadian Nurse*, Vol. 73, No. 1, pp. 28–30, Jan. 1977.

Galloway, Karen, "The Uncertainty and Stress of Hi-Risk Pregnancy," *Maternal Child Nursing*, Vol. 2, pp. 294–299, Sept./Oct. 1976.

Kitay, David, "Bleeding Disorders in Pregnancy," *Contemporary Ob/Gyn*, Vol. 7, pp. 87–94, Jan. 1976.

McQueen, Annabel, "Termination of Pregnancy Using Extra-Amniotic Prostaglandins," *Nursing Mirror*, pp. 45–47, June 17, 1976.

Paul, Eve, Harriet Pelpel, and Nancy Wechsler, "Pregnancy, Teenagers and the Law," *Nursing Digest*, Vol. 3, pp. 61–62, Sept.–Oct. 1975.

Pritchard, Jack and Paul MacDonald: *Williams Obstetrics*, 15th ed., Appleton-Century-Crofts, New York, 1976.

Spellacy, William: *Management of the High Risk Pregnancy*, University Park Press, Baltimore, Md., 1976.

Toppozaba, Mokhtai, "Aberrant Uterine Responses to Prostaglandins E_2 and a Possible Etiologic Factor in Function Infertility," *Fertility and Sterility*, Vol. 28, No. 4, p. 434, April 1977.

PRETEST ANSWERS

1. Termination of the pregnancy before the viability of the fetus   2. Stressors within the maternal and/or fetal homeodynamic systems   3. Mechanical or medicinal agents   4. Abnormalities of the ovum and/or placenta   5. Hormonal imbalances; ingestion of heavy metals; infections; uterine abnormalities; severe malnutrition; psychiatric problems   6. A spontaneous abortion, in lay terms   7. Vaginal bleeding that may or may not result in the termination of pregnancy   8. Bleeding and cervical dilatation that will end in an abortion   9. Before the tenth week   10. Placenta   11. She has had three consecutive spontaneous abortions   12. Dilatation and curettage; dilatation and suction; hysterotomy   13. The introduction of hypertonic saline into the amniotic cavity, stimulating contractions so that the products of conception are expelled   14. Intravenous infiltration; peritoneal spill; injection into the bladder   15. Urea; prostaglandins E_2, F_{2A} 16. Nausea; vomiting; diarrhea

POST-TEST ANSWERS

1. T   2. T   3. F   4. T   5. T   6. T   7. T   8. F   9. T   10. T   11. T   12. F   13. T   14. T   15. T   16. F   17. T   18. T   19. T

CHAPTER TWO
ECTOPIC PREGNANCY

OBJECTIVES   *Define the term "ectopic pregnancy."*

Identify factors that predispose to the development of ectopic pregnancies.

Identify the types of ectopic pregnancies.

Identify the signs of a tubal rupture or abortion.

Identify the nursing intervention when the mother develops an ectopic pregnancy.

GLOSSARY   *Ectopic pregnancy:* A pregnancy located outside the endometrium of the uterine cavity
Salpingectomy: The surgical removal of a fallopian tube

PRETEST In the spaces provided, fill in the word or words that best complete(s) the statements. Then turn to page 117 and check your answers.

1. An ectopic pregnancy is _____

_____.

2. Major factors that predispose to the development of an ectopic pregnancy are _____, _____

_____, _____, _____

_____, and _____

_____.

3. Three types of tubal pregnancies are _____, _____, and _____.

4. The signs of tubal rupture are _____

_____, _____, _____

_____,

and _____.

5. The treatment for a tubal rupture is _____

_____.

An *ectopic pregnancy* is defined as any pregnancy that is located outside the endometrium of the uterine cavity. Stressors that operate to cause the pregnancy to implant outside of the uterine cavity are the following: factors that slow or prevent the ovum from traveling to the uterine endometrium, such as endosalpingitis; abnormalities of the fallopian tubes; and adhesions of the tube following infections, tumors in the tubes, and previous surgery on or near the tubes. The other factor that seems to be conducive to slowing or stopping the passage of the ovum is increased receptivity of the lining of the tubes to the fertilized ovum. Age may also be a factor. A majority of ectopic pregnancies occur in the twenty to twenty-nine year age group.

An ectopic pregnancy is _____ _____ _____.

any pregnancy located outside the endometrium of the uterine cavity

Factors that predispose towards the development of an ectopic pregnancy are _____, _____ _____, _____, _____, ____ _____, _____ _____, and _____.

endosalpingitis; abnormalities of the tube; adhesions; tumors, previous surgery; increased receptivity; age

There are four types of ectopic pregnancies: tubal, abdominal, ovarian, and cervical. The most common one is the tubal pregnancy. There are three areas of the tube where the pregnancy may implant: the *ampullar* part, closest to the fimbriated end; the *isthmic* section, which is the middle part of the tube; and the *interstitial* area, which is at the junction of the tube and the uterus. The most common place in the fallopian tubes for the ovum to implant and begin to grow is the ampullar region.

The four types of ectopic pregnancies are: _____, _____, _____, and _____. The ampullar portion of the tube is the part _____ _____. The isthmic part of the tube is the part _____ _____.

tubal; abdominal; ovarian; cervical nearest the fimbriated end in the middle of the tube

The interstitial part of the tube is the part _____ | at the
_____ | junction of the tube and the
_____. | uterus

The most common site for the tubal pregnancy is the
_____. | ampullar portion

If a mother has a tubal pregnancy, because of the hormonal alterations, during the first six to twelve weeks she may experience many of the changes associated with pregnancy. Amenorrhea, breast changes, and morning sickness may be experienced, but most of the mothers also experience some vaginal spotting or bleeding. Since the tube can expand to only a certain size, the pregnancy soon outgrows its supporting structure and a rupture of the tube or a tubal abortion occurs, usually between the sixth and the twelfth week. When the tube ruptures, the contents are spilled into the peritoneal cavity; if a tubal abortion occurs, the contents of the products of conception can be extruded either into the peritoneal cavity or into the uterine cavity.

In a tubal pregnancy the mother will experience signs and symptoms of pregnancy and often _____ | some vaginal
_____. | bleeding or spotting

Usually between the sixth and the twelfth week the pregnancy ends by _____ or _____ | tubal rupture; tubal
_____. | abortion

A tubal rupture or tubal abortion produces a crisis state, and the only treatment is immediate surgery and removal of the tube involved (salpingectomy). The mother will experience severe sudden pain in the lower abdomen, often radiating to the shoulder, and vaginal tenderness upon examination due to the pressure of the blood and products of conception in the peritoneal cavity. Shock may occur depending on the amount of blood loss, and some bleeding may be apparent. A pelvic mass can be palpated, and the uterus shows changes of pregnancy; this finding helps to confirm the diagnosis.

Interstitial pregnancies are not frequent occurrences but are more dangerous to the mother than are ampullar, isthmic, ovarian, cervical, and abdominal pregnancies since the major uterine and ovarian blood vessels are tapped. At the time of rupture, hemorrhage is so severe that it often is life-threatening. The treatment is the removal of the uterus—hysterectomy.

Abdominal and ovarian pregnancies are rare occurrences. Usually fetal death occurs early. Abdominal pregnancies go to term very infrequently. Cervical pregnancies are not frequent, and if they do occur, there is much bleeding because the blood vessels are tapped. Surgical intervention is necessary to terminate this pregnancy.

Signs and symptoms that indicate that the mother has a tubal rupture or abortion are: _____

_____, _____,

_____, _____, _____,

and _____.

sudden severe

pain; vaginal tenderness;

shock; bleeding; pelvic mass;

uterine changes

Treatment of an ampullar or isthmic rupture is _____

_____.

removal

of the tube (salpingectomy)

Treatment following the rupture of an interstitial pregnancy is

_____

_____.

removal of the uterus

(hysterectomy)

The occurrence of a tubal rupture or abortion usually is unexpected, and occasionally the mother does not realize that she is pregnant since she may have experienced spotting at the usual time of her menstrual period. When this sudden occurrence develops, the mother and family have no time for preparation and often are overwhelmed by the situation. Later they will want to know the prospects for another pregnancy following salpingectomy. Their chances for normal fertility are lower than usual, since the factors that operated originally still are present and there is only one tube for passage. It is important to help the family understand and deal with this situation as they make plans for the future.

POST-TEST Indicate whether each statement is true or false by circling the appropriate letter. Then turn to page 117 and see how well you have done.

1. Stressors that slow the traveling of the ovum to the uterine cavity predispose to the occurrence of ectopic pregnancy.   T   F

2. The interstitial section of the tube is the part that is in the middle of the tube.   T   F

3. The mother who has an ectopic pregnancy may experience many of the early signs of a normal pregnancy.   T   F

4. In a tubal abortion the contents of the products of conception are extruded into either the peritoneal or the uterine cavity.   T   F

5. Treatment of an interstitial pregnancy is a hysterectomy.   T   F

6. The mother always is aware that she is pregnant when she has an ectopic pregnancy.   T   F

In the specific areas with which you had difficulty, return to the material and review.

BIBLIOGRAPHY

Dickason, Elizabeth and Martha Schult: *Maternal and Infant Care, A Text for Nurses*, McGraw-Hill Book Co., New York, 1975, Table 22.2, p. 408.

Hallatt, Jack, "Ectopic Pregnancy Associated with the Intrauterine Device: A Study of Seventy Cases," *American Journal of Obstetrics and Gynecology*, Vol. 125, No. 6, p. 754, July 15, 1976.

Pritchard, Jack and Paul MacDonald: *Williams Obstetrics*, 15th ed., Appleton-Century-Crofts, New York, 1976, Chap. 21.

Rengachary, Donna, et al., "Ovarian Pregnancy," *Obstetrics and Gynecology*, Vol. 49, No. 1 (Supplement), p. 765, Jan. 1977.

Schonberg, Leonard, "Ectopic Pregnancy and First Trimester Abortion," *Obstetrics and Gynecology*, Vol. 49, No. 1 (Supplement), p. 735, Jan. 1977.

Tatum, Howard and Frederick Schmidt, "Contraception and Sterilization Practice and Extrauterine Pregnancy: A Realistic Perspective," *Fertility and Sterility*, Vol. 28, No. 4, pp. 407–421, April 1977.

PRETEST ANSWERS

1. Any pregnancy located outside the endometrium of the uterine cavity   2. Abnormal fallopian tubes; infections of the tubes; tumors; surgery of the tube; altered receptivity of the tubes   3. Ampullar; isthmic; interstitial   4. Pain often radiating to the shoulder; bleeding; pressure and a mass in the peritoneal cavity; shock   5. Immediate surgery and removal of the affected tube (salpingectomy)

POST-TEST ANSWERS

1. T   2. F   3. T   4. T   5. T   6. F

CHAPTER THREE
HYDATIDIFORM MOLE

OBJECTIVES   *Identify the characteristics of a hydatidiform mole.*

Identify the clinical signs and symptoms experienced by the mother.

Identify the kind of treatment and follow-up care after the mole is removed.

Identify the nursing intervention when the mother has a hydatidiform mole.

GLOSSARY   *Hydatidiform mole:* An abnormal pregnancy with chorionic villi changing into clear cystic vesicles resembling clusters of grapes
Hysterotomy: The removal of contents from the uterine cavity

PRETEST In the spaces provided, fill in the word or words that best complete(s) the statements. Then turn to page 123 and check your answers.

1. A hydatidiform mole is _____

   _____

   _____

   _____

   _____.

2. The factor that has been associated with the development of the mole is

   _____.

3. During the first three months, the size of the uterus _____

   _____

   _____.

4. The mother has uterine bleeding and spotting and may develop

   _____.

5. If there is no spontaneous abortion, the treatment is _____

   _____.

6. Careful medical follow-up of the mother is important since _____

   _____

   _____.

A *hydatidiform mole* is an abnormal pregnancy resulting from a defective ovum. It is a condition in which the embryo usually dies and the chorionic villi change into masses of clear vesicles. These vesicles are described as grapelike clusters; they are rampant in growth and take over the uterine cavity.

A hydatidiform mole is not a common occurrence, but the age of the mother is associated with its development. The mole often is found in young mothers under twenty and even more frequently in older mothers over forty. Significant stressors that cause this mole to develop have not been identified.

A hydatidiform mole would be described as an _____   abnormal

_____ occurring because of a _____   pregnancy; defective

_____ so that _____   ovum; the embryo dies

_____   and the chorionic villi become

_____.   vesicles

The incidence of the mole seems to be related to _____   the age

_____.   of the mother

Since the growth of the chorionic vesicles is fast, the size of the uterus increases rapidly so that when the mother would be considered three months pregnant, the size of the uterus is that of a five- or six-month pregnancy. The chorionic vesicles produce high levels of chorionic gonadotrophins which may be responsible for severe nausea and vomiting. The mother has uterine bleeding or spotting and may pass some of the vesicles; as a result of this, anemia often develops. Symptoms of preeclampsia frequently appear before the time when they usually occur, at 20 weeks. These symptoms are increased blood pressure, edema or weight gain, and proteinuria. At 18 weeks the mother may have a spontaneous abortion of the mole. If this does not occur, then surgical intervention is needed because of the hemorrhaging. Infection and uterine perforation can complicate this surgery.

The symptoms experienced by a mother who has a mole are

_____,   increased size of the uterus;

_____,   nausea and vomiting;

_____, _____,   bleeding or spotting; anemia;

and signs of _____.   preeclampsia

The concerns and fears of the mother are heightened as the tests and examinations are being done to determine if she has a mole. If the mother is in the older age group, many other anxieties may contribute to her feelings; if this is her first pregnancy or if the pregnancy was not planned, she may have more difficulty resolving her feelings. The mother also may have feelings about the abnormality of the pregnancy and possible guilt feelings that she has done something wrong to contribute to this development. Nursing intervention can help the mother to express her concerns. If surgical intervention is needed in the older mother, a hysterectomy is often performed rather than a hysterotomy (removal of the contents of the uterine cavity). The nurse can help the mother resolve her feelings about her sexual identity as a result of the surgery.

Extensive follow-up of the mother who has a hysterotomy is necessary since the incidence of choriocarcinoma following the development of the mole is high. Urines are tested for chorionic gonadotrophins, and, if these are found, a D and C is performed and the mother is observed closely for a year. If the urine is positive again for chorionic gonadotrophins, a hysterectomy is performed. Further follow-up is important to determine if there has been any metastasis. It is necessary for the nurse to reinforce the importance of this follow-up care.

It is important to help the mother express ___ ___ and ___ about the mole.

feelings, anxieties

If a surgical removal of the uterus is necessary, the nurse can help the mother deal with her feelings about ___ and ___.

surgery; sexual identity

Follow-up care is important to rule out ___.

choriocarcinoma

Follow-up tests determine the levels of the hormone ___.

chorionic gonadotrophin

POST-TEST   Indicate whether each statement is true or false by circling the appropriate letter. Then turn to page 123 and see how well you have done.

1. The embryo usually dies with the development of the hydatidiform mole.   T   F

2. High levels of chorionic gonadotrophins are produced by the chorionic vesicles.   T   F

3. The mother usually has no signs of edema or increased blood pressure.   T   F

4. Infection and uterine perforation often complicate the surgical removal of the mole.   T   F

5. After the removal of the mole, the mother's urine level of chorionic gonadotrophins is watched carefully.   T   F

6. It is important for the nurse to explain the follow-up care to the mother.   T   F

In the specific areas with which you had difficulty, return to the material and review.

BIBLIOGRAPHY   Jensen, Margaret, Ralph Bensen, and Irene Bobak: *Maternity Care, the Nurse and the Family*, C. V. Mosby Co., St. Louis, Mo., 1977, pp. 231–232, 245.

Kaplan, Hans G. and Myroslaw M. Hreshchyshyn, "Estetrol in Molar Pregnancies Quantitated by Rapid Gas Chromatographic Method in Conjunction with Estrone, Estradiol 17$_B$, Estriol and Pregnanediol," *American Journal of Obstetrics and Gynecology*. Vol. 115, No. 6, pp. 803–810, March 15, 1973.

Pritchard, Jack and Paul MacDonald: *Williams Obstetrics*, 15th ed., Appleton-Century-Crofts, New York, 1976.

PRETEST ANSWERS   1. An abnormal pregnancy resulting from the death of the ovum with the chorionic villi taking over and filling the uterine cavity with vesicles   2. The age of the mother   3. Increases rapidly to a five- or six-months-pregnant size   4. Anemia   5. Surgical removal   6. Often choriocarcinoma develops after the presence of the mole

POST-TEST ANSWERS   1. T   2. T   3. F   4. T   5. T   6. T

CHAPTER FOUR

HYPEREMESIS GRAVIDARUM

OBJECTIVES   *Identify the signs and symptoms of hyperemesis gravidarum.*

Identify the specific nursing intervention for the mother and family.

PRETEST In the spaces provided, fill in the word or words that best complete(s) the statements. Then turn to page 133 and check your answers.

1. Hyperemesis gravidarum occurs when the mother _____ _____.

2. As a result of the severe nausea and vomiting, the mother is _____, _____, and _____.

3. Exhaustion results from _____.

4. The signs of severe involvement are _____ _____, _____, and _____.

5. Treatment with intravenous fluids and electrolytes will assist in the restoration of the _____.

6. The mother's room should be _____ and _____ _____.

7. Explanations about pregnancy, labor, and delivery will _____ _____ _____.

8. The prognosis once treatment has started is _____.

Hyperemesis gravidarum, also called "pernicious vomiting," is a state in which the mother has severe nausea and vomiting that is uncontrollable, so that the adaptive resources are unable to respond. Dehydration, electrolyte imbalance, and starvation occur. This condition is found between the second and fourth months of pregnancy, and no specific stressors have been identified other than, possibly, high levels of chorionic gonadotrophins, psychological difficulties, abnormalities in the metabolic changes of pregnancy, and the decrease in the motility of the gastrointestinal system which occurs during the pregnant state.

The mother who has hyperemesis gravidarum has _____ _____.

  uncontrolled

  nausea and vomiting

This condition produces _____, _____ _____, and _____.

  dehydration; imbalance

  of electrolytes; starvation

Some stressors thought to possibly produce this condition are _____ and _____ during pregnancy.

  high chorionic gonadotrophins;

  psychological difficulties

The specific signs and symptoms the mother has, other than constant and persistent nausea and vomiting, are exhaustion due to inability to sleep; signs of dehydration; and decreased urine output, with acetone, albumin, casts, and bile often found in the urine. If the condition has persisted without treatment, the mother will have a fever and increased pulse rate, jaundice, and if the condition is very severe, peripheral nerve involvement. The mother must be treated before signs of acidosis or alkalosis appear.

The first signs the mother shows are _____, _____, _____, _____, and _____ _____.

  nausea;

  vomiting; dehydration;

  exhaustion; decreased urine

  output

The progression of signs indicating more serious changes are _____, _____, _____, _____ and _____ or _____.

  fever; increased pulse;

  jaundice; nerve involvement;

  acidosis; alkalosis

Intervention begins when the mother is hospitalized and given antiemetics and intravenous fluids of glucose with vitamins and necessary electrolytes to assist the restoration of the homeodynamic balance. A nasal tube often is used to give additional calories and proteins to reverse the starvation. The mother is placed in a quiet room and given sedatives to assist her to relax. Psychotherapy has been found to be very beneficial in assisting the mother to identify and work through her problems with support.

Dehydration is reversed by _____ and _____.

antiemetics; fluids

Starvation is reversed by giving the mother _____,

carbohydrates;

_____, and _____.

proteins; vitamins

Exhaustion is altered by _____ and _____.

quiet; sedation

Good ventilation of the room is important. You should have a quiet and positive attitude, since often the mother feels that she will not get better. Often visitors are restricted; it is important to explain to the mother and her visitors that this is the regulation since the mother needs rest and no psychological stress. The mother often has many concerns about the pregnancy and many feelings that she finds difficult to deal with. Explanation about the phenomena involved in pregnancy and discussion of her various fears, especially about labor, can be very helpful to her.

The feelings of the father also should be explored so that any guilt or anger can be handled effectively. It is important to help the father understand about pregnancy and discuss the possible ways in which he can be supportive to the mother now and after discharge.

The mother's room should be _____ and _____

quiet; well

_____.

ventilated

The mother's concerns about pregnancy and labor are often sources of stress; thus it is helpful if the nurse _____

explores the

_____

mother's feelings and concerns

_____.

and provides information

The immediate prognosis with treatment is good, and no effects on the fetus have been identified. However, it is not uncommon for the condition to reappear after discharge from the hospital if the predisposing stressors are primarily psychosocial.

Now let us examine a situation you may face in the clinic. You are in an antepartum clinic when Lila DiSesso comes in. Upon taking the admission history, you find that Lila thinks that she is about nine weeks pregnant. She appears tired, pale, and listless. She states that she was feeling okay until about three days ago, when she started vomiting, and that since then she has been unable to eat or drink anything. When you test her urine, you find that it is very scanty, is concentrated, and shows protein and acetone. She has lost 3 pounds. The doctor suspects hyperemesis gravidarum. You would counsel Lila in the following way:

A. "Nausea and vomiting are very common occurrences in pregnancy. You should stay in bed and eat dry crackers until you feel better."

Go to page 129.

B. "You seem to be having difficulty. Is there some emotional problem that is upsetting you?"

Go to page 130.

C. "You seem to be very uncomfortable with all this nausea and vomiting. I can understand this. It must be overwhelming to you right now. With medication to stop the vomiting, and rest, you will feel better soon."

Go to page 131.

Your choice of *A* indicates that you have not clearly understood the material in this chapter.

Return to page 126. Review the material and choose another response from page 128.

Your choice of *B* indicates that you lack sensitivity to the mother. You are not supportive of the mother but rather accusing her of causing this difficulty.

Return to page 126. Review the material and choose another response.

Your choice of *C* indicates that you have recognized that there often is the feeling that one will never be better. You have been supportive by indicating to the mother that help is available and that she will feel better.

Advance to page 132 and take the post-test.

POST-TEST   Indicate whether each statement is true or false by circling the appropriate letter. Then turn to page 133 and see how well you have done.

1. Stressors possibly associated with the development of hyperemesis gravidarum are high levels of chorionic gonadotrophins and psychological difficulties.   T   F

2. The mother is able to sleep well; her only difficulty is that she is unable to eat.   T   F

3. Often one of the signs the mother will have is decreased urine output.   T   F

4. The mother often feels that she will not get better.   T   F

5. The mother usually has no concerns about the pregnancy or labor and delivery.   T   F

6. The father should be included in the treatment.   T   F

In the specific areas with which you had difficulty, return to the material and review.

BIBLIOGRAPHY Clark, Ann and Dyanne D. Alfonso: *Childbearing: A Nursing Perspective*, F. A. Davis Co., Philadelphia, 1976, pp. 633–634.

Clausen, Joy, Margaret Flook, and Bonnie Ford: *Maternity Nursing Today*, 2d ed., McGraw-Hill Book Co., New York, 1977, pp. 716–717.

Pritchard, Jack and Paul MacDonald: *Williams Obstetrics*, 15th ed., Appleton-Century-Crofts, New York, 1976, pp. 633–634.

PRETEST ANSWERS   1. Experiences severe and uncontrolled nausea and vomiting   2. Dehydrated; in electrolyte imbalance; in a state of starvation   3. Lack of sleep   4. Increased temperature and pulse rate; jaundice; peripheral nerve involvement   5. Homeodynamic balance   6. Quiet; well-ventilated   7. Help to alleviate some of the mother's fears and concerns   8. Good

POST-TEST ANSWERS   1. T   2. F   3. T   4. T   5. F   6. T

CHAPTER FIVE

INFECTIONS DURING PREGNANCY

OBJECTIVES *Identify the effects of venereal disease in pregnancy.*

Identify the effects of rubella during early pregnancy.

Identify the effects of herpes simplex during pregnancy.

Identify two common vaginal infections often seen during pregnancy.

PRETEST In the spaces provided, fill in the word or words that best complete(s) the statements. Then turn to page 142 and check your answers.

1. The incidence of venereal disease is _____.

2. If the mother has syphilis before the sixteenth week, _____
_____
_____.

3. When the mother is treated, it is important that _____
_____.

4. If the mother has syphilis late in pregnancy, _____
_____.

5. If the mother contracts gonorrhea early in pregnancy, the infection
_____
_____.

6. The treatment for gonorrhea is _____.

7. In the adult, rubella is _____.

8. If the mother is in early pregnancy when she contracts rubella, _____
_____.

9. The incidence of rubella has been decreased because of
_____.

10. During pregnancy the herpes simplex virus has been found to _____
_____.

11. If at delivery time the mother has a herpes lesion on the generative tract,
then _____.

12. If the neonate contracts herpes simplex, the infection can _____
_____.

13. *Trichomonas vaginalis* is a _____ organism.

14. The discharge that is characteristic of *Trichomonas vaginalis* infection is
_____.

15. *Candida albicans* is a _____ organism.

16. The discharge that is characteristic of *Candida albicans* infection is
_____.

VENEREAL DISEASE

Venereal diseases continue to occur at an alarming rate of frequency both in this country and abroad. Syphilis, caused by the *treponema*, is spread through direct sexual contact with infected individuals. It is found in all socioeconomic groups. Before the sixteenth week of pregnancy the fetus does not have the inflammatory or antibody response developed. Thus no signs of infection are present. After this time infection can be seen in the fetus as congenital syphilis. However, if early maternal diagnosis is made before pregnancy and treatment is instituted, the mother will be cured, eliminating the problem of congenital infection. When a mother is treated, it is important that her sexual partner also be treated so that she will not become reinfected. Should the mother contract syphilis in pregnancy, the fetus will be affected. Although penicillin does cross into the fetal circulation, often the baby at birth has a positive VDRL (venereal disease research laboratory). The nurse is instrumental in disease control through case-finding activities. These include gathering a complete sexual history, assuring that laboratory tests are done, educating individuals and families, maintaining a supportive confidential atmosphere, and ensuring that all identified cases are reported to the appropriate community agency with the knowledge of the individual(s) involved. The mother/family can be assured that prompt treatment will protect the individual, contact person, and fetus. For further discussion, see the chapter entitled "Infections in the Neonate."

The organism *Treponema pallidum* will cross over and affect the fetus _____.

> if the mother is affected

When the mother is being treated, it is important that

_____.

> her sexual partner be treated

Gonorrhea will travel up the mother's reproductive tract and affect the tubes and endometrium very early in pregnancy. During pregnancy it sometimes is difficult to recognize that the mother has been infected if the infection is high in the genital tract. Treatment consists of administering high doses of penicillin to the mother and her contact. The intracellular gram-negative diplococcus *Neisseria gonorrhoeae* can cause such inflammation of the fallopian tubes that the mother will be sterile. Gonorrhea also has been known to become a widespread pelvic infection. Should the mother have to undergo a cesarean section, this infection can become so extensive that it is overwhelming to the mother. The effects of the gonococcus on the baby are discussed on page 500.

If the mother is infected with gonorrhea during the early months of pregnancy, _____ _____ _____.

the infection may travel and affect the tubes and endometrium

Treatment of gonorrhea is _____ _____.

high doses of penicillin

The infection can be widespread and become _____ _____.

overwhelming to the mother

RUBELLA (GERMAN MEASLES)

Rubella is a mild infection in the adult. It often can go without notice, causing a slight fever, malaise, and a mild rash. This virus in early pregnancy crosses the placental barrier and interrupts the growth and development of the fetus so that the child can be born with any or all of the following: blindness; deafness; cardiac problems; and retardation, either physical or mental.

If a pregnant woman suspects that she either has been exposed to or has developed rubella, she should report it to her doctor or clinic immediately. A blood test called the hemagglutination-inhibition antibody (HAI) test will identify HAI titers indicating possibility of disease (a titer less than 1:8) or nonsusceptibility (a titer 1:16 or more). If the mother has antibodies, that is, is not susceptible to the disease, the fetus will not be in danger.

A vaccine has been developed and has been given to young school-age children in the hope that the immunization of children will stop the infection of mothers. This procedure has lessened the prevalence of the infection. If women of childbearing age wish to take the vaccine before they are pregnant, they must wait over three months before becoming pregnant after being vaccinated.

In the adult, rubella is _____.

a mild infection

If the mother contracts rubella in early pregnancy, _____ _____.

the fetus is severely affected

The incidence of rubella has been lessened by _____ _____.

vaccination of school-age children

HERPES SIMPLEX

Herpes simplex is a common infection found among the general public, but when the mother is affected during pregnancy, the effects on the fetus are dramatic. Recent studies have indicated that the herpes virus is able to alter the pattern of growth and development of the fetus with such results as microcephaly. If the mother at the time of delivery has a herpes lesion on her generative tract, a cesarean section is performed to eliminate the possible fetal contact. If the newborn contracts herpes simplex, the infection is so overwhelming that infant mortality is high.

Herpes simplex has been found to affect fetal _____ _____.

growth and development

If the newborn contracts herpes virus, _____ _____ _____.

the infection can be overwhelming and cause death

If at term the mother has a herpes lesion on her generative tract, the delivery is _____.

by cesarean section

VAGINAL INFECTIONS

Trichomonas vaginalis is a parasitic organism that causes an infection characterized by irritation, itching, and a profuse yellowish green discharge. This infection is seen frequently during pregnancy but is only symptomatic in a small percentage. The treatment should involve both the mother and her partner so that she will not become reinfected. The treatment with the medication Flagyl is *not* administered during the first trimester because of possible teratogenic effects and then is given later only if the mother is experiencing severe symptoms during pregnancy.

Trichomonas vaginalis produces a _____ _____.

profuse yellowish green discharge

The mother often feels uncomfortable because of the _____.

irritation and itching

The drug Flagyl used to treat this infection is _____ _____ _____.

not administered in the first trimester

Candida (Monilia) albicans is a yeast organism that causes an infection found in the vagina and seen during pregnancy as the changes of the vaginal secretions include more glycogen. The discharge is a profuse, white, curdlike substance that often is irritating. The treatment is an antibiotic, Mycostatin, used locally as vaginal tablets. Gentian violet is occasionally used, and the mother should be prepared for the purple staining. The baby can contract this infection. See page 499.

⇩

Candida albicans produced a _____ | white, curdike

_____. | discharge

The usual treatment is _____ | Mycostatin vaginal

_____. | tablets

POST-TEST Indicate whether each statement is true or false by circling the appropriate letter. Then turn to page 142 and see how well you have done.

1. If the mother's syphilis is treated during early pregnancy, there is no problem for the fetus.   T   F

2. The fetus is not affected by syphilis until the time of delivery.   T   F

3. It sometimes is difficult to determine that the mother has gonorrhea during pregnancy.   T   F

4. Gonorrhea cannot be treated during pregnancy.   T   F

5. Rubella is dangerous to both the mother and fetus during early pregnancy.   T   F

6. If women of childbearing age take the rubella vaccine, they should not become pregnant for at least three months.   T   F

7. Herpes simplex can affect the growth and development of the fetus.   T   F

8. If the mother has a herpes lesion on the labia, the delivery is vaginal.   T   F

9. *Trichomonas vaginalis* is a yeast organism.   T   F

10. The drug used to treat *Trichomonas vaginalis* in the first trimester is Flagyl.   T   F

11. *Candida albicans* produces a yellowish green, profuse discharge.   T   F

12. *Candida albicans* infection is seen in pregnancy as glycogen is increased in the vaginal secretions.   T   F

In the specific areas with which you had difficulty, return to the material and review.

BIBLIOGRAPHY   Amstey, Marvin S., Michael A. Nasello, and Charles J. Hochberry, "Multiple Virus Isolations from a Pregnant Patient," *American Journal of Obstetrics and Gynecology*, Vol. 115, No. 7, pp. 897–900, April 1, 1973.

———— and Kenneth Steadman, "Asymptomatic Gonorrhea and Pregnancy," *Journal of the American Venereal Disease Association*, Vol. 3, No. 1, p. 14, Sept. 1976.

Avery, Gordon: *Neonatology, Pathophysiology and Management of the Newborn*, J. B. Lippincott Co., Philadelphia, 1975, pp. 568–611.

Clausen, Joy, Margaret Flook, and Bonnie Ford: *Maternity Nursing Today*, 2d ed., McGraw-Hill Book Co., 1977, pp. 699–706.

Florman, Alfred L., et al., "Intrauterine Infection with Herpes Simplex Virus–Resultant Congenital Malformations," *Journal of the American Medical Association*, Vol. 225, No. 2, pp. 129–132, July 9, 1973.

Friedrich, Edward G., "Relief for Herpes Vulvitis," *Obstetrics and Gynecology*, Vol. 41, No. 1, pp. 74–77, Jan. 1973.

Gall, Stanley, "Maternal Immune System During Human Gestation," *Seminars on Perinatology*, Vol. 1, p. 119, April 1977.

Lukas, T. and Lawrence Corey, "Genital Herpes Simplex Virus Infection, An Overview," *The Nurse Practitioner*, Vol. 2, No. 5, pp. 7–9, May–June 1977.

Whalley, Peggy and F. Gary Cunningham, "Short-Term Versus Continuous Antimicrobial Bacteruria in Pregnancy," *Obstetrics and Gynecology*, Vol. 49, No. 3, pp. 262–265, March 1977.

PRETEST ANSWERS

1. Increasing rapidly   2. No symptoms are evident in the fetus   3. Her partner be treated
4. The fetus will exhibit congenital syphilis   5. May travel high in the generative tract
6. Penicillin   7. A mild infection   8. The fetus will be adversely affected
9. Immunization of school-age children   10. Affect fetal growth and development   11. A cesarean section is performed   12. Become overwhelming   13. Parasitic   14. Yellowish green, profuse, and irritating   15. Yeast   16. White, curdlike, and often irritating

POST-TEST ANSWERS

1. F   2. F   3. T   4. F   5. F   6. T   7. T   8. F   9. F
10. F   11. F   12. T

CHAPTER SIX
CHRONIC HYPERTENSION

OBJECTIVES   *Identify the signs and symptoms of chronic hypertension.*

Identify the nursing intervention with the family.

PRETEST In the spaces provided, fill in the word or words that best complete(s) the statements. Then turn to page 149 and check your answers.

1. The mother is hypertensive when her blood pressure is _____ _____.

2. The mother's hypertension is seen _____ _____ _____.

3. The mothers who tend to develop hypertension are _____, _____, and _____.

4. During pregnancy a mother's blood pressure _____.

5. After the pregnancy is over, a mother with chronic hypertension will find that her blood pressure _____ _____.

6. If the mother's blood pressure is severely elevated, the chances for the fetus's survival are _____.

7. The treatment and intervention that are helpful for this mother are _____, _____, _____, and _____.

Chronic hypertension results from a disruption of the vascular system that causes blood pressure of 140/90 or greater. In order to be considered a chronic hypertensive, the mother must have had evidence that her blood pressure was at least at this level prior to the pregnancy and the identification of the elevation must be made prior to the twentieth week of gestation. There are instances, however, in which a woman's blood pressure elevates only during pregnancy and returns to a normal reading between pregnancies; this is important information to obtain during an obstetrical history.

Chronic hypertension may be difficult to recognize if the mother is not seen in early pregnancy, before the twentieth week, because the hypertension can be confused with preeclampsia. The alterations of blood volume that occur during the pregnancy place an increasing stressor on the vascular system. When hypertension is present before the pregnancy, the adaptation of the vascular system is limited and so blood pressure increases, especially during the third trimester of the pregnancy. The mothers who are usually found in this group are older, often obese, and multiparous.

Some of the accompanying physiologic disturbances that may be found during pregnancy, the possibility of which should be investigated, are diseases of the kidney and urinary tract; collagen diseases, such as lupus erythematosis and scleroderma; polycystic disease; and vascular changes due to diabetes mellitus

After delivery the blood pressure of the hypertensive mother does not return to the previous prepregnancy level, but rather remains somewhat elevated. This happens because the stress during the pregnancy causes the vascular system to lose some of its adaptive ability. Successive pregnancies continue to increase the amount of hypertension so that the condition becomes life-threatening to the mother and the baby.

Chronic hypertension is _____
_____
_____. | a disruption of the vascular system resulting in increased blood pressure

The onset of chronic hypertension is _____
_____. | before pregnancy

Pregnancy affects the mother who has hypertension by _____. | increasing her blood pressure

After the pregnancy the mother's blood pressure _____
_____. | remains somewhat elevated

If the mother's blood pressure is severely elevated, the prognosis for the baby is poor. The placental circulation often is inadequate because of the hypertension, and early fetal death or premature delivery results. Abruptio placenta (see Unit IV, Chapter Seven) also may occur in a number of these mothers.

Once the mother's status has been assessed medically, it is important that she and the father understand the significance of the problem, since frequently the mother feels fine, with only an occasional headache. The mother should see the physician frequently throughout the pregnancy; every two weeks during the first half of the pregnancy and then every week.

The nurse can help the family to plan when the mother can rest for one hour in the morning and one hour in the afternoon. If there are children in the family, neighbors or friends can help the mother by taking the youngsters for one or two hours. If the children are not in school, they may be eligible for day care or nursery school, and in this way the mother will be able to find more time to relax. The mother often is given sedation, and it is important that alcohol not be taken with this medication or that she not drive a vehicle for at least three hours after taking the sedation.

The mother's diet is watched closely. The nurse can help the mother plan meals that are not high in salt. The mother should use lemon juice and spices to flavor foods. It is important that the mother not cook with salt; rather she should let each member of the family salt his or her own food. The mother often is placed on diuretic and anti-hypertensive therapy. It is important that the mother understand the importance of eating foods high in potassium to replace the loss through the kidneys due to the diuretics. Also, the mother should take the diuretic in the morning so that her sleep will not be interrupted during the night because of increased urinary frequency. A diet high in potassium is necessary to maintain the normal potassium level when the mother is taking a diuretic.

The mother may have difficulty in realizing the severity of the hypertension because _____.

she feels fine

The mother sees the doctor _____ _____ during the first half of the pregnancy and then _____.

every two

weeks

every week

The nurse can help the family plan for time during the day _____.

when the mother can rest

Anxiety of the mother can be reduced by _____.

The diet of the mother is low in _____.

Excess fluid in the body is removed by _____.

The family needs much support and encouragement to follow the medical regimen in order to decrease the operating stressor.

sedation

sodium

diuretics

POST-TEST   Indicate whether each statement is true or false by circling the appropriate letter. Then turn to page 149 and see how well you have done.

1. Proteinuria often is associated with chronic hypertension.   T   F

2. Chronic hypertension occurs after the twentieth week of pregnancy.   T   F

3. Pregnancy acts as a stressor for the maternal vascular system.   T   F

4. After pregnancy the blood pressure returns to the prepregnancy level.   T   F

5. The hypertension can be severe enough to be life-threatening for both the mother and the fetus.   T   F

6. Premature delivery is thought to be due to decrease of the placental function.   T   F

7. The hypertensive mother often feels seriously ill during the pregnancy.   T   F

8. The mother should be seen frequently during the pregnancy.   T   F

9. The mother's diet should be low in sodium.   T   F

10. The family can help by planning how the mother can rest.   T   F

In the specific areas with which you had difficulty, return to the material and review.

BIBLIOGRAPHY Christianson, Roberta, "Studies on Blood Pressure During Pregnancy: Influence of Parity and Age," *American Journal of Obstetrics and Gynecology*, Vol. 125, No. 4, pp. 509–513, June 15, 1976.

Pritchard, Jack and Paul MacDonald: *Williams Obstetrics*, 15th ed., Appleton-Century-Crofts, New York, 1976.

Speroff, Leon, "Pregnancy-Induced Hypertension," *Contemporary Ob/Gyn*, Vol. 9 (Symposium) Jan. 1977.

PRETEST ANSWERS
1. 140/90 or greater of pregnancy   2. Before the twentieth week of pregnancy and often before the onset   3. Multiparous; older; obese   4. Rises   5. Lowers but not to the prepregnancy level   6. Poor   7. Rest; sedation; diet; diuretics

POST-TEST ANSWERS
1. T   2. F   3. T   4. F   5. T   6. T   7. F   8. T   9. T   10. T

Student _____

ANTEPARTUM

Secondary Care

While caring for a high-risk pregnant woman, the student will:

			Satisfactory						Unsatisfactory					
*	1.	Identify the reasons for the hospitalization												
*	2.	Assist the mother in exploring feelings regarding the hospitalization												
A	3.	Understand the maternal physiologic process that is occurring with this interruption												
A	4.	Understand the fetal physiologic process that is occurring with this interruption												
*	5.	Gather all data pertinent to setting nursing priorities of care:												
		a. Chart												
		b. Textbook or other reference description												
		c. Health team members												
		d. Nursing observations												
		e. Laboratory results												
		f. Mother (family) interpretation of the interruption												
*	6.	State priorities for nursing care by synthesizing accumulated data												
A	7.	Make referrals to appropriate members of the health team as need is identified												
*	8.	Appropriately communicate information and record the needs identified on the mother's chart												
B	9.	Interpret data pertinent to the status of the mother and fetus												
*	10.	Give data to mother/parents regarding the status of the mother												
B	11.	Obtain feedback from mother/parents regarding understanding of the high-risk situation												
*	12.	Carry out care of the mother based on identified needs												
*	13.	Monitor the well-being of the fetus												

Instructor Comments:

Student _____

			Satisfactory					Unsatisfactory				
*	14.	Identify the characteristics of medications ordered for the mother										
*	15.	Administer medications safely										
B	16.	Recognize need for anticipatory guidance										
A	17.	Initiate anticipatory guidance appropriately (timing: level of understanding)										
B	18.	Alter priorities as needs change										
B	19.	Prepare the mother/family for discharge to the home by evaluating their ability to carry out priorities of care										
A	20.	Evaluate the sociocultural influences regarding the reasons for the high-risk situation										

Instructor Comments:

**UNIT III
EXAMINATION** The following multiple-choice examination will test your comprehension of the material covered in the third unit of this program. Remember, you are not competing with anyone but yourself. Therefore, do not guess in order to answer the questions; if you are unsure, this means that you have not learned the content. Return to the areas that give you difficulty and review them before going on with the examination.

Circle the letter of the best response to each question. After completing the unit examination, check your answers on page 541 and review those areas of difficulty before proceeding to the next unit.

1. A common cause of spontaneous abortions is:
    a. Trauma
    b. Mother's emotional response
    c. Abnormalities of the placenta
    d. Nausea and vomiting of the mother

2. Treatment for a threatened abortion is:
    a. Dilatation and curettage
    b. Vitamin supplement
    c. Rest and sedation
    d. Leutenizing hormone

3. If the mother is admitted to hospital with a threatened abortion, it is important to inform her that:
    a. Everything will be all right
    b. The baby is definitely dead
    c. She need not worry about the pregnancy
    d. The outcome is unknown but everything possible is being done

4. A mother who is admitted with a diagnosis of inevitable abortion rather than threatened abortion will exhibit which of the following signs?
    a. Bleeding, nausea, and headache
    b. Cramps, diarrhea, and bleeding
    c. Bleeding, pain, ruptured membranes
    d. Bleeding, backache, and flushing

5. Nursing assessment of the mother who is having an inevitable abortion should include:
    a. The fetal heart rate
    b. The assessment of fetal movements
    c. A perineal pad count
    d. The strength of contractions

6. If the mother is bleeding and the cervix is dilated at the twelfth week of pregnancy, you as the nurse would expect that this will be a (an):
    a. Incomplete abortion
    b. Complete abortion
    c. Missed abortion
    d. Threatened abortion

7. Complications associated with spontaneous abortions include:
   a. Toxemia and uremia
   b. Hemorrhage, shock, and infection
   c. Aspiration pneumonia
   d. Leukorrhea and puritis

8. A mother who is an habitual aborter is one who has had:
   a. A threatened abortion, an induced abortion, and a spontaneous abortion
   b. A threatened abortion and two induced abortions
   c. One incomplete abortion and two complete abortions
   d. Five induced abortions consecutively

9. A medical abortion done during the first twelve weeks is:
   a. A major procedure in which the mother is hospitalized for several days after surgery
   b. Often complicated so that a hysterectomy must be performed
   c. A relatively simple procedure in which the mother is admitted for the day only
   d. A simple procedure if the mother has had this procedure done before

10. If the mother is Rh negative, after the abortion it is important to:
    a. Give her RhoGam
    b. Watch her for the danger of a blood reaction
    c. Watch her carefully since she may hemorrhage more readily than an Rh positive mother
    d. Give her Benadryl

11. During a saline abortion it is important that signs of which of the following be watched for?
    a. Drug withdrawal
    b. Nystagmus
    c. Intravascular injection of saline
    d. Sugar intolerance

12. Often large doses of oxytocins are used during the saline abortion. One side effect you may observe is:
    a. Uterine contractions
    b. Hypotension
    c. Frequency of urination
    d. Water intoxication

13. The most common type of ectopic pregnancy is:
    a. Tubal
    b. Ovarian
    c. Cervical
    d. Abdominal

14. The mother experiences which of the following signs after a tubal rupture?
    a. Severe sudden pain and signs of shock

b. A bad taste in her mouth and sleepiness
c. Hunger and a mild itching of the skin
d. Tingling of her arms and hunger

15. A hydatidiform mole develops when:
a. The decidua of the uterus changes and becomes hyperplastic
b. The ovum dies and the chorionic villi become vesicles
c. The spore of a bacterium implants and begins to develop
d. A number of sperm group together and form a mass

16. The signs that the mother experiences as the hydatidiform mole develops are:
a. Shrinking of the breasts
b. Nausea, vomiting, and an increased size of the uterus
c. Heartburn and fetal movement
d. Quickening and oliguria

17. Careful follow-up of the mother who has had a hydatidiform mole is important since she:
a. Will have difficulty becoming pregnant
b. Will have dysmenorrhea
c. May develop choriocarcinoma
d. Probably will develop moles on the skin

18. A mother who has hyperemesis gravidarum will:
a. Be dehydrated and in a state of starvation
b. Be hypertensive
c. Have had many children
d. Probably not carry the pregnancy to term

19. The room you would select for the mother who was admitted with the diagnosis of hyperemesis gravidarum would be:
a. Cheery with lots of other people to distract her
b. Dark and closed to prevent drafts
c. Quiet, with good ventilation
d. Far away from the nurse's station because isolation is important

20. If the mother contracts syphilis during the twenty-second week of pregnancy:
a. The fetus is protected
b. The fetus is affected with congenital syphilis
c. The mother will have only a mild case and the fetus is not involved
d. The mother cannot be cured during the pregnancy

21. Gonorrhea:
a. Is not contagious during pregnancy
b. Can be treated only during the postpartum period
c. Can be treated before delivery so that the baby is not affected
d. Can be treated, but the baby will be affected

22. Rubella during pregnancy is:
    a. An infection that can have deleterious effects on fetal development
    b. A serious infection for the mother, but the baby is not affected
    c. A mild infection in the mother, and the fetus is not affected
    d. Life-threatening to the mother

23. If the mother has herpes simplex on the labia, the delivery of the baby will be:
    a. Normal, spontaneous vaginal delivery
    b. Attempted forceps vaginally, then possibly cesarean section
    c. Cesarean section
    d. Low forceps

24. *Candida (Monilia) albicans* is:
    a. A parasite that causes vaginal infection
    b. A virus
    c. A yeast
    d. A bacterium

25. Chronic hypertension develops:
    a. After the twenty-fourth week of pregnancy
    b. After the thirteenth week of pregnancy
    c. Before the pregnancy begins
    d. Only after the fifth pregnancy

26. If the mother has chronic hypertension during pregnancy, the fetus:
    a. Is not affected
    b. Has a poor prognosis because of the inadequacy of the placental circulation
    c. Is larger than normal because it tends to be postmature
    d. Often is hypertensive

UNIT IV

INTERRUPTIONS IN HEALTH IN LATE PREGNANCY

CHAPTER ONE

THE DIABETIC MOTHER

OBJECTIVES   *Identify the physiological alterations of pregnancy which are sources of stress for the diabetic mother.*

Identify the stressors capable of producing crisis during pregnancy, labor, and delivery for the diabetic mother and fetus.

Identify the specific intervention needed by the mother and family.

Identify the nursing aspects in the care and support of the family.

PRETEST   In the spaces provided, fill in the word or words that best complete(s) the statements. Then turn to page 175 and check your answers.

1. Pregnancy alters the _____ and _____ metabolism.

2. Class A diabetic mothers are _____
_____
_____
_____
_____.

3. During pregnancy, class A diabetic mothers are treated _____
_____.

4. The effect of insulin is lessened during pregnancy because _____
_____
_____ and _____
_____.

5. The mother's regulation of insulin is difficult since the urine _____
_____.

6. Nausea and the vomiting of pregnancy can produce _____
_____
_____
_____.

7. Common infections during pregnancy in the diabetic mother _____
_____
_____.

8. In the diabetic mother the incidence of toxemia is _____
_____
_____.

9. Fetal abnormalities are found _____
_____
_____.

10. During the last six weeks of pregnancy, the fetus _____
_____.

11. In the diabetic mother the size of the fetus is _____.

12. Delivery of the diabetic mother usually takes place _____ _____.

13. After delivery the blood sugar level of the baby is _____.

14. The baby is considered to be _____ because of its size and development.

15. After delivery the care the baby receives is _____.

⬇

Pregnancy often produces a diabetogenic effect in the mother who has no diabetes or endocrine disorder. Carbohydrate and lipoid metabolisms alter because of the different hormones, such as human placental lactogen (HPL), estrogen, and progesterone, and enzymes produced in pregnancy. Thus the diabetic mother's homeodynamics are significantly altered during pregnancy.

White classified mothers who are diabetic as follows: Class A mothers are women who have an abnormal glucose tolerance test (GTT) during pregnancy and often a history of a large baby over 4,500 grams. Class B mothers are those who have developed diabetes when they were over twenty years of age. Class C diabetic mothers are those who have had the disorder over ten years, and class D mothers are those who had juvenile diabetes and beginning vascular involvement. Classes E, F, and R indicate more progressive deterioration of the vascular system.[1]

Class A diabetics are watched and treated by diet only and often have no problems. All the other classes of mothers are treated with insulin throughout the pregnancy and need very close supervision from both the obstetrician and the internist.

Pregnancy alters the _____ and _____ metabolism.
    carbohydrate; lipoid

Class A diabetics are determined by _____ _____ _____ _____.
    an abnormal glucose tolerance test and often a history of a large baby, over 4,500 grams

Vascular changes indicate the severity of the diabetes, and the classes of mothers involved are _____, _____, _____, and _____.
    D; E; F; R

Those mothers who are regulated on diet are _____.
    class A

The classes of mothers who need insulin for regulation are _____.
    B, C, D, E, F, and R

After pregnancy class A mothers do not have an abnormal GTT, but often five to ten years later they develop diabetes and so they often are termed "prediabetic."

Many of the normal alterations of pregnancy are sources of stress for the diabetic mother, since because of her endocrine disorder, her adaptive ability is more limited and interruptions of her health status are more prevalent. In early pregnancy, as the hormonal levels of estrogen, progesterone, and chorionic somatomammotrophins increase, the metabolism changes so that the effectiveness of insulin is lessened. The placenta produces an enzyme that destroys insulin. The amount of replacement therapy the mother is on before pregnancy increases because of these alterations of pregnancy and the needs for growth. Regulation of the mother's insulin coverage becomes more difficult because of the increased glomerular filtration rate and slowed reabsorption in the tubules of sugar from the urine.

It has been found that during the first two trimesters, insulin regulation is a problem. The mother's labile condition produces an undetermined and changing insulin need. She and her family must be made aware of the necessity for constant surveillance. During the third trimester the mother's insulin needs increase drastically. No upper limit for adequate control has been shown in any studies. It has been recommended that a combination of intermediate and short-acting insulin be utilized for best control. The amounts and times of administration are determined according to individual needs.

The effectiveness of insulin during pregnancy is lower than in nonpregnancy because of _____

_____

_____   _____

and _____

_____.

high levels of estrogen, progesterone, chorionic somatomammotrophins; destruction of insulin by an enzyme

During pregnancy the amount of insulin taken by the mother

_____.

increases

Regulation of insulin coverage is difficult since _____

_____

_____.

sugar
can normally be found in the urine of a pregnant woman

Insulin requirements are determined according to the mother's _____. Both _____ and _____ insulin are often used in combination. The most difficult times in pregnancy to adequately control the diabetic state are during the _____ and _____

_____.

needs; intermediate; short-acting

first; second trimesters

The frequent nausea and vomiting of early pregnancy can become a severe stressor for the diabetic mother, and she can easily go into a state of insulin shock. If the mother is nauseated and goes without nourishment for a period of time, she may develop ketoacidosis, which is a crisis state. Common infections such as cystitis, found in pregnancy, if not medically diagnosed and treated, produce alterations in the mother's metabolism which increase the need for insulin, and the infection readily becomes widespread. Healing of any skin lesions requires a longer time than normal, and any infection can modify the metabolism of insulin, causing difficulty in regulation. The diabetic mother seems to have less resistance against infections than nondiabetic mothers have, and once the infection begins, it produces serious interferences within the homeodynamic state.

Nausea and vomiting of pregnancy in the diabetic mother can cause _____ and, if prolonged, _____.

insulin shocks;
ketoacidosis

Infections, such as cystitis, often become _____ and alter the metabolism of _____.

serious (severe);
insulin

Infections often are seen in the diabetic mother since _____ _____.

she has lower resistance or
slower adaptive response

Stressors associated with the diabetic state are capable of producing crisis states during the pregnancy, labor, and delivery periods. The source of some of these stressors has been identified, while for other stressors more research is necessary to determine the specific interactions.

The diabetic mother has an increased probability of developing preeclampsia or eclampsia during the last half of the pregnancy. It has been theorized that the placental function is limited and that the production of the hormones is reduced, precipitating the development of preeclampsia. Eclampsia can become life-threatening to both mother and fetus.

There also is an interference with amniotic fluid dynamics so that there is an increased amount, over 1,000 cubic centimeters, of fluid; this condition is termed "hydramnios." It causes much respiratory discomfort to the mother and also causes the uterine muscles to become very stretched.

The incidence of fetal abnormalities is higher when the mother has diabetes, but it is not affected if it is the father who has the diabetes. The high incidence of congenital problems is partly responsible for the higher fetal death rate in utero. The other factor that produces the significantly high fetal loss in the last six weeks of pregnancy has not been identified but may be due in part to the placental function.

In diabetic mothers, during the last half of pregnancy, the mother often develops _____ _____ , which can become life-threatening to both mother and fetus.

> preeclampsia or
>
> eclampsia

Hydramnios frequently is found in the diabetic mother; this is _____ _____ _____ .

> an increased amount of
>
> amniotic fluid, over 1,000
>
> cubic centimeters

In the last six weeks of pregnancy there is a high _____ _____ .

> fetal
>
> death rate

The fetus is larger than the average term baby, and because of the increased size and weight, often there is cephopelvic disproportion, making vaginal delivery impossible.

The medical intervention is committed to delivering a live baby who will have a good chance of surviving. The mother often is admitted to hospital around the thirty-sixth or thirty-seventh week so that close observation can be made. In some institutions, studies are being done in which daily estriol levels are used as an indicator, and if there is a significant drop (50 percent), then the baby is delivered. In other institutions, physicians may bring the mother in and deliver her at thirty-seven weeks. Sonography helps in the determination of whether there is cephopelvic disproportion, before a trial labor with Pitocin is started. Often, because of the baby's large size, the mother has a cesarean section. If the mother's state of health is severely interrupted with toxemia, severe hydramnios, or circulatory problems, delivery is performed earlier, around the thirty-fourth week. Postpartum hemorrhage is seen frequently because of the overstretching of the uterus.

Cephopelvic disproportion frequently is seen when the mother has diabetes because _____ _____ .

> fetal size and weight
>
> are increased

Delivery often is effected by _____ _____ .

> cesarean
>
> section

If the estriol levels drop 50 percent, then _____ _____ .

> the baby
>
> is delivered immediately

The type of insulin the mother is on at the time of delivery is _____ .

> regular

It is extremely important to observe the mother postpartally for

_____.

⬇

hemorrhage

The baby has its own problems after delivery. A higher incidence of respiratory distress syndrome is seen in these children (see page 474). The babies are hypoglycemic shortly after birth, a reaction thought to be due to the hyperglycemia of the mother stimulating the production of insulin by the baby and the sudden drop of blood sugar levels after delivery. Hypocalcemia and hyperbilirubinemia are conditions commonly found in the neonate of the diabetic mother. If the delivery was vaginal, then often difficulties such as brachial palsy are encountered. The baby also has a higher probability of having an anomaly.

Observation of the baby's respiratory adaptation is important since the infant may develop _____

_____.

respiratory
distress

The mother's hyperglycemia is thought to be responsible for the baby's _____ shortly after birth.

hypoglycemia

If the delivery was vaginal, often the baby shows signs of

_____

_____

_____.

the difficulty of passing
through the pelvis, e.g.,
brachial palsy

At the time the mother becomes pregnant, the family needs to know that many of the maternal difficulties and complications can be lessened or prevented with ongoing frequent care by both the obstetrician and the internist. The nurse can help the mother plan her activities, diet, and changes in insulin coverage necessary with the pregnancy. It is important for the mother to understand that sugar in the urine often is normally found in pregnancy. The mother should be instructed to see the physician promptly should she develop any infection.

Along with these concerns, the parents are worried about the chance of transmission of diabetes to the offspring. There is a 25 percent chance that the child will develop diabetes if one parent has the disorder.

When the diabetic mother becomes pregnant, the nurse can encourage the parents by informing them that the difficulties for the mother will be minimal if _____

_____.

she regularly sees
the doctors

The parents realize that they can transmit this problem to their offspring because there is a _____ chance that the child will develop diabetes.

25 percent

Since the stressors for the diabetic mother produce a crisis state for her and the family, it is important for the nurse to identify their strengths and provide support for the family when needed. Should the pregnancy terminate with a stillbirth, grief, loss, guilt, and feelings of inadequacy are emotions often experienced by the parents. Nursing intervention can help that family deal with these feelings and resolve their conflicts. If the mother is critically ill, the father often feels very responsible and guilty, i.e., that he caused this. Allowing him to express his fears and providing support so that he can help the mother are important.

The baby is not premature by weight or postmature by dates but rather is considered dysmature because many of the systems are still immature and interruptions in functioning are present in some. This means that the infant is placed in the high-risk nursery and often is put under intensive care. The parents should be kept informed of the status of the baby so that they will not become unduly alarmed by the various procedures. The parents' concerns and fears about the well-being of the baby need to be expressed, and the nurse can be very helpful with this.

The family may be in a crisis state because of complications during the pregnancy. Nursing intervention can help the family by _____, _____, and _____ _____.

identifying strengths;

providing support;

allowing for verbalization of

feelings

At birth the baby is considered _____.

The baby often is in a special nursery because _____ _____ _____.

dysmature

intensive

care measures may be needed

due to interruptions of the

systems

Molly and Gerald Lamont have been married for three years and recently decided that they would like to start a family. Molly currently is ten weeks pregnant. Molly has a history of diabetes mellitus and is classified as a class B diabetic. You are with Molly and Gerald during their prenatal visit. The physician asks you to confer with the family about the course of early pregnancy. Your best response would be:

A. "Molly, you may experience nausea and occasional vomiting, but don't worry, this usually passes in a few hours. It is important to rest more. Continue taking insulin with the same coverage as you were using before you were pregnant."

Go to page 171.

B. "Molly, you must recognize that it is very important that you do not contract any type of infection because of the danger to you at this time. Your insulin coverage should be regulated according to the result of the urine testing."

Go to page 173.

C. "Molly, pregnancy causes a stress, especially if you experience any nausea and vomiting. Call the doctor because you can have difficulty if you don't eat. Your insulin coverage is altered during pregnancy, and the urine testing is unreliable now. Follow the schedule given to you by the doctor."

Go to page 172.

No, your choice of *A* is poor. Remember about the kinds of difficulty the diabetic mother can get into if she experiences nausea and vomiting. Your advice about more rest is good, but then you give her incorrect information about her insulin dosage.

Return to page 165. Review the material and choose another response from page 170.

Your choice of *C* is excellent. You have identified for Molly an area of possible difficulty, nausea and vomiting, but you also have given her a way of seeking help to cope with this problem. You also have explained about the changes of pregnancy altering the reliability of urine testing, and you again have provided her with a way of dealing with the situation.

Advance to page 174 and take the post-test.

Incorrect. Your choice of *B* demonstrates you do not clearly understand the way of providing information while at the same time being supportive. Look at the counseling you gave about infection. That was enough to raise the mother's level of anxiety. You also gave misinformation about the insulin coverage.

Return to page 165. Review the material and choose another response from page 170.

POST-TEST   Indicate whether each statement is true or false by circling the appropriate letter. Then turn to page 175 and see how well you have done.

1.   Pregnancy produces a diabetogenic effect in the normal mother.   T   F

2.   Class A diabetics are regulated on insulin during pregnancy.   T   F

3.   Estrogen and progesterone affect the metabolism of insulin.   T   F

4.   The need for insulin is increased during pregnancy.   T   F

5.   The diabetic mother has a good resistance against infections.   T   F

6.   Eclampsia is seen more frequently in diabetic mothers than in non-diabetic mothers.   T   F

7.   Hydramnios is seen often in these mothers; it causes difficulty with respiration.   T   F

8.   The incidence of congenital abnormalities is higher when the father is a diabetic than when the mother is.   T   F

9.   There is a high rate of fetal loss, especially in the last weeks of pregnancy.   T   F

10. The mother often rests at home until term and then is admitted to the hospital.   T   F

11. The size of the fetus often causes cephalopelvic disproportion.   T   F

12. The incidence of respiratory distress syndrome is high in the infants.   T   F

13. The baby's blood sugar levels often show hyperglycemia.   T   F

14. The baby is considered to be premature because delivery is early. T   F

15. The parents should be kept informed of the baby's status.   T   F

In the specific areas with which you had difficulty, return to the material and review.

REFERENCE 1. Jack Pritchard and Paul MacDonald: *Williams Obstetrics*, 15th ed., Appleton-Century-Crofts, New York, 1976, p. 622.

BIBLIOGRAPHY Avery, Gordon: *Neonatology, Pathophysiology and Management of the Newborn*, J. B. Lippincott Co., Philadelphia, 1975.

Cohen, M., F. Haour, M. Dumont, and J. Bertrand, "Prognostic Value of Human Chorionic Somatomammotrophin Plasma Levels in Diabetic Patients," *American Journal of Obstetrics and Gynecology*, Vol. 115, No. 2, pp. 202–210, Jan. 15, 1973.

Coustan, Donald and Stephen Lewis, "Clinical Approaches to Diabetes in Pregnancy," *Contemporary Ob/Gyn*, Vol. 7, pp. 27–32, May 1976.

———, "Does Maternal Diabetes Predispose the Neonate to RDS?" *Contemporary Ob/Gyn*, Vol. 7, pp. 113–114, April 1976.

Duhring, John L., "Diabetes in Pregnancy: How to Diagnose and Treat It," *Contemporary Ob/Gyn*, Vol. 9, pp. 117–120, Feb. 1977.

Goebelsman, Uew, et al., "Estriol in Pregnancy, Daily Urinary Estriol Assays in the Management of the Pregnant Diabetic Woman," *American Journal of Obstetrics and Gynecology*, Vol. 115, No. 6, pp. 795–802, March 15, 1973.

Kofi, S., et al., "The Incidence of Gestational Diabetes," *Obstetrics and Gynecology*, Vol. 49, No. 4, April 1977.

Murata, Yuji and Chester B. Martin, Jr., "Growth of the Biparietal Diameter of the Fetal Head in the Diabetic Pregnancy," *American Journal of Obstetrics and Gynecology*, Vol. 115, No. 2, pp. 252–256, Jan. 15, 1973.

Pritchard, Jack and Paul MacDonald: *Williams Obstetrics*, 15th ed., Appleton-Century-Crofts, New York, 1976.

PRETEST ANSWERS 1. Carbohydrate; lipoid   2. Those with an abnormal glucose tolerance test during pregnancy and/or a history of a large baby, 4,500 grams or over   3. By diet alone   4. The hormones interfere with the action of insulin; an enzyme destroys some of the insulin   5. Normally can contain sugar during pregnancy   6. Insulin shock and ketoacidosis after prolonged episodes of nausea and vomiting   7. Alter the insulin metabolism and easily become widespread   8. More frequent than in the nondiabetic mother   9. More often in the diabetic mother than in the nondiabetic mother   10. May die in utero   11. Increased   12. Earlier, around the thirty-eighth week   13. Low   14. Dysmature   15. Intensive

POST-TEST ANSWERS 1. T   2. F   3. T   4. T   5. F   6. T   7. T   8. F   9. T   10. F   11. T   12. T   13. F   14. F   15. T

CHAPTER TWO

THE CARDIAC MOTHER

Identify the classifications of cardiac mothers.

Identify the alterations of pregnancy which become serious stressors for the cardiac mother.

Identify the medical care of the cardiac mother in pregnancy, labor, and the postpartum period.

Identify the nursing intervention with the family.

PRETEST In the spaces provided, fill in the word or words that best complete(s) the statements. Then turn to page 185 and check your answers.

1. Class I mothers are those who _____

    _____

    _____.

2. Class II mothers can perform normal activity but _____

    _____.

3. If the mother has had cardiac failure, she is considered to be class

    _____.

4. Anemia in the cardiac mother _____

    _____

    _____.

5. Around the twenty-eighth week the mother may experience difficulty due

    to the _____

    _____.

6. The prognosis for the cardiac mother during pregnancy is dependent on the

    _____

    _____, _____, _____

    _____, and _____.

7. Signs of early cardiac difficulty are _____

    _____, _____

    _____, _____,

    and _____.

8. Class III and IV mothers often are restricted in their activity and often are

    _____.

9. Fetal death can occur from _____ and _____

    _____.

10. The mother's diet often is limited in _____, _____

    _____, and _____.

11. The mother frequently is admitted early before labor to _____

    _____.

12. During labor the mother's vital signs are taken _____

    _____.

13. If the mother should become dyspneic, it is important to have _____
     _____ .

14. Anesthesia during labor and delivery is _____ .

15. During the second stage of labor, the mother _____
     _____ .

16. The postpartum period can be a critical time for the mother since this is
     when the _____
     _____ .

17. As the mother plans for discharge, it is important for the nurse to
     _____
     _____
     _____ .

Normal alterations of the cardiovascular system in pregnancy produce stressors capable of causing interruptions of the homeodynamics of mothers with cardiac disorders. The cardiac disorders are classified according to the New York Heart Association's criteria: Class I cardiac mothers have a functional heart murmur but no limitation on physical activity, and class II mothers have discomfort with heavy or strenuous activity but are comfortable with ordinary activity. Class III mothers are comfortable at rest but experience discomfort with exercise, whereas class IV mothers experience discomfort even at rest. Any mother who has had cardiac failure during the past or during the present pregnancy is automatically placed in class III.[1]

Class I and II mothers can perform normal activities and exercises and experience _____. **no discomfort**

Class III mothers experience discomfort during _____ **normal**
_____ and Class IV _____. **activity; at rest**

If there is any history of cardiac failure, the mother is considered class _____. **III**

Alterations of pregnancy may be of sufficient force to produce interruptions in the homeodynamics of the mother since her adaptive ability is lessened by her cardiac conditions.

During the second trimester the blood volume _____. **increases**

The increased blood volume results in an increased cardiac output, which places more stress on the heart. As the blood plasma increases, the hematocrit level lowers because _____ **the red**
_____ **blood cells do not increase**
_____. **corresponding to volume**

Although in the past rheumatic heart disease was the major culprit, good prophylaxis with antimicrobial agents has decreased that threat. More often, congenital heart disease is indicated as the predisposing factor to cardiac difficulty in pregnancy.

Let us review some of the normal cardiovascular problems that make a definitive diagnosis difficult in pregnancy and that also increase cardiac stressors. If anemia is present with a hemoglobin of 8 or lower, then the mother probably will go into cardiac failure. As the metabolic rate increases during the second trimester, the heart rate increases, and the need for oxygenation of the tissues of both mother and fetus is increased.

The rate of increase in blood volume is greatest around the twenty-eighth week, which may be an especially difficult time for the mother. The volume does not drop significantly until about ten days postpartum, and close observation through the entire period is necessary.

During the pregnancy, alterations that occur and which often cause difficulty for the cardiac mother are _____ _____ , _____ _____ , _____ , and the need for increased _____ .

increased blood volume; physiological anemia; increased metabolism; oxygenation

The prognosis for the mother during the childbearing period is dependent on the functional status of her cardiac condition, any complicating infections, proper medical care, and the psychological reactions and financial resources of the family. The mother should see both the obstetrician and the cardiologist frequently throughout the pregnancy.

Most mothers in classes I and II do very well during the childbearing period when they are under good supervision to prevent episodes of cardiac embarrassment or failure. Extra rest is very important following meals and at night. Heavy work and climbing of stairs are to be avoided; this restriction includes much of the housework. The mother should avoid any crowd or persons who have colds or infections.

Signs of beginning cardiac difficulty are things such as inability to do normal activity; increased pulse rate, often with rales; and progressive edema. The mother should go to bed immediately and call the physician.

Class III and IV mothers are often in bed throughout the pregnancy and sometimes are hospitalized if rest is limited at home. These mothers are often on digitalis, diuretics, and diets restricted in sodium and calories. The pregnancy can be life-threatening for both mother and baby.

Episodes of hypoxia or hypotension are known to cause fetal death resulting in an abortion early in pregnancy or a stillbirth late in pregnancy.

The prognosis for the cardiac mother depends on the adaptive resources available; thus the outcome is dependent on _____ , _____ , _____ , and _____ _____ .

functional status; infection; medical care; family resources and responses

Class I and II mothers who are supervised closely during pregnancy usually have a _____ outcome.

good

Class III and IV mothers during pregnancy must _____ _____ throughout the pregnancy.

Fetal death can occur from _____ or

_____ .

> stay
>
> in bed
>
> hypoxia;
>
> hypotension

Nursing intervention with the family during pregnancy is geared to assisting the family in making the special adaptation necessary because of the mother's limited adaptive cardiac response. Class III and IV mothers, once they are pregnant, frequently are offered a therapeutic abortion because of the inherent dangers of pregnancy and the severe limitations on activity which are necessary. The nurse can be very helpful to the mother and father as they make their decision, weighing the factors. The nurse can explain and reinforce the information given the parents and help them plan for the pregnancy or abortion. While the parents plan for the activities during the pregnancy, referrals to agencies such as homemakers are required. Helping the parents share their feelings about the added responsibilities on top of the normal alterations occurring during pregnancy is very helpful. The severe limitations of activity may be difficult for the mother, and encouraging interest in activities and hobbies that are quiet and restful can help. Often the mother can make lists and plan family shopping needs and in this way not abandon her family responsibilities. If she is home with other children, then activities such as reading and crafts can be shared with the children.

Encouraging the family members to get enough rest and relaxation so that they do not develop colds and other such infections is important as is discouraging visitors who have any infectious conditions.

Diet is very important for the mother; often carbohydrates, sodium, and fluids are limited. The family may need dietary counseling in this area.

The family should be alert to signs of impending cardiac failure; they should have the mother go to bed immediately and notify the physician. If the mother is on bed rest throughout the pregnancy, often a crisis state is produced within the family itself. Thus nursing intervention must involve the whole family since they frequently need support during this period of crisis.

Nursing intervention assists the family as they adapt to the limitations of activity of the mother and to their added responsibilities. Also, the nurse provides counseling about _____,

_____, and _____

_____ .

> rest;
>
> diet; avoidance of
>
> infections

Support of the family can be provided by inviting

_____

_____ and by _____.

verbalization of feelings and

problems; referrals

Usually the mother is admitted to the hospital several weeks before delivery so that her cardiac status can be assessed before she undergoes the strenuous time of labor and the rapid changes occurring in the postpartum period. At this time the mother may be digitalized. During labor the mother is kept in a semi-Fowler's position so that the pressure on the heart is decreased and any hypotension is prevented from developing. Oxygen is available in the room should the mother become dyspneic. Vital signs are monitored every 15 to 20 minutes, and an increase in pulse rate above 100 or respiratory rate over 28 is indicative of the beginning of cardiac failure. Should this condition develop, morphine, digitalis, and a diuretic are given and rotating tourniquets are applied.

An epidural or caudal may be given to provide local anesthesia during labor, to lessen the discomfort and help the mother to relax. Hypotension must be avoided. Nursing support with explanations about what treatments are being done and what to expect as labor progresses should be constant during labor.

General anesthesia and cesarean section are contraindicated for the cardiac mother. During delivery she is alert and needs much encouragement and reinforcement of previous instruction. Usually she is not allowed to push during the second stage because pushing increases the load on the heart. Frequently forceps are used to shorten the second stage.

During labor the position the mother is in is _____.

semi-Fowler's

Frequent observation of _____

vital signs;

is important to identify signs of _____.

cardiac failure

Equipment in the delivery room includes _____.

oxygen

If local anesthesia is given, _____ must be avoided.

hypotension

During the second stage the mother _____

is not

_____.

allowed to push

Explanations and encouragement are very important since they

_____.

reduce anxiety

During the postpartum period there is a great shift in the body fluids, so _____

there is a sudden

_____.

increase in the blood volume

It is very important at this time to observe the mother for signs of cardiac failure, which can develop during the first five days. Following the third stage of labor, there is an increase in blood volume due to the emptying of the blood supply previously delivered to the uterus into the systemic circulation. There are, however, adaptive mechanisms that aid in establishing a state of equilibrium. Some adaptation occurs through the moderate blood loss due to delivery and following placental separation and the increased postpartal urinary output. Any of the postpartum complications can produce a crisis for the cardiac mother. Care must be taken so that the mother does not develop hemorrhage, infection, or phlebitis. Often during the early postpartum period, the mother is on restricted activity and does not care for the baby, so it is important that she know how the baby is feeding and doing. If possible, short visits by the baby will be very helpful in reassuring the mother that everything is all right.

During the first three months of the postpartum period, the mother is still on restricted activity as her body readjusts to the nonpregnant state. Often, because of the pregnancy, the cardiac status of the mother has worsened.

A careful assessment by the nurse of the family's needs is very important. Referrals for an infant care technician often are necessary as part of the plan for the mother's discharge. Family members need support as they adapt to the new infant and its demands. Rest is extremely important for the mother. If there is extended family living nearby, these people can be of help to the family members and can share some of the responsibility, helping the family to adapt successfully to the new member.

During the postpartum period it is important to observe for signs of _____ due to _____ _____.

cardiac failure; shift of body fluids

Since the mother does not care for the infant immediately, it is important for the nurse to _____ _____.

inform her of the baby's activity and feeding

When the family is preparing for discharge, the nurse helps by _____ _____ and _____.

assisting in planning daily activities; making referrals

POST-TEST   Indicate whether each statement is true or false by circling the appropriate letter. Then turn to page 185 and see how well you have done.

1. Class I cardiac mothers have no physical limitation of activity.   T   F

2. Class III mothers experience discomfort at rest.   T   F

3. Normal alterations of pregnancy can produce interruptions in the health status of the cardiac mother.   T   F

4. During the last trimester the mother should be watched closely should she experience any difficulties due to the increases in blood volume.   T   F

5. The prognosis for the mother is dependent on her cardiac status alone.   T   F

6. It is important that the mother rest after meals.   T   F

7. If the mother has difficulty doing normal activities, this means that she has not had enough sleep.   T   F

8. Class III and IV mothers are often in bed throughout the pregnancy.   T   F

9. The family should be alert to the signs and symptoms of cardiac failure.   T   F

10. General anesthesia is given to the cardiac mother during delivery to lessen the pain and anxiety.   T   F

11. During labor the cardiac mother is in a semi-Fowler's position.   T   F

12. The cardiac mother usually is not allowed to push during the second stage.   T   F

13. During the first five days of the puerperium, it is important that the mother be watched for signs of cardiac failure.   T   F

14. It is important to keep the mother informed of the baby's progress.   T   F

In the specific areas with which you had difficulty, return to the material and review.

REFERENCE 1. Jack Pritchard and Paul MacDonald: *Williams Obstetrics,* 15th ed., Appleton-Century-Crofts, New York, 1976, p. 610.

BIBLIOGRAPHY Clark, Ann and Dyanne D. Alfonso: *Childbearing: A Nursing Perspective,* F. A. Davis Co., Philadelphia, 1976, pp. 604–607.

Clausen, Joy, Margaret Flook, and Bonnie Ford: *Maternity Nursing Today,* 2d ed., McGraw-Hill Book Co., New York, 1977, pp. 755–756.

Gerber, Albert, ''Management of Heart Disease Complicated by Pregnancy,'' *Hospital Medicine,* Vol. 1, No. 16, June 1965.

Oakley, Celia, ''Heart Disease in Pregnancy,'' *Nursing Times,* pp. 1923–1924, Dec. 9, 1976.

Pritchard, Jack and Paul MacDonald: *Williams Obstetrics,* 15th ed., Appleton-Century-Crofts, New York, 1976, pp. 608–618.

Ueland, Kent, Miles J. Novy, and James Metcalfe, ''Cardiorespiratory Responses to Pregnancy and Exercise in Normal Women and Patients with Heart Disease,'' *American Journal of Obstetrics and Gynecology,* Vol. 115, No. 1, pp. 4–10, Jan. 1, 1973.

PRETEST ANSWERS 1. Have a functional heart murmur but no limitation of activities   2. Experience discomfort with strenuous activities   3. III   4. Is a serious condition causing more work load for the heart, possibly cardiac failure   5. Rapid rate of increasing blood volume   6. Functional status of her heart; infection; medical care; family reactions, attitudes, and finances   7. Inability to do normal activity; increased pulse rate; cough; progressive edema   8. On bed rest throughout the pregnancy   9. Hypoxia; hypotension   10. Carbohydrates; sodium; fluids   11. Assess her status   12. Every 15 to 20 minutes   13. Oxygen readily available   14. Local only   15. Is not allowed to push   16. Body fluids shift occurs, rapidly increasing the blood volume   17. Make appropriate referrals and help the family plan realistically

POST-TEST ANSWERS 1. T   2. F   3. T   4. T   5. F   6. T   7. F   8. T   9. T   10. F   11. T   12. T   13. T   14. T

CHAPTER THREE

MULTIPLE PREGNANCY

OBJECTIVES   *Identify the characteristics of monozygotic and dizygotic twins.*

Identify the alterations of the childbearing cycle as a result of multiple pregnancy.

Identify the possible interruptions in the maternal health status due to the multiple pregnancy.

Identify the nursing intervention with the family when there is a multiple pregnancy.

Describe possible interruptions in the health state of the twins.

GLOSSARY   *Monozygotic twins:* Two fetuses developing from one fertilized ovum
Dizygotic twins: Two fetuses developing from two fertilized ova

PRETEST   In the spaces provided, fill in the word or words that best complete(s) the statements. Then turn to page 194 and check your answers.

1.   Monozygotic twins are formed from _____.

2.   Dizygotic twins develop from _____.

3.   It is possible to diagnose that the mother is carrying twins at the _____ week.

4.   In a monozygotic pregnancy there are _____ amnions and _____ chorions.

5.   The increased size of the uterus makes it difficult for the mother to _____ and _____.

6.   The mother often goes into labor _____ _____.

7.   The twins frequently weigh around _____ each.

8.   Analgesia during labor is _____.

9.   The twin who has the most difficulty during delivery is the _____,

10   The risk to the mother during the postpartum period is _____.

11.   After delivery the twins are often placed in a _____ _____.

12.   The mother frequently is discharged _____ the twins are.

13.   During the pregnant state mothers carrying a twin pregnancy are more prone to _____ and _____ and may have an abnormal amount of _____.

14.   Following the delivery of twins, mothers must be watched carefully for _____ due to the overdistension of the uterus during pregnancy.

Multiple pregnancies that are naturally occurring, not medically induced by administration of hormones to increase fertility, are rather infrequent occurrences. Twins are seen in the general population at the rate of about 1 percent of the total number of live births, whereas triplets, quadruplets, and quintuplets are seen with decreasing frequency.

The term *twinning* means "dividing in half" and refers to one fertilized ovum splitting in half and becoming two individuals. This division produces *monozygotic twins*, who are identical in all characteristics. As the fertilized ovum divides, the usual structures that are produced are the following: one chorion, one placenta, two umbilical cords, two amnions, and two fetuses. It is theorized that if the division of the ovum takes place very early in development, each twin will have all the structures of a single fetus, so there will be two chorions, two placentas (occasionally just one), two amnions, two cords, and two fetuses.

Monozygotic twins develop from _____.   one ovum

Monozygotic twins have _____ amnions and   two;

_____ chorions.   one or two

Dizygotic twins usually result from the fertilization of two ova at relatively the same time. This means that there are two separate fetuses with all the structures of a single fetus, developing concurrently, with different characteristics and often different sexes. Dizygotic twins also are known as "fraternal twins."

Thus, dizygotic twins have _____ chorions,   two;

_____ amnions, _____ placentas; and   two; two

two umbilical cords.

During pregnancy the location of each twin and the attachment to its placenta (one, two, or often fused) will determine the amount of nutrition each twin receives. Sometimes one twin is larger by several pounds than the other due to better exchange through the placenta. There have been occasional instances of one twin transfusing the other in utero. This occurrence is caused by vascular shunting. In other words, during fetal development an "anastamosis" between the vascular systems of both fetuses occurs. At birth it is very easy to identify the recipient twin and the donor twin. The fetus that received the extra blood supply may appear to have edema; its skin is often flushed and its pulse rate feels fuller; the donor twin, however, is usually the smaller of the two, is pale in contrast to its sibling, and appears to be dehydrated. Blood studies will also identify anemia in the donor twin.

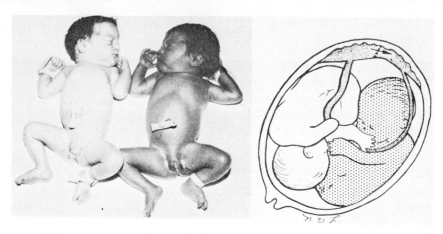

Feto-fetal transfusion syndrome in identical twins. (*A*) Larger twin on right, hematocrit 87 percent (anemic twin, 32 percent). (*B*) Placental arteriovenous shunt (anemic twin on right). (*From Comprehensive Pediatric Nursing by G. Scipien et al. Copyright © 1975 by McGraw-Hill Book Company.*)

It is rare that each twin weighs as much as 7 pounds at birth. On the average twins weigh about 5 pounds each. The total weight and combined size of twins is larger than the dimensions of the single pregnancy. Before term the uterus becomes very stretched, so that frequently the mother goes into labor at about the thirty-seventh week. Approximately half of the time there is recognition and diagnosis of the fact that the mother has twins.

The size of each twin depends upon _____ _____.

the nutrition

from the placenta

The combined weight of both fetuses in relationship to that in a single pregnancy is _____.

greater

The average weight of each twin is _____.

5 pounds

A twin pregnancy usually terminates about the _____.

thirty-seventh week

A diagnosis of twins can easily be made by the twentieth week of gestation. At the time the parents are informed, there often is much surprise, and a great deal of readjustment must take place before the parents can accept and deal with the reality of two children instead of one. It is important for the nurse to accept the parents' initial response and to help them adapt effectively to the fact. During the pregnancy, often the mother experiences nausea and vomiting more frequently and the incidence of anemia is greater and more severe than with a single pregnancy. The mother is placed on iron supplement and sometimes folic acid in order to relieve this condition. Toxemia and hydramnios occur more frequently in multiple pregnancies than in single pregnancies. Therefore, prenatal care is extremely important for the mother, for early diagnosis and treatment of toxemia. Toward the latter part of pregnancy, the mother may have difficulty with eating and may be more comfortable eating small meals more often than eating a few larger meals. Also, her increased size makes it difficult for her to sleep at night, and it is important for her to have her head elevated so that she can breathe more easily. Since the mother often goes into labor prematurely, she is advised not to work after the thirtieth week. If the mother's cervix begins to dilate prematurely, then she may be placed on bed rest so that hopefully labor will not begin for several weeks.

Upon learning that they are going to have twins, the parents are often _____.

surprised and overwhelmed

If the mother has nausea and vomiting, you would recommend that she _____
_____
_____.

eat dry crackers before arising, and take small meals of liquids and then solids

If the mother obtains prenatal care, then early treatment is possible should _____ develop.

toxemia

The mother's extremely large size toward the end of pregnancy may cause discomfort when _____ and _____.

eating; sleeping

The mother may be restricted from working early in her pregnancy because _____.

prematurity is a problem

Labor and delivery are more complicated because there are two infants to be delivered and, for a vaginal delivery, one must precede the other. The overdistended uterus does not contract as effectively during labor as it does in a single pregnancy, and during the postpartum period there is a very high incidence of hemorrhage. The amount of analgesia given the mother is minimal because of the usual prematurity of the infants. Once the membranes have been ruptured, there is no contraindication to the use of an oxytocin if carefully monitored. The twins often are in a breech and vertex presentation, and the time of labor tends to be somewhat shorter due to the smaller size of the infants. Problems that may be encountered are prolapsed cord and closing down of the cervix after the delivery of the first twin. The ideal time between the delivery of the first twin and the second is 5 to 15 minutes. There often are more difficulties delivering the second twin than the first since this twin has to be brought down from the upper part of the uterus so that engagement can take place. Occasionally there is difficulty with the presentations of the twins and cesarean section is the method of delivery.

After the delivery of the second twin, the placentas are delivered.

It is extremely important that the cord is clamped after the first twin is delivered because the second twin might possibly bleed to death if the circulations through the placenta had fused. Immediately after the delivery of the placenta, high doses of oxytocin are given intravenously to the mother to prevent the occurrence of postpartum hemorrhage. Nursing assessment of the mother during the first part of the postpartum period is essential to determine the mother's status and to report any significant change.

Only light analgesia is used during labor since _____ _____.

the
twins usually are premature

The length of labor in a multiple pregnancy as compared with that of a single pregnancy is _____.

shorter

Problems that may occur during labor and delivery are _____ and _____ _____.

prolapsed cord; early closing
of the cervix

The twin who undergoes the most difficulty during delivery is the _____.

second

After the first twin is delivered, it is especially important to clamp the cord attached to the placenta to prevent _____ _____.

hemorrhage
of the second twin

In the immediate postpartum period the nurse must observe closely for signs of _____.

postpartum hemorrhage

After the delivery the infants often are placed in a special premature nursery for intensive care. A careful newborn evaluation is important since there is a higher frequency of congenital problems in a multiple pregnancy than in a single pregnancy.

The family during the postpartum period needs help and guidance as they plan to go home and assume the care of two newborns. Since the mother may be discharged before the infants are ready to leave the hospital, much support of the family is needed as they assume their parental roles with this interruption of time and space.

After delivery the infants often are in _____ _____.

a special
or premature nursery

When preparing for discharge the family needs help in _____.

planning care for two

Should the twins remain longer in the hospital, the parents need _____.

much support

It is essential that the parents be involved with seeing, touching, and caring for the infant as soon as possible for the binding mechanism to take place. The parents will need to be told about the premature nursery, the incubator, and any equipment that is attached to the infant. They will need the opportunity to discuss their anxieties, fears, and feelings of responsibility. It is a nursing responsibility to use good communication techniques and to provide a supportive atmosphere in which this can take place.

POST-TEST Indicate whether each statement is true or false by circling the appropriate letter. Then turn to page 194 and see how well you have done.

1.   Identical twins are dizygotic. T   F

2.   If early division occurs with the monozygotic twins, the structures formed are the same as those found with the single pregnancy. T   F

3.   Monozygotic twins have different characteristics. T   F

4.   The size of each twin is dependent on the amount of nutrition received from the placenta. T   F

5.   Twins can be born unequal in size and weight. T   F

6.   Anemia is more severe in the mother with a multiple pregnancy. T   F

7.   Toxemia is seen more frequently in the mother who is carrying twins. T   F

8.   The mother is not restricted from working during the pregnancy. T   F

9.   The labor is longer for the mother because there are two infants to be delivered. T   F

10. Prolapsed cord is a problem encountered because of the baby's small size. T   F

11. The second twin can bleed to death if the cord from the first twin is not clamped. T   F

12. Postpartum hemorrhage is a danger that often occurs as a complication for the mother. T   F

In the specific areas with which you had difficulty, return to the material and review.

BIBLIOGRAPHY   Dickason, Elizabeth and Martha Schult: *Maternal and Infant Care, A Text for Nurses*, McGraw-Hill Book Co., New York, 1975.

Jensen, Margaret, Ralph Benson, and Irene Bobak: *Maternity Care, The Nurse and the Family*, C. V. Mosby Co., St. Louis, Mo., 1977.

Pritchard, Jack and Paul MacDonald: *Williams Obstetrics*, 15th ed., Appleton-Century-Crofts, New York, 1976.

PRETEST ANSWERS   1. One ovum   2. Two ova   3. Twentieth   4. Two; one or two   5. Eat; sleep   6. Prematurely, at around the thirty-seventh week   7. 5 pounds   8. Minimal   9. Second   10. Hemorrhage   11. Special intensive-care nursery   12. Before   13. Toxemia; anemia; amniotic fluid   14. Postpartal hemorrhage

POST-TEST ANSWERS   1. F   2. T   3. F   4. T   5. T   6. T   7. T   8. F   9. F   10. T   11. T   12. T

CHAPTER FOUR

TOXEMIA

OBJECTIVES   *Identify the three classifications of toxemia.*

Identify the signs and symptoms of mild preeclampsia, severe preeclampsia, and eclampsia.

Identify the types of treatment indicated.

Identify the nursing intervention with the mother and family.

GLOSSARY   *Apnea:* Cessation of breathing
Tracheostomy: An incision into the trachea made in order to ensure ventilation
Hyperreflexia: A state or condition occurring when alterations in the nervous system produce an overreaction of reflex movement to a stimulus
Oliguria: A state in which little or no urine is secreted by the kidney
Polydipsia: A state of excessive thirst

PRETEST   In the spaces provided, fill in the word or words that best complete(s) the statements. Then turn to page 210 and check your answers.

1.   The three cardinal signs of toxemia are _____, _____ _____, and _____.

2.   Mild preeclampsia occurs when the mother has _____ _____, _____ _____, and _____.

3.   Severe preeclampsia is present when the mother has _____ _____, _____ _____, and _____ _____.

4.   Eclampsia occurs when the mother _____.

5.   Prenatal care is geared to _____ _____.

6.   If the mother has mild preeclampsia, she feels _____.

7.   The treatment for mild preeclampsia is _____.

8.   The mother's room should be dark and _____.

9.   The mother's nutritional intake should contain _____ _____ and _____.

10.   The mother's vital signs are taken _____.

11.   The aim of the treatment of severe preeclampsia is to _____ _____ and to _____ _____.

12.   Magnesium sulphate is used to _____.

13.   Toxic effects of magnesium sulphate are _____ _____ and _____.

14.   The antidote for magnesium sulphate is _____ _____.

15.   If the mother develops severe preeclampsia, her vital signs are monitored _____.

16.   The urinary output of the mother is measured _____.

17. As well as checking the mother's vital signs, it is important to check
    _____.

18. Restlessness may be a sign of _____.

19. Signs of an impending convulsion are _____, _____
    _____, _____
    _____, _____
    _____, _____
    _____, and _____.

20. The convulsions of eclampsia are first _____ then
    _____.

21. Careful observation of the mother is important during the early postpartum
    period since _____.

Toxemia is a specific entity found only in pregnancy and described only by signs and symptoms. There are three cardinal signs and symptoms: *hypertension*, *edema*, and *proteinuria*. Toxemia appears in the latter part of pregnancy, after the twentieth week.

The classification of mild preeclampsia is made when the mother's blood pressure is above 140/90 or the systolic has risen 30 millimeters of mercury and the diastolic 15 millimeters of mercury from the mother's previous status. The blood pressure often will rise if the mother is anxious or apprehensive about the prenatal visit, so the initial reading should be repeated twice within a six-hour period for the elevation to be meaningful. Edema, especially in the hands and face, may be observable, but many times it is not since it is a generalized edema. Thus the mother's weight gain is indicative if there is a gain of more than 1 pound per week; this usually is caused by fluid retention. Proteinuria is significant when found in a midstream clean catch or a catheterized specimen.

The mother is said to have mild preeclampsia when her blood pressure is above _____ or has risen _____ _____ _____.

140/90; 30 millimeters systolic and 15 millimeters diastolic

Edema may be generalized and may not be seen but is present if the mother has _____ _____.

gained more than 1 pound per week

A clean catch urine specimen when tested will show _____.

proteinuria

Severe preeclampsia is identified when the mother's blood pressure is 160/110 or either systolic or diastolic is above this when the mother is on bed rest. Readings should be taken twice, six hours apart, to rule out a transitory rise. Edema and hypertension can cause cerebral disturbance such as severe headaches. Often visual disturbances—double vision and blurring of images—are present. Pulmonary edema also may be present and to such a degree that cyanosis results. The amount of protein found in the urine is 3 to 4+, and if there is severe kidney involvement, oliguria is present, so the urinary output can drop to 240 cubic centimeters in a 24-hour period.

Severe preeclampsia occurs when the mother's blood pressure is _____ or _____ _____.

160/110; either is above

As the blood pressure rises and the edema increases, there are
_____.

Edema also can produce limited pulmonary function due to
_____ and can produce
_____.

Kidney function is interrupted as indicated by _____
_____ and _____.

cerebral and visual disturbances

pulmonary edema;

cyanosis

protein

of 3–4+ in the urine; oliguria

Eclampsia is a further progression of the disorder to the point where the mother, with no diagnosed neurological disease, convulses. The mother may have one or more convulsions, often followed by a period of coma that lasts for a few minutes or until the next convulsion.

The mother's condition is described as eclamptic when
_____. Convulsions are often followed
by _____.

she convulses;

coma

The cause of toxemia is unknown, although there are several theories offered. Recent literature seems to indicate that the symptomatology may be caused by stressors that for some reason precipitate less than the normal increase in blood plasma volume. This phenomenon plus arteriole and capillary constriction that may be intermittent or prolonged decreases blood and oxygen supply to vital organs including the uterus. Thus one of the primary symptoms, hypertension, is caused. There is also a concomitant decrease in kidney function and glomerular filtration, causing sodium retention and edema. Other researchers still adhere to the theory that malnutrition, including poor protein intake, is a causative factor in the development of preeclampsia-eclampsia since the highest incidence has been thought to be in lower socioeconomic individuals.

Research on the clinical findings indicates that there is generalized vascular involvement, with vasospasm of the kidney, eyes, and peripheral arterioles as well as changes in the heart, brain, and liver.

The cause of toxemia is _____.
Clinical findings indicate _____
_____.

not known

widespread vascular

changes

All prenatal care is geared to the detection of preeclampsia since at each visit the _____,

_____, and

_____.

blood pressure is taken;

the mother is weighed;

urine is tested

The signs and symptoms of mild preeclampsia are so subtle that the mother does not recognize them and she feels fine. The mother's feeling of well-being makes it very difficult for her to understand the seriousness of her condition. Mild preeclampsia can be effectively treated so as to stop the progression to severe preeclampsia.

The treatment of mild preeclampsia is *bed rest*, and this regimen may be carried out at home if the symptoms are very mild or may require hospitalization. The mother is kept in bed on her side, a position that increases the circulation through the kidneys. The room should be dark and quiet so that the mother will rest and begin to relax. Often the mother is given sedation such as phenobarbital. Supportive nursing measures include providing information to mother and family, restricting visitors, and assisting the family to make provision for the other members at home.

Assessment of the mother's blood pressure is done every four hours during the day and through the night only if there is a change and a rise. The mother is weighed daily to assess the amount of edema. It is now felt that a sodium-restricted diet is unnecessary, since a decrease in sodium intake will not decrease an elevated blood pressure due to vascular constriction. The diet should have sufficient protein, and the fluid intake should be 2,500 cubic centimeters every 24-hour period. The fluid intake is measured along with the urinary output, and each time the mother voids, the urine is tested for protein and the specific gravity is measured. Explanations about diet and the frequency of the vital signs are an important means of allaying the mother's apprehensions and gaining her cooperation in following the regimen.

It has been found that diuretics are of little help. If used at all they should be given for only five days. The physician checks daily for hyperreflexia of the reflexes, which would indicate cerebral involvement, and checks the retina for indications of vascular spasm or hypertension.

The main treatment for the mother with mild preeclampsia is

_____.

The mother can be helped to relax by _____

_____,

_____, and _____.

bed rest

keeping her

in a quiet, dark room;

explanations; sedation

Nursing assessment of the mother's status includes _____

_____, _____,

and _____

and tests for _____.

The mother's diet includes _____

and a total of _____

_____.

In order to gain the mother's cooperation and participation in the treatment, it is important to _____

_____

_____.

daily

weights; blood pressure;

fluid intake/output;

protein in the urine

sufficient protein;

2,500 cubic centimeters

of fluids

explain why the diet

and rest are important and why

vital signs are taken frequently

Should the mother's condition worsen or the signs and symptoms indicate that she has severe preeclampsia, the nursing and medical intervention becomes intensive. The aim of the treatment is to prevent convulsions and deliver the baby who is capable of surviving. Often these two criteria are at odds since the only cure for preeclampsia is delivery and the baby may be premature with the problems of high morbidity and mortality inherent.

Medication is used to prevent the development of convulsions. Magnesium sulphate is the agent used, and it is effective because it depresses the activity at the neuromuscular junctions. Magnesium sulphate also increases the urinary output and lowers the blood pressure. This drug is administered in very high dosages, so it is extremely important to be aware of the toxic effects. Respiratory depression and cardiac arrest will develop with overdosage, so the antidote, calcium gluconate, must be on hand at all times. Before a repeated dosage of magnesium sulphate is given, the knee jerks must be present and the respiratory rate must be above 16 per minute.

Other signs of toxicity are a sudden large decrease in blood pressure, polydipsia, flushing of the skin, sweating, and depressed reflexes. Careful nursing observations must be made while the mother is receiving this chemical therapy. Since mothers can become comatose, level of consciousness must also be assessed.

Magnesium sulphate can be administered intravenously or intramuscularly. If given intramuscularly, xylocaine is given with it to decrease the discomfort and the Z technique is used since a large amount is given.

Decreased stimulation is very important since jarring of the bed or sudden noises can cause the mother to convulse. The room should be darkened and quiet and only the treatments necessary carried out. Sedation also is important, and often phenobarbital is used.

The prevention of convulsions is important in the treatment of the preeclamptic mother, and the medication used is _____ _____.

magnesium
sulphate

The repeated dosage of magnesium sulphate is given when _____ and _____.

the knee jerks are present;
respirations are above 16

The antidote necessary to have on hand when giving magnesium sulphate is _____.

calcium gluconate

Sudden stimulation of the mother may cause _____.

a convulsion

Phenobarbital is often given for _____.

sedation

The mother's blood pressure is monitored every 15 minutes to every hour depending on the mother's status. Any significant change should be reported.

An accurate hourly measurement of urine output is very important. Therefore an indwelling catheter is used; it causes less stimulation from attempts to void than using a bedpan does, and it allows a more precise measurement of kidney function. The use of hypertonic dextrose 20 to 50 percent or mannitol to reduce cerebral edema and increase urinary output has been questioned since their effectiveness is difficult to measure.

The fetal heart rate must be checked regularly, and the mother should be observed closely for signs of labor. Often the mother's restlessness may be an indication of labor; always check the perineum since the labor usually progresses very quickly.

The nursing care of the mother is constant, and the mother should never be left alone. Symptoms such as throbbing headache, nausea and vomiting, severe epigastric pain, blurring or temporary loss of vision, extreme apprehension or somnolence, and hyperreflexia are a prelude to a convulsion. The physician should be notified immediately, and more sedation is given to allay convulsions.

Other medications that may be ordered by the physician include hypotensive agents and anticonvulsive drugs.

The mother's blood pressure is monitored frequently according to _____ _____.

her status; *q* 15 minutes
to *q* 1 hour

The urinary output is measured _____.

every hour

The fetal heart rate is checked _____.

regularly

If the mother becomes restless, this may be a sign of _____.

labor

Certain signs and symptoms may occur before the onset of convulsions. These are _____, _____, _____, _____, _____, _____, _____, and _____.

throbbing headache; nausea and vomiting; severe epigastric pain; blurring or loss of vision; apprehension; somnolence; hyperreflexia

Eclampsia, the most severe form of this disorder, is marked by convulsions that often produce a life-threatening situation for both the mother and the baby. The statistics indicate that if the mother convulses there is a 50 percent chance that the fetus will survive and a mortality rate of 10 percent for the mother.

The convulsions that occur in eclampsia at first are tonic and then become clonic; they often are so violent that the mother is thrown out of bed or sustains injury by hitting the siderails. The period of apnea usually lasts over a minute before the mother starts to breathe again. The coma that follows the convulsions lasts for a few seconds or until the next convulsion. Suction should be available in the room, and oxygen is administered following the convulsion. A tracheostomy set and mouth gag are important to have in the room. If the mother is comatose it is important to turn her from side to side every two hours, and the siderails are padded to protect her from injury. Drugs are given in an attempt to stabilize the mother's status so that no further convulsions occur. Delivery is effected either by induction or by cesarean section.

Eclampsia is characterized by _____.

convulsions

Once eclampsia develops, the mortality rate _____.

increases

The convulsions begin first as _____ and then become _____.

tonic;

clonic

The siderails are padded to _____ during the convulsion, and with the onset you would insert _____.

prevent injury

a mouth gag or airway

If the mother vomits during the convulsion or has a lot of fluid in her mouth, it is important to _____ and then administer _____.

suction;

oxygen

Signs that indicate that the mother's adaptive forces are decreasing progressively and her status has worsened are repeated convulsions, an increase in cardiac and/or respiratory rate, an increase in temperature, a decrease in urinary output, a falling blood pressure and pulse pressure, and pulmonary edema or cyanosis. If palliative treatment is not able to support the maternal systems, death ensues.

In the immediate postpartum period the mother may convulse, especially during the first 24 hours, even if she has not done so before delivery. Careful observation during the first several days is very important.

Indications that the maternal systems' functioning and adaptive ability have greatly decreased are _____,
_____
_____, _____
_____, _____
_____, _____
_____,
and _____.

repeated convulsions; increased cardiac and/or respiratory rate; increased temperature; decreased urinary output; falling blood pressure and pulse pressure; pulmonary edema or cyanosis

Constant assessment and observation of the mother are extremely important during the postpartum period, especially during the first 24 hours, because _____.

the mother may convulse

The need for antepartum care throughout the pregnancy is essential so that early diagnosis and treatment of mild preeclampsia will prevent the development of eclampsia. The nurse is instrumental in encouraging and explaining the importance of medical care throughout pregnancy and providing a pleasant and positive atmosphere so that the mother and family will keep appointments and continue with their care.

Follow-up studies done on women who have had preeclampsia-eclampsia in first pregnancy indicate little indication of essential hypertension later in life. However, if women have hypertensive disorders in more than one pregnancy it is felt that there is an underlying hypertensive problem, exacerbated by pregnancy, that may become chronic later in life.

Let us look at the following situation. Jennifer and Jay Berman are excited about the prospect of their first child, who is due in five weeks. You meet them during their prenatal visit and note that Jennifer's blood pressure is 160/100, her urine shows 1+ protein, and she has gained 4 pounds since her visit two weeks ago. The physician decides to admit Jennifer for observation. You find the couple upset and anxious about the doctor's findings. Jennifer states, "I feel fine. Why do I have to stay in the hospital?"

Your initial response would be:

A. "Your blood pressure has risen so it is important to watch this carefully. Often with rest the blood pressure goes down. Also, your weight gain has increased. This may be due to a change in your diet, or it may mean that you are retaining fluids. With close observation we can better assess your status and prevent any further problems."

Go to page 206.

B. "Your blood pressure is high, and your urine test is abnormal; these with the additional weight gain could mean trouble for you and the baby unless you do as the doctor says."

Go to page 207.

C. "I can understand your feelings about there being no need for hospitalization. Well, we are going to let you rest here for a little while and then probably discharge you—so there is no real problem."

Go to page 208.

Excellent. Your choice of *A* demonstrates your ability to provide clear information and explanations to the mother. In this manner you have supported her and have stressed the positive aspects. Her hospitalization will be easier for her, and she will be able to relax better.

Advance to page 209 and take the post-test.

In your choice of *B*, you do not seem to understand the meaning you are conveying to the mother. You are, in essence, threatening the mother if she does not do as the doctor says. This response will arouse a high level of anxiety in the family, making the rest and relaxation very difficult to achieve.

Return to page 200. Review the material and choose another response from page 205.

Your choice of *C* is poor. Although you are accepting the mother's feelings, you are not clarifying the reasons for the hospitalization but are adding to the vagueness. How do you plan to obtain the mother's cooperation so that she can rest and relax as needed?

Return to the situation on page 204 and choose another response from page 205.

POST-TEST Indicate whether each statement is true or false by circling the appropriate letter. Then turn to page 210 and see how well you have done.

1. Toxemia occurs after the twentieth week of pregnancy.   T   F

2. If the mother has mild preeclampsia, she feels ill.   T   F

3. In mild preeclampsia, edema may be seen in the hands and face.   T   F

4. If the mother gains $\frac{1}{2}$ pound a week then this would indicate generalized edema.   T   F

5. If the mother has severe preeclampsia, her blood pressure is 160/110.   T   F

6. Edema and hypertension can produce cerebral disturbances.   T   F

7. If the kidneys are severely involved, then often oliguria is present.   T   F

8. The mother who has mild preeclampsia must rest and relax.   T   F

9. The diet the mother has should be low in protein.   T   F

10. The mother's fluid intake should be 3,000 cubic centimeters per day.   T   F

11. Magnesium sulphate lowers the blood pressure and increases the urinary output.   T   F

12. Before a repeated dose of magnesium sulphate is administered, it is important to count the respiration and check the knee jerks.   T   F

13. It is important to ensure that the mother has sufficient stimulation.   T   F

14. Hourly urine samples will indicate the kidney function.   T   F

15. If the mother is restless, it is important to give more sedation.   T   F

16. Hyperreflexia indicates that a convulsion may be imminent.   T   F

17. Convulsions are life-threatening for both the mother and the baby.   T   F

18. There is no period of coma after the convulsion.   T   F

19. After delivery there is no worry that the mother may convulse.   T   F

20. Good prenatal care can reduce the incidence of toxemia.   T   F

In the specific areas with which you had difficulty, return to the material and review.

BIBLIOGRAPHY Butts, Priscilla, "Magnesium Sulfate in the Treatment of Toxemia," *American Journal of Nursing*, Vol. 77, pp. 1294–1298, Aug. 1977.

Chelsey, Leon, "What Is the Long-Term Prognosis for Eclamptic Patients?" *Contemporary Ob/Gyn*, Vol. 7, pp. 137–141, June 1976.

Clark, Ann and Dyanne D. Alfonso: *Childbearing: A Nursing Perspective*, F. A. Davis Co., Philadelphia, 1976.

Duncan, Margaret, Ralph Benson, and Irene Bobak: *Maternity Care, The Nurse and the Family*, C. V. Mosby Co., St. Louis, Mo., 1977, pp. 248–252.

Galloway, Karen, "Placental Evaluation Studies: Their Procedures, Their Purposes, and the Nursing Care Involved," *Maternal Child Nursing*, Vol. 1, pp. 300–306, Sept./Oct. 1976.

Goodlin, Robert, "Severe Pre-Eclampsia: Another Great Imitator," *American Journal of Obstetrics and Gynecology*, Vol. 125, No. 6, pp. 747–751, July 15, 1976.

Karbakri, Dilip, John Harrigan, and Robert LaMagra, "The Supine Hypertensive Test as a Predictor of Incipient Pre-Eclampsia," *American Journal of Obstetrics and Gynecology*, Vol. 127, No. 6, pp. 620–621, March 15, 1977.

Marshall, George and Robert Newman, "Roll-Over Test," *American Journal of Obstetrics and Gynecology*, Vol. 127, No. 6, pp. 623–625, March 15, 1977.

———, John Annitto, and Robert Cosgrove, "The Remote Prognosis of Eclamptic Women," *American Journal of Obstetrics and Gynecology*, Vol. 124, No. 5, pp. 446–459, March 1, 1976.

Pritchard, Jack and Paul MacDonald: *Williams Obstetrics*, 15th ed., Appleton-Century-Crofts, New York, 1976.

Speroff, Leon, "Pregnancy-Induced Hypertension," *Contemporary Ob/Gyn*, Vol. 9 (Symposium), pp. 137–166, Jan. 1977.

PRETEST ANSWERS

1. Hypertension; edema; proteinuria   2. Blood pressure of 140/90 or above; weight gain of 1 pound or more a week; proteinuria   3. Blood pressure of 160/110; generalized edema; proteinuria of 3–4+ (plus)   4. Convulses   5. The early detection of toxemia   6. Fine   7. Bed rest   8. Quiet   9. Adequate protein; restricted sodium   10. Every four hours   11. Prevent convulsions; deliver a viable baby   12. Prevent convulsions   13. Respiratory depression; cardiac failure   14. Calcium gluconate   15. Every 15 minutes   16. Hourly   17. The fetal heart rate   18. Labor   19. Headache, nausea and vomiting; epigastric pain; blurring or loss of vision; apprehension or somnolence; hyperreflexia   20. Tonic; clonic   21. The mother can convulse

POST-TEST ANSWERS

1. T   2. F   3. T   4. F   5. T   6. T   7. T   8. T   9. F   10. F   11. T   12. T   13. F   14. T   15. F   16. T   17. T   18. F   19. F   20. T

CHAPTER FIVE
MISSED ABORTIONS

OBJECTIVES   *Define the term "missed abortion."*

Identify the signs and symptoms of a missed abortion.

Identify some of the responses to the missed abortion.

Identify the nursing intervention with the family when there is a missed abortion.

GLOSSARY   *Hypofibrinogenemia:* Low fibrinogen in the blood with the result that bleeding and hemorrhage may occur

Macerated fetus: A fetus that has undergone change so that all tissues become soft

Mummified fetus: A fetus that has undergone change so that it loses fluid and becomes very dried

PRETEST   In the spaces provided, fill in the word or words that best complete(s) the statements. Then turn to page 216 and check your answers.

1. A missed abortion is a condition in which _____

_____

_____

_____.

2. Signs of a missed abortion are _____

_____, _____

_____, and _____

_____.

3. A condition that is associated with the missed abortion is _____

_____, which contraindicates surgical intervention.

4. Saline and/or prostaglandins may be used to _____

_____.

A *missed abortion* occurs when the fetus dies in utero and the products of conception are retained within the uterine cavity for a period of *eight* weeks or longer. The pregnancy begins normally, and the mother experiences the normal phenomena of breast changes, enlargement of the uterus, amenorrhea, and morning sickness during the first several months. The mother then becomes aware that the fetus is not moving, the size of the uterus is not increasing, and her breasts are beginning to shrink in size. She may experience fatigue, depression, an unpleasant taste in her mouth.

Some theorize that the placenta continues to function after the death of the fetus and that this is the reason why the products are retained in utero so long. However, the factors that cause this death of the fetus have not been clearly identified.

A missed abortion is defined as _____

_____

_____.

the retention of the products of conception eight weeks after the fetus dies

When a missed abortion occurs, the mother becomes aware of signs that are not seen in the normal pregnancy. These signs are

_____ _____, _____

_____, and _____

_____.

no fetal movement; no increase of uterine size; shrinking of breasts

The mother often becomes concerned and visits her physician, and a fetal electrocardiogram or other measure is done to determine whether the fetal heart is functioning. Frequently associated with the missed abortion is the condition of *hypofibrinogenemia* (low fibrinogen in the maternal blood). This means that any surgical intervention is contraindicated because of bleeding problems. Since the mother and family find this a difficult, morbid, and depressing state, rather than waiting for a spontaneous abortion of the products to occur, termination of this state can be accomplished by the use of oxytocins alone or in combination with prostaglandins or intrauterine hypertonic saline. The fetus may be macerated or mummified by the time it is expelled.

Nursing intervention is aimed at providing support and information to the family. The mother should not be left alone in this crisis situation when the difficult and often frightening outcome is known. Fears and fantasy can be very disturbing to the family, so explanations should be clear and reassurance given when possible. If large doses of oxytocins are used, signs of water intoxication should be watched for (see pages 102–103).

Analgesia is important, and the mother should be kept comfortable. Following the abortion, care includes checking for hemorrhage, infection, and the retention of any clots. Since the baby had become more of a reality after quickening, the mother and father must deal with the grief of the loss of a baby. The nurse can be very helpful by reassuring the parents that their feelings are normal and that they were not guilty of causing the death of their child either by wishes or by actions.

When the mother has a missed abortion, the associated bleeding problems are due to _____.

hypofibrinogenemia

Termination of the missed abortion can be spontaneous or induced by use of _____, _____,

oxytocins; prostaglandins

or _____.

intrauterine hypertonic saline

Nursing support can be provided by _____

staying with the

_____, _____,

mother; making her comfortable;

_____, and _____

giving information; allowing

_____.

for expression of feelings

POST-TEST Indicate whether each statement is true or false by circling the appropriate letter. Then turn to page 216 and see how well you have done.

1. In a missed abortion the pregnancy begins normally. T F

2. If the mother has a missed abortion, the fetus has been dead for at least eight weeks in utero. T F

3. The retention of the products of conception may be due to the fact that the placenta continues to function for some time after the fetus dies. T F

4. The mother does not often suspect that the fetus has died. T F

5. Hypofibrinogenemia means that surgery is contraindicated because of the possibility of hemorrhage. T F

6. The fetus may be mummified or macerated. T F

7. After the expulsion of the fetus, the parents are glad that the state is over and do not have any feelings of grief. T F

In the specific areas with which you had difficulty, return to the material and review.

BIBLIOGRAPHY   Breuer, J., "Sharing a Tragedy," *American Journal of Nursing*, Vol. 76, No. 5, pp. 758–759, May 1976.

Grubb, Caroline, "Body Image Concerns of a Multipara in the Situation of Intrauterine Fetal Death," *Maternal-Child Nursing Journal*, Vol. 5, No. 2, pp. 93–115, Summer 1976.

————, "Is the Baby Alive or Dead: Psychological Work of a Woman with Intrauterine Fetal Death," *Maternal-Child Nursing Journal*, Vol. 5, No. 1, pp. 25–37, Spring 1976.

Kitay, David, "Bleeding Disorders in Pregnancy," *Contemporary Ob/Gyn*, Vol. 7, pp. 88–90, Jan. 1976.

Pritchard, Jack and Paul MacDonald: *Williams Obstetrics*, 15th ed., Appleton-Century-Crofts, New York, 1976.

PRETEST ANSWERS   1. The fetus is dead and is retained in utero for a period of eight weeks or longer   2. Absence of fetal movement; cessation of uterine growth; shrinkage of the mother's breasts   3. Hypofibrinogenemia   4. Induce labor to expel the contents

POST-TEST ANSWERS   1. T   2. T   3. T   4. F   5. T   6. T   7. F

CHAPTER SIX
PLACENTA PREVIA

OBJECTIVES　*Identify the three types of placenta previa.*

Identify the signs and symptoms that characterize placenta previa.

Identify the nursing intervention with the mother and family.

PRETEST   In the spaces provided, fill in the word or words that best complete(s) the statements. Then turn to page 223 and check your answers.

1. Placenta previa occurs when _____
    _____
    _____
    _____.

2. The three types of placenta previa are _____, _____
    _____, and _____.

3. Stressors associated with the development of placenta previa are _____
    and _____.

4. The major symptom of placenta previa is _____
    _____.

5. The diagnosis of placenta previa is _____
    _____.

6. A pelvic examination of the mother _____
    _____
    _____.

7. The danger to the fetus is _____.

8. The danger to the mother is _____.

9. The usual treatment for placenta previa is _____
    _____.

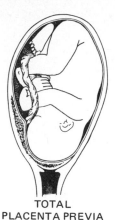 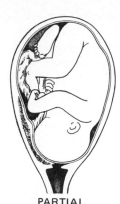 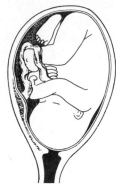

| TOTAL PLACENTA PREVIA | PARTIAL PLACENTA PREVIA | LOW OR MARGINAL IMPLANTATION |

Placenta previa.

Placenta previa describes the position of the placenta when it is found *over or near the internal cervical os*. This means that the placenta is below the fetus and during labor would be the first part that is delivered, a situation causing severe anoxia and often death to the fetus.

The three types of placenta previa describe the degree to which they cover the internal os. *Total placenta previa* completely covers the cervical os, while *partial placenta previa* covers only a portion of the cervical os. The last type, *marginal or low Implantation* of the placenta, refers to the placenta that encroaches on the cervical os. The placenta is found at the edge of the os and can be palpated on digital exam, so that as the cervix begins to dilate, the placenta is apparent.

Placenta previa refers to the _____
_____
_____.

position of the placenta over or near the cervical os

The three types of placenta previa are _____,
_____, and _____
_____.

total; partial; marginal/low implantation

Two stressors associated with the development of placenta previa are multiparity and increased age. One theory that attempts to explain why the placenta is implanted low in the uterine cavity suggests that the endometrium in the upper portion is not capable of providing enough nourishment and therefore the ovum attaches to the lower segment and spreads out more to obtain adequate nutrition.

The major symptom experienced by the mother is *painless* bleeding. The mother feels fine and then suddenly begins to hemorrhage. The onset of this bleeding is usually after the seventh month, as the cervix begins to dilate and the maternal blood vessels are torn away from the placental surface. Often the bleeding ceases for a period of time, to reoccur when least expected, or the mother may have a continuous spotting or bloody discharge. This sudden and continuous loss of blood produces a physical and psychological state of stress for the mother because there is no way that the mother or family can prevent this hemorrhage. Another hemorrhage can produce a crisis state of shock, and without immediate intervention death of both the mother and the fetus may result.

Two factors that are seen associated with the development of placenta previa are _____ and _____.   age; multiparity

The main sign of placenta previa is _____   painless

_____.   bleeding

Before the onset the mother experiences _____   no

_____.   symptoms

The hemorrhage may stop completely, or _____   continuous

_____.   spotting may occur

The difficulty is to determine a definite diagnosis. A pelvic examination that would confirm the diagnosis is contraindicated, since the digital examination is likely to cause massive hemorrhage if the placenta is over the os. The most reliable test is the sonogram, which will outline the location of the placenta and the degree to which the cervical os is covered. Other tests, such as soft tissue x-rays and radioactive uptake of iodine which collects where the blood pools, have not been highly reliable.

Once the diagnosis has been made or it is suspected that the mother has placenta previa, the mother often is hospitalized because of the danger of another unexpected hemorrhage. The gestational maturity of the fetus is determined. If the mother is close to her expected date of confinement, a pelvic exam is performed in the operating room with a double setup. A *double setup* means that preparations for both an immediate vaginal delivery and cesarean section are made.

If the mother is earlier in the pregnancy, then she is watched carefully, and should labor begin and should the pelvic exam confirm the diagnosis, a cesarean section usually is performed. A vaginal delivery may be possible if the placenta is marginal, if the cervix dilates rapidly so that the danger of hemorrhage is not great, and if the fetal heart tones are good so that there is no indication of fetal anoxia.

A definite diagnosis of placenta previa is difficult to make since

_____.   a pelvic exam is contraindicated

A pelvic exam is done _____ in the _____.

with a double setup; operating room

If placenta previa is diagnosed early in the eighth month, the mother _____.

is hospitalized

If the diagnosis of placenta previa is definite, the delivery is _____.

usually cesarean section

The mother and family often are in a state of emotional shock when the first signs of hemorrhage begin because there has been no indication of any interruption in the health state. Fear and anxiety about the mother's well-being develop. The nurse can assist the family to understand the various tests that are being conducted to attempt to determine the diagnosis. There may be limited time to prepare the family for the pelvic exam, which is conducted with many people about and much equipment. Simple explanations and reassurance that everything possible is being done for the mother and baby will help the mother and family as they deal with this crisis situation.

If the mother is hospitalized for a period of time before the delivery, a homemaker often is needed to look after the children and financial assistance may be necessary. The mother may have many questions about the cesarean section which should be discussed with her. If this is the mother's first pregnancy she may be very upset at missing the birth of her baby and may feel she is inadequate. Allowing her to verbalize these feelings is helpful. Also, informing the mother that having a cesarean section does not mean that a cesarean section will be necessary the next time she delivers may provide some reassurance.

POST-TEST Indicate whether each statement is true or false by circling the appropriate letter. Then turn to page 223 and see how well you have done.

1. Placenta previa occurs when the placenta separates early from the decidua.   T   F

2. Low implantation of the placenta means that it does not cover the internal os but is very near it.   T   F

3. The mother feels well and then experiences painful bleeding.   T   F

4. Continuous spotting or vaginal bleeding makes the mother vulnerable to shock should another episode of bleeding occur.   T   F

5. Once the diagnosis of placenta previa is suspected, the mother usually is hospitalized.   T   F

6. If the fetus is at maturity, a cesarean section is usually performed once the diagnosis of placenta previa is confirmed.   T   F

7. It is important to allow the mother to express her feelings about the delivery by cesarean section.   T   F

In the specific areas with which you had difficulty, return to the material and review.

BIBLIOGRAPHY   Duncan, Margaret, Ralph Benson, and Irene Bobak: *Maternity Care, The Nurse and the Family*, C. V. Mosby Co., St. Louis, Mo., 1977.

Galloway, Karen, "Placenta Evaluation Studies: Their Procedures, Their Purposes, and the Nursing Care Involved," *Maternal-Child Nursing*, pp. 300–306, Sept.–Oct. 1976.

Goodman, D. J., "The OCT: Implementation and Protocol," *Journal of Obstetrics and Gynecological Nursing*, Vol. 6, pp. 28–34, Jan.–Feb. 1977.

Louka, M. H., "Obstetric and Gynecologic Bleeding," *Hospital Medicine,* Vol. 12, p. 44, Aug. 1976.

Pritchard, Jack and Paul MacDonald: *Williams Obstetrics*, 15th ed., Appleton-Century-Crofts, New York 1976.

Roberts, A., "Systems of Life," *Nursing Times*, p. 73, March 3, 1977.

de Tornay, Rheba, "Nursing Decisions: Experiences in Clinical Problem Solving—An Occurrence of Placenta Previa," *RN*, Vol. 39, No. 4, pp. 43–48, April 1976.

PRETEST ANSWERS   1. The placenta is implanted in the lower segment of the uterus over or near the internal os   2. Total; partial; marginal/low implantation   3. Age; multiparity   4. Painless bleeding   5. Difficult to confirm   6. Is contraindicated unless done in the operating room with a double setup   7. Anoxia   8. Hemorrhage   9. Cesarean section

POST-TEST ANSWERS   1. F   2. T   3. F   4. T   5. T   6. T   7. T

CHAPTER 7
ABRUPTIO PLACENTA

OBJECTIVES   *Identify the types of abruptio placenta.*

Identify the signs and symptoms of abruptio placenta.

Identify the nursing intervention with the mother and family.

GLOSSARY   *Abruptio placenta:* Premature separation of the placenta

PRETEST   In the spaces provided, fill in the word or words that best complete(s) the statements. Then turn to page 230 and check your answers.

1. Abruptio placenta is _____

_____

_____.

2. The degrees of separation are _____ and _____.

3. The bleeding that occurs can be either _____ or _____

_____.

4. The mother experiences _____ with the bleeding.

5. If abruptio placenta occurs, the uterus when palpated feels _____

_____.

6. The mother may rapidly develop _____

_____.

7. The fetus often suffers from _____.

8. The condition often associated with abruptio placenta is _____

_____.

9. Initial treatment of abruptio placenta is _____

_____.

10. Delivery is by _____ or _____

_____.

Abruptio placenta is the condition in which the normally implanted placenta separates from the uterine wall before delivery of the baby. This premature separation can be found to occur at any time after the twentieth week until the delivery of the infant. The separation can be of the complete placenta, as seen with *total abruptio placenta*, or of only a portion of the placenta, as occurs with *partial abruptio placenta*. As the placenta separates, there is maternal bleeding between the surface of the placenta and the uterine wall as the mother's arterioles become unattached from the villi.

If the blood escapes by passing through the cervix, then the blood loss is *apparent*. Less frequently the blood is contained between the uterine wall and the placenta and membranes. This *concealed* hemorrhage or internal hemorrhage is more often associated with the complete separation of the placenta.

Abruptio placenta occurs when the _____ _____ _____.

placenta separates prematurely or before the delivery of the fetus

The types of abruptio placenta are _____ and _____.

total;
partial

The bleeding occurring with abruptio placenta can be either _____ or _____.

apparent; concealed

The stressors that are thought to be associated with the development of abruptio placenta are eclampsia and preeclampsia, chronic hypertensive vascular disorders, endocrine imbalances, placenta previa in a previous pregnancy, pressure on the inferior vena cava by the

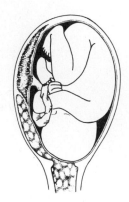

PARTIAL ABRUPTIO
WITH
APPARENT HEMORRHAGE

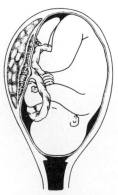

TOTAL ABRUPTIO
WITH
CONCEALED HEMORRHAGE

Abruptio placenta.

distended uterus, and poor nutrition. Also, the greater the mother's parity, the more frequent the development of abruptio placenta.

The separation of the placenta creates a crisis state for the maternal systems, because the amount of bleeding often produces shock. The bleeding also causes *pain* as the uterus becomes contracted with such *rigidity* that it is often described as "boardlike." The uterus is very tender to the touch, and the amniotic fluid is blood-tinged. Depending on the degree of shock, kidney function is interrupted and oliguria may be found. Also associated with abruptio placenta is hypofibrinogenemia.

The sudden and dramatic symptoms often produce an overwhelming fear for the mother and baby. If the mother is in the hospital, this emergency situation brings all the medical personnel to intervene. The fear of death of both herself and the baby often is apparent in the mother and the family. The fetal heart tones are monitored continuously. Often if the separation is a major portion of the placenta, the anoxia is sufficient to produce fetal death, which will be indicated by an absence of the fetal heart tones.

Abruptio placenta is found more frequently in mothers _____ | with
_____ parity | high

The bleeding produces maternal _____, and, if severe, causes interruptions of the kidney function. | shock

When the uterus is palpated it is _____, and the | rigid;
mother complains of _____. | pain

Often the blood does not clot well due to _____ | low
_____. | fibrinogen

The mother and family often fear _____. | death

If a large portion of the placenta is separated, the fetus usually _____. | dies from anoxia

The treatment of abruptio placenta is to immediately replace the blood loss and to give fluids to maintain kidney function and reverse the state of shock. Also, determining the fibrinogen level is necessary, and fibrinogen is administered as needed. At this time the membranes are ruptured, and an oxytocin is given with the hope of accomplishing delivery vaginally within six hours. If this is not possible, then a cesarean section is performed. The maternal outcome is good with prompt treatment, and the fetus does well if the separation is a small portion and the amount of blood loss small.

Nursing intervention is geared to support of the maternal systems. The nurse may be the first person to recognize the signs and symptoms of abruptio placenta if the mother is in the hospital. Explanations of examinations and treatments are important, and if the fetal heart tones are good, the mother should be encouraged, while if the fetal heart tones are absent, it is important not to falsely reassure the mother. Reassuring that all is being done and keeping the family informed are essential.

The father's presence often is helpful to the mother if the mother is out of shock. It is important for the nurse to assist the mother through the labor and help her relax as much as possible, and the nurse is continuously assessing the physical status of the mother and the fetus.

Immediate treatment of abruptio placenta is _____ _____ _____.

replacement
of blood and fluids and
fibrinogen

If possible, delivery is _____.

vaginal

Nursing intervention assesses the _____ _____.

maternal and
fetal status

Support is provided to the family by _____ and _____.

explanations;
reassurance

POST-TEST Indicate whether each statement is true or false by circling the appropriate letter. Then turn to page 230 and see how well you have done.

1. In abruptio placenta the normally implanted placenta separates prematurely. T F

2. If the separation of the placenta is complete, the bleeding often is concealed. T F

3. There always is a warning before abruptio placenta occurs. T F

4. The mother may be in shock within a short period of time. T F

5. If the fetal heart rate is absent, it is important not to tell the mother this fact. T F

6. The mother often has bleeding problems because of hypo-fibrinogenemia. T F

7. The nurse can be supportive by explaining the procedures and treatments. T F

In the specific areas with which you had difficulty, return to the material and review.

BIBLIOGRAPHY   Galloway, Karen, "Placenta Evaluation Studies: Their Procedures, Their Purposes, and the Nursing Care Involved," *Maternal Child Nursing*, pp. 300–306, Sept.–Oct. 1976.

Goodman, D. S., The OCT: Implementation and Protocol," *Journal of Obstetric and Gynecological Nursing*, Vol. 6, pp. 28–34, Jan.–Feb. 1977.

Kitay, David, "Bleeding Disorders in Pregnancy," *Contemporary Ob/Gyn*, Vol. 7, pp. 87–89, 1976.

Louka, M. H. "Obstetric and Gynecologic Bleeding," *Hospital Medicine*, Vol. 12, p. 44, Aug. 1976.

Pritchard, Jack and Paul MacDonald: *Williams Obstetrics*, 15th ed., Appleton-Century-Crofts, New York, 1976.

Roberts, A. "Systems of Life," *Nursing Times*, p. 73, March 3, 1977.

de Tornay, Rheba, "Nursing Decisions: Experiences in Clinical Problem Solving—An Occurrence of Placenta Previa," *RN*, Vol. 39, No. 4, pp. 43–48, April 1976.

PRETEST ANSWERS   1. The separation of the placenta before the delivery of the fetus   2. Total; partial   3. Apparent; concealed   4. Pain   5. Rigid or boardlike   6. Symptoms of shock   7. Anoxia   8. Hypofibrinogenemia   9. Replacement of blood and plasma   10. Vagina; cesarean section

POST-TEST ANSWERS   1. T   2. T   3. F   4. T   5. F   6. T   7. T

CHAPTER EIGHT

INTERRUPTIONS IN HEALTH DURING PREGNANCY DUE TO MATERNAL ANEMIA

OBJECTIVES   *Identify the problems associated with anemia during pregnancy.*

Identify the types of hemorrhage.

Identify the characteristics of iron deficiency anemia.

Identify the characteristics of megaloblastic anemia.

Identify the hemoglobin disorder associated with sickle cell anemia.

Identify the hemoglobin disorder associated with thalassemias.

Identify nursing needs and intervention with mothers and families when anemia is present.

GLOSSARY   *Anemia:* A decrease in hemoglobin and/or in the number of erythrocytes
Hemoglobin: A molecule made up of heme (or iron) and globin, formed by four polypeptide chains, two beta and two alpha. Hemoglobin transports oxygen throughout the system.
Iron deficiency anemia: A decrease in the number of erythrocytes due to a lack of iron
Megaloblastic anemia: A decrease in the number of erythrocytes usually due to a lack of folic acid when seen in this country
Sickle cell: A disorder of hemoglobin in which S hemoglobin is formed

Thalassemia: A disorder of hemoglobin production in which there is less hemo-
globin than normally
Hypochromic erythrocyte: Pale red blood cell
Microcyte: Small red blood cell
Macrocyte: Large red blood cell

PRETEST In the spaces provided, fill in the word or words that best complete(s) the statements. Then turn to page 242 and check your answers.

1. Anemia means that there is a _____
   _____.

2. The most common cause of anemia during pregnancy is _____
   _____.

3. The anemia caused by a folic acid deficiency is called _____
   _____ anemia.

4. Folic acid is necessary for the synthesis of _____
   _____.

5. Sickle cell anemia is transmitted by _____.

6. When the red blood cells sickle, this produces clumping and does not allow them to carry adequate _____ to the tissues.

7. The resulting lack of oxygen supply to small blood vessels causes severe pain, commonly called _____.

8. Pregnant, sickle cell women have a high incidence of maternal and perinatal _____ and _____.

9. Thalassemia major is also known as _____ anemia.

10. Thalassemia is a _____ transmitted _____ disorder.

11. Supplemental _____ is given prophylactically to pregnant women who are known to have thalassemia minor.

Anemia results from a decrease in the number of erythrocytes and/or in the amount of hemoglobin. Anemia in pregnancy may be due to interruptions in maternal health status that occur when there is loss of blood, as with abortions and abruptio placenta, or it may develop from a deficient intake or utilization of nutrients. While some anemias result from slow production of red blood cells, due to infection, in other instances there is hemolysis, or destruction of the erythrocytes. Finally, the genetic disorders that lead to alterations of the synthesis of hemoglobin often mean that the life of the erythrocyte is decreased and cause the mother to enter pregnancy with an already anemic status.

The alterations of blood volume in pregnancy may cause a normal lowering of the hemoglobin level to a range of 11 to 13 grams per 100 milliliters, whereas *a hemoglobin level of less than 10 grams per 100 milliliters* is considered to define anemia of pregnancy. Fetal problems such as growth retardation and an increased incidence of fetal morbidity and mortality may occur when anemia is present. The maternal problems associated with anemia include abortion, infection, toxemia, premature labor, and congestive heart failure if very severe anemia is present.

Anemia of pregnancy is defined by a _____ _____ _____. Anemia predisposes to fetal problems such as _____ and maternal problems such as _____, _____, _____, _____, and even _____.

hemoglobin of

less than 10 grams per 100

milliliters;

growth retardation;

abortion; infection;

toxemia; premature labor;

cardiac failure

The most common occurrences that predispose to anemia are hemorrhage and iron deficiency. *Hemorrhage* if severe is treated by blood replacement, and the nursing responsibilities include making sure that the blood to be hung is of the correct type and Rh and being alert for any reaction to the transfusion, such as chills, pallor, urticaria, increased temperature, and shock. If the blood loss is mild then often the treatment is iron supplements given orally or intramuscularly. Oral iron ingestion may produce the side effects of severe gastric irritation with nausea and vomiting, cramping, and diarrhea or constipation, which may mean that the mother will be given the intramuscular preparation. This route, too, has side effects: local irritation at the site. The medication is given in a Z track to reduce this problem. Sometimes the sudden increase of iron in the system causes not only gastric irritation but also central nervous system problems such as encephalopathy as well as cardiac failure. The nurse must explain to the family the current status of the mother and the reason for the treatment. The nurse should inform a mother who is receiving oral medication that she should tell the physician if she cannot tolerate the oral iron. If she is having problems of constipation, the mother should increase her intake of fluids and roughage. Iron is absorbed better if it is taken before meals, but the gastric irritation may be increased so the mother may try taking it after meals if necessary. The mother also needs an adequate intake of vitamin C to absorb the iron.

If the mother is receiving a transfusion of blood, it is important that the nurse observe for _____.
Oral iron may produce side effects affecting _____

_____.

signs of a reaction;

the

gastrointestinal tract

The technique used to administer intramuscular iron preparations is the _____. Central nervous system side effects of intramuscular iron include _____.

Z track;

encephalopathy

Iron deficiency anemia develops when there is an inadequate intake of iron. During pregnancy there is an estimated need for 800 milligrams of iron to ensure fetal use and storage and to maintain the mother's stores. Since only a small part of the ingested iron is absorbed, the above amount of iron is difficult to ingest with the normal balanced diet and most women are given a supplement of 30 to 60 milligrams daily during pregnancy.

The mother who is prone to developing iron deficiency anemia is one whose stores at the beginning of pregnancy are low, often due to previous pregnancies. Also, the mother who does not take the supplemental iron and whose diet has a low content of iron may develop anemia. The decreased amount of iron in the maternal system interrupts the synthesis of hemoglobin. If the iron depletion is severe then changes are seen in the erythrocytes, which become pale (hypochromic) and small (microcytic). The symptoms the mother exhibits are usually seen in the last trimester, as the fetal stores increase at the expense of the maternal system. The mother tires easily, feels weak, and if severe anemia is present, may have dyspnea. Looking at the mother's nail beds, you will see that they are pale, as are the conjunctiva.

The treatment of mild iron deficiency is the administration of oral iron in the amount of 200 milligrams daily. If the mother is not able to tolerate this, then the iron is given by the intramuscular route. If the iron deficiency is severe, then a series of intramuscular injections is administered. The nursing implications for the drug therapy are as above (see page 234). It is important for you to give careful explanations of why the mother needs the therapy, since not many people enjoy injections. The mother should understand and be able to explain to you why these shots are necessary. You can also inform her that she will feel less tired and weak in five to ten days, since this is when the response to the therapy occurs, although normal hemoglobin levels are not reached for several months.

Mothers who are prone to develop iron deficiency anemia during pregnancy are those who _____ stores are low;

and _____. dietary intake is poor in iron;

The anemia develops around the _____. third trimester;

If you look at the mother who has iron deficiency, you will see

_____ and _____. pale nail beds; conjunctiva

Megaloblastic anemia, although not a common occurrence, when it occurs in this country is usually due to a deficiency of folic acid. There is evidence that many mothers have low folic acid values during pregnancy, but since anemia is a later sign of the deficiency, the lack of folic acid is not always identified. Folic acid is one of the essential components necessary to form the nucleic acids, along with vitamins B_{12} and C. During pregnancy the fetal need for growth takes priority and the folic acid is utilized by the fetus; thus if the mother has inadequate levels then her production of nucleic acids is reduced and in turn, the production of erythrocytes is reduced. Instead of being normal erythrocytes they may be macrocytic or larger than normal. The bone marrow usually shows megaloblastic changes. The mothers who are prone to develop megaloblastic anemia are multiparous women whose diet is poor in leafy greens and liver. In some instances, mothers with absorption problems or liver damage are predisposed to low folic acid levels. It is during the third trimester that the mother exhibits symptoms of megaloblastic anemia, such as diarrhea, soreness of the tongue, edema of the feet, bruising, retinal and mucous membrane hemorrhages, and enlarged liver and spleen. The treatment is the administration of folic acid, usually 30 milligrams daily, and a response is seen in two to six weeks.

The nursing implications are to take a good diet history and, with the mother, plan to incorporate liver and leafy greens in her diet. If there are greens in the diet it is important that these not be overcooked because overcooking destroys folic acid. Since megaloblastic anemia occurs increasingly with successive pregnancies, the nurse can counsel the mother and father about spacing children. The nurse can also help the parents select suitable family planning methods by providing any needed information.

A lack of folic acid produces an anemia called _____

_____. Mothers who develop this anemia usually

are _____ or have _____

_____.

Folic acid is utilized in the body for _____

_____. Sources of folic acid are

_____, liver, and yeast. Before giving any counseling

it is important that the nurse take _____ in-

cluding cultural and economic factors.

megaloblastic

anemia;

multiparous; absorption

problems or liver damage

production

of nucleic acids;

leafy greens;

a diet history

Alterations of the hemoglobin from the normal are termed *hemo-globinopathies*. The problems mothers experience with these vari-ations of hemoglobin depend on the degree, i.e., how much of the hemoglobin is affected and if there are combinations of several vari-ations. The adult normally has hemoglobin A constituting about 95 percent of the total hemoglobin. The rest is hemoglobin A_2, a normal variant, and hemoglobin F, termed "fetal hemoglobin."

The variant that is seen with *sickle cell* is hemoglobin S. This hemoglobin S is formed because one of the amino acids on the beta chains forming the globin is altered (valine is substituted for glutamic acid). This alteration produces a change in the structure of the eryth-rocyte under lowered oxygen tension, so that the cell becomes rigid rather than flexible and assumes the characteristic sickle shape, which in turn occludes the small blood vessels. Once the cells have sickled and stay this shape for any period of time, they usually do not return to their original shape but rather they are picked up by the liver and spleen, where hemolysis takes place, causing further anemia.

Hemoglobin S is an autosomal dominant characteristic; thus a heterozygous person has hemoglobin A and hemoglobin S while a homo-zygous person has hemoglobin S-S. If an individual has hemoglobin A-S, his or her condition is "sickle cell trait." Such an individual has only about 35 percent of the S hemoglobin. In this instance there is enough A hemoglobin so that the erythrocytes do not change structure unless there are extreme conditions, such as shock, severe dehydration, or severe lack of oxygen. If the individual has S-S hemoglobin, the con-dition is termed "sickle cell anemia." Such an individual has between 75 and 95 percent hemoglobin S with the remaining portion made up of hemoglobin F. The problem of sickle cell is found predominantly among the black population in this country. The sickle cell variant is thought to have evolved as a protection against malaria.

Hemoglobin S is formed because there is an alteration of

⇩

_____   one of the amino acids on the

_____.   beta chain of the globin;

Hemoglobin S is inherited and is an _____   autosomal

_____ characteristic.   dominant

Under conditions of dehydration, acidosis, and _____ low

_____ the erythrocytes will   oxygen tension

sickle.

A person who has sickle cell trait has hemoglobin _____,   A-S;

while a person with sickle cell anemia has hemoglobin _____.   S-S

During pregnancy the mother with sickle cell trait has a normal hemoglobin level and there are no problems encountered during pregnancy except the possible increased incidence of pyelonephritis. Should the mother go into shock or receive general anesthesia, there could be problems of intravascular sickling; otherwise there are no interruptions in health status. The family may be concerned about the infant's chance of developing either the trait or the anemia. No means are available to detect these conditions in utero. If both parents have the trait, then in each pregnancy there is a 25 percent chance that the child will have anemia, a 50 percent chance that the child will have the trait, and a 25 percent chance that the child will not be affected.

The mother with sickle cell trait will have a healthy pregnancy with no anemia but may have _____.   pyelonephritis;
If both parents have the trait, the chance that the child will have

the trait is _____.   50 percent

Sickle cell anemia is a much more severe interruption in health, resulting in a sharply reduced life expectancy. It is estimated that around 50 percent of persons with sickle cell anemia will survive past the age of twenty and may live to about forty years of age. The fertility rate is decreased, and for the mother who does become pregnant there is a high incidence, around 50 percent, of abortion, stillbirth, and neonatal death. Other problems encountered are cardiac failure, infection, and pyelonephritis. Most women enter pregnancy with a hemoglobin of 8 grams per 100 milliliters, and pregnancy often lowers this level even further. These mothers then are more prone to crises of both the sequestration type, in which blood is suddenly sequestered in the spleen, and the painful crisis in which there is intravascular sickling. When sequestration crises develop, the mother is apt to go into cardiac failure. Prompt treatment with blood transfusions and oxygen is necessary.

When the painful crisis occurs, the intravascular sickling occludes the blood vessels and there are often infarcts in the kidney, spleen, brain, and bones. These painful crises are often precipitated by infection or dehydration, exposure to cold, or physical exercise. The treatment for the painful crisis is rest, fluids, analgesia, and sometimes the administration of oxygen. There are studies being conducted to determine whether the administration of red blood cells that do not contain hemoglobin S to the mother during pregnancy will reduce the incidence of crises and fetal problems. The preliminary outcomes seem encouraging.

Mothers with sickle cell anemia begin pregnancy with a hemoglobin level of about _____.

The treatment for sequestration crisis is _____

_____.

Painful crisis may be precipitated by _____,

_____, and

_____.

8 grams per 100 milliliters;

blood

transfusion and oxygen

infection;

exposure to cold;

physical exercise

During pregnancy, the mother with sickle cell anemia must have careful medical supervision. It is the nurse's responsibility to assist the family in recognizing the need for good nutrition and prenatal visits. Most of these women are also given folic acid supplements. It is a nursing responsibility to explain the necessity for this medication to the parents.

It is imperative that nurses do not assume that abdominal pain in a sickle cell mother is sickle cell crisis. There is a danger of late diagnosis of polynephritis, appendicitis, or ectopic pregnancy when such pain is not reported and steps are not taken for a definitive diagnosis.

It is a nursing responsibility to adequately supervise the mother during the pregnancy experience and to make the family aware of the need for genetic counseling. There is also a need for guidance and teaching in the area of conception control. The parents may also need information concerning sterilization techniques. Repeated pregnancies in a woman with sickle cell disease increase chronic problems. There is also research that supports the finding of a shortened life span for these women.

The *thalassemias* are a group of genetic disorders of the hemoglobin in which there is an interference with the production of the chains of globin (the polypeptide chains) so that a decreased amount of hemoglobin A is produced. In this country, those primarily affected are families from Italy and Greece, who have the thalassemia that affects the beta chain; whereas the form that affects the alpha chain is found in Southeast Asia and China. The altered hemoglobin has shown an increased resistance to malaria.

Thalassemia affects the production of the _____ _____ with the result that there is a decreased amount of _____.

globin
chains;
hemoglobin A

The person with homozygous thalassemia (beta), also called Cooley's anemia, has severe anemia that is treated with frequent transfusions. Life expectancy is rarely into the second decade, and no pregnancy has been reported in this group.

The heterozygous form (beta), called thalassemia minor or trait, produces a chronic anemia and the erythrocytes are hypochromic and microcytic. The mother enters pregnancy with a hemoglobin of 10 to 12 grams per 100 milliliters. There is some increased destruction of the erythrocytes, probably due to their mechanical fragility. Hemoglobin levels during pregnancy may range as low as 8 grams per 100 milliliters in the second trimester and increase to 9 grams per 100 milliliters in the third trimester. Iron therapy is not usually recommended, but folic acid supplements are a must. As in all anemia, it is important that the mother does not let any infection go untreated.

The mother who has thalassemia minor has _____ anemia. In pregnancy the hemoglobin level may drop to a low of _____.

The mother must take a supplement of _____ during pregnancy. Infection increases _____, and early treatment is necessary.

chronic;

8 grams per 100 milliliters;

folic acid;

the anemia

When there are combinations of the variant hemoglobins, the mother may have sickle thalassemia. The severity of the disorder varies from no symptoms to severe anemia. There are also some individuals who have hemoglobin C and hemoglobin S, and the problems encountered are similar to but not as severe as with hemoglobin S-S.

POST-TEST   Indicate whether each statement is true or false by circling the appropriate letter. Then turn to page 242 and see how well you have done.

1. Infection predisposes an individual to develop anemia.   T   F

2. Megaloblastic anemia is caused by an insufficient number of red blood cells.   T   F

3. Megaloblastic anemia is a fatal complication of pregnancy.   T   F

4. Sickling of the red blood cells produces intravascular occlusion.   T   F

5. Ectopic pregnancy is sometimes mistaken for sickle cell crisis.   T   F

6. Thalassemia is a genetically transmitted condition.   T   F

7. Females with thalassemia minor never get pregnant.   T   F

8. Genetic counseling is an important referral for nurses to make in cases of sickle cell anemia and thalassemia.   T   F

In the specific areas in which you had difficulty, return to the material and review.

BIBLIOGRAPHY   Barber, Janet, Lillian Stokes, and Diane Billings: *Adult and Child Care; A Client Approach to Nursing*, C. V. Mosby Co., St. Louis, Mo., 1977, p. 819.

Dickason, Elizabeth and Martha Schult: *Maternal and Infant Care, a Text for Nurses*, McGraw-Hill Book Co., New York, 1975, pp. 395–397.

McFarlane, Judith, "Sickle Cell Disorders," *American Journal of Nursing*, Vol. 77, No. 12, p. 1948, Dec. 1977.

Morrison, J. C. and S. A. Fish, "Sickle Cell Hemoglobinopathies and Pregnancy: Current Concepts," *Ob/Gyn Digest*, Jan. 1976.

————, W. D. Whybrew, E. T. Bercovag, and W. L. Wiser, "Fluctuations of Fetal Hemoglobin in Sickle Cell Anemia," *American Journal of Obstetrics and Gynecology*, Vol. 125, No. 8, pp. 1085–1088, Aug. 15, 1976.

Pritchard, Jack and Paul MacDonald: *Williams Obstetrics*, 15th. ed., Appleton-Century-Crofts, New York, 1976, pp. 602–607.

Romney, Seymore, et al.: *Gynecology and Obstetrics: The Health Care of Women*, McGraw-Hill Book Co., New York, 1975.

Scipien, Gladys, Martha Barnard, Marilyn Chard, Jeanne Howe, and Patricia Phillips: *Comprehensive Pediatric Nursing*, McGraw-Hill Book Co., New York, 1975, pp. 618–622.

Shafer, Kathleen, Janet Sawyer, Audrey McCluskey, Edna Beck, and Wilma Phipps: *Medical-Surgical Nursing*, C. V. Mosby Co., St. Louis, Mo., 1975, pp. 414–415.

**PRETEST
ANSWERS**
1. Low hemoglobin or erythrocytes   2. Hemorrhage   3. Megaloblastic   4. Nucleic acids   5. Genes   6. Oxygen   7. Painful crisis   8. Morbidity; mortality
9. Cooley's   10. Genetically; hemoglobin   11. Folic acid

**POST-TEST
ANSWERS**
1. T   2. F   3. F   4. T   5. T   6. T   7. F   8. T

UNIT IV EXAMINATION The following multiple-choice examination will test your comprehension of the material covered in the fourth unit of this program. Remember, you are not competing with anyone but yourself. Therefore, do not guess in order to answer the questions; if you are unsure, this means that you have not learned the content. Return to the areas that give you difficulty and review them before going on with the examination.

Circle the letter of the best response to each question. After completing the unit examination, check your answers on page 541 and review those areas of difficulty before proceeding to the next unit.

1. Physical alterations of pregnancy create often severe stressors for the diabetic mother. Some of these alterations are:
   a. The increased hormonal production of estrogen and progesterone
   b. The increased need for oxygen
   c. The frequency of urination
   d. Backache, due to the mobility of the joints

2. If the diabetic mother experiences nausea and vomiting, you would instruct her to:
   a. Increase her insulin dosage to deal with this stress
   b. Stop taking her insulin
   c. Take only clear fluids and remain on the same dosage of insulin
   d. Call the physician and inform him/her of the symptoms because of the danger of going into insulin shock

3. The diabetic mother may have discomfort with respirations, especially when she lies down, because of:
   a. The cardiac involvement during the last months
   b. The hydramnios that often is present
   c. The increased blood volume
   d. The decreased basal metabolic rate

4. The diabetic mother often is delivered earlier than the EDC because:
   a. The diabetes becomes very unstable at the end of pregnancy
   b. The insulin has adverse effects on the fetus
   c. The mother often has placenta previa
   d. There is a high incidence of fetal loss during the last weeks

5. The delivery of the baby when the mother is diabetic is often by cesarean section because:
   a. Vaginal delivery is too stressful for the mother because of the time it takes
   b. The mother's tolerance for pain is too low
   c. The baby is too large
   d. The baby will have fewer side effects from the insulin

6. After the delivery of the diabetic mother, the baby is watched carefully since often the baby develops:
   a. Hyperglycemia
   b. Hypoglycemia

    c.   Hypercalcemia

    d.   Anemia

7.   The baby of the diabetic mother is considered:

    a.   Premature

    b.   Postmature

    c.   Mature

    d.   Dysmature

8.   If one parent has diabetes, the chance of the offspring developing or inheriting the disorder is:

    a.   10 percent

    b.   20 percent

    c.   25 percent

    d.   50 percent

9.   Stressors during pregnancy for the cardiac mother are often a result of normal alterations. One of these stressors is:

    a.   A decrease in metabolic rate

    b.   An increase in the hematocrit

    c.   A decrease in oxygen consumption

    d.   An increase in blood volume

10.   During pregnancy the danger for the cardiac mother is:

    a.   Nausea and vomiting

    b.   Insomnia

    c.   Cardiac failure

    d.   Frequency

11.   The prognosis for the cardiac mother during pregnancy is dependent on:

    a.   The length of time she has had the cardiac problem

    b.   The kind of food she eats

    c.   The amount of common discomforts she experiences

    d.   The functional status of her heart

12.   You would prepare the family to watch for signs of cardiac embarrassment. Some of these are:

    a.   Cough that rattles and inability to do normal activity

    b.   Frequency of urination and lack of appetite

    c.   Hiccups and headache

    d.   Headaches and loss of weight

13.   The fetal life is threatened should the mother develop:

    a.   Hypotension

    b.   Nausea and vomiting

    c.   Hyperorexia

    d.   Increased cardiac output

14.   During labor the mother who is a cardiac will:

    a.   Have no problems and be treated as normal

    b.   Be kept in a semi-Fowler's position and be monitored carefully

    c.   Be kept in a recumbent position and be given an epidural

    d.   Have a problem only if she has not eaten within the last six hours

15.   During the delivery of the cardiac mother:
    a.   She is given general anesthesia to reduce the discomfort
    b.   She participates by pushing during the second stage
    c.   She is given general anesthesia because forceps are used
    d.   She is given local anesthesia, and forceps are used to shorten the second stage

16.   It is important to watch the cardiac mother during the postpartum period because:
    a.   She may develop urinary frequency
    b.   The fluid shift rapidly increases the circulating volume
    c.   She often becomes depressed
    d.   She may experience signs of nausea and vomiting

17.   Monozygotic twins are:
    a.   Those twins who arise from two ova and have different characteristics
    b.   Those twins who arise from one ovum and have different characteristics
    c.   Those twins who arise from two ova and have the same characteristics
    d.   Those twins who arise from one ovum and have the same characteristics

18.   During pregnancy a mother with twins often will experience:
    a.   Increased energy levels due to her high hemoglobin
    b.   Increased difficulty in breathing due to size near term
    c.   Decreased difficulty in breathing since both drop sooner
    d.   Decreased blood pressure, making her tired

19.   At the delivery of the twins, the most difficulty arises:
    a.   With the delivery of the first twin
    b.   With the delivery of the second twin
    c   With the delivery of the first placenta
    d.   With the delivery of the second placenta

20.   A mother who is considered a mild preeclamptic will have:
    a.   Edema of the hands and feet
    b.   A blood pressure of 165/95
    c.   3+ proteinuria
    d.   A blood pressure of 134/84

21.   The mother has eclampsia when:
    a.   The blood pressure is 180/110
    b.   She convulses
    c.   She has 4+ proteinuria
    d.   She has generalized edema

22.   The aim of the treatment for the mother who has severe preeclampsia is to:
    a.   Stabilize her vital signs

    b.   Reduce the number and severity of her headaches

    c.   Increase her urinary output

    d.   Prevent convulsion and deliver a viable baby

23.   Magnesium sulphate is one of the drugs ordered for the mother. This medication:

    a.   Effectively increases the circulation through the placenta

    b.   Induces the contractions of labor

    c.   Reduces the activity at the neuromuscular junctions

    d.   Increases the blood pressure through vasoconstriction

24.   The occurrence of which of the following would be the *first* indication of the need to administer the antagonist of magnesium sulphate?

    a.   Tetanic contractions

    b.   Convulsions

    c.   Absent knee jerk reflex

    d.   Depressed respirations

25.   A vaginal examination is contraindicated in a mother who is bleeding during the last trimester. This is because:

    a.   The examination may dislodge a low-lying placenta, causing hemorrhage

    b.   The examination is painful and will stimulate labor

    c.   There is a danger of infection being introduced

    d.   The membranes may rupture prematurely

26.   When abruptio placenta occurs, you would observe which of the following signs?

    a.   A soft, boggy uterus

    b.   A hard, boardlike uterus

    c.   A distended bladder and hypertension

    d.   Mild contractions lasting only 30 seconds

27.   Associated often with abruptio placenta is which of the following conditions?

    a.   Thrombosis

    b.   Increased urinary output

    c.   Hypofibrinogenemia

    d.   Convulsions

28.   The mother in her thirty-second week of pregnancy suddenly develops vaginal bleeding. She appears to be in no discomfort when the uterus is palpated, and her tentative diagnosis is placenta previa. The mother is admitted and observed for changes in her status, which has stabilized, and the bleeding has stopped. Delivery should be scheduled:

    a.   Immediately, before any changes occur

    b.   Only if the mother should hemorrhage again; then an emergency cesarean section will be performed

    c.   In a day or two

    d.   Following labor, which will be induced within a week

29. If the mother has abruptio placenta, the major sign she will exhibit is:
    a. Painful bleeding
    b. Painless bleeding
    c. Hypertension
    d. Nausea and vomiting

UNIT V

INTERRUPTIONS IN HEALTH IN THE INTRAPARTUM PERIOD

Chapter 8
Operative Obstetrics

Chapter 9
Uterine Rupture and Amniotic Fluid Embolism

Chapter 10
Resuscitation of the Neonate

Chapter 11
Early Postpartum Hemorrhage

INTRODUCTION   At times conditions may emerge which seriously threaten the life of the mother and the viability of the fetus by interrupting the normal processes or mechanisms of labor. Serious taxing of adaptive mechanisms and constant draining of maternal energy reserves give rise to crisis situations requiring adept and immediate intervention measures to ensure prevention of death and to support restorative processes.

The processes and mechanisms of labor may be complicated or interrupted by any number of situations: membranes may rupture prematurely, labor may begin prematurely, there may be dysfunction or inertia of the uterine muscles, or a fetal part other than a vertex may be presenting. In the following chapters we will discuss the major and most common situations leading to interruptions in the progression of labor and affecting the lives of both the mother and the baby.

Throughout pregnancy the parents have focused on how they would handle the stress of labor, pain being their primary concern. They usually have strengthened their adaptive resources by either becoming informed, learning techniques of active participation, or eliciting promises of sedation from their physicians. When, as in the case of an unexpectedly difficult or painful labor, the parents are called upon to utilize further adaptive mechanisms, the stressor may be more than they can handle alone.

The nurse must identify the meaning of this occurrence to them. Are they afraid of a dire outcome to the mother or baby? Or is it the unexpectedness that creates the crisis? Are they the kind of parents who expect to be told in detail everything that is occurring and will occur, or would they rather have a cursory explanation of what is occurring and details about the condition of the mother and baby? Who is in the supportive role? What strengths can the nurse draw upon in this family unit to help with their adaptive mechanisms? The nurse must call upon the skills of observation, assessment, and communication so that intervention is meaningful in this situation to this family.

CHAPTER ONE
FETAL DISTRESS

OBJECTIVES   *Identify signs of intrauterine fetal distress.*

Differentiate between patterns of deceleration in fetal heart rate.

GLOSSARY   *Fetal bradycardia:* A fetal heart rate of under 120 beats per minute
Fetal tachycardia: A fetal heart rate of over 160 beats per minute

PRETEST   In the spaces provided, fill in the word or words that best complete(s) the statements. Then turn to page 258 and check your answers.

1. A type I dip, or early deceleration, that occurs simultaneously with the onset of a contraction is considered _____.

2. If a type II dip, or late deceleration occurs more than once consecutively, it is an indication of possible _____.

3. Fetal tachycardia is defined as _____ _____.

4. Fetal bradycardia is defined as _____ _____.

5. Meconium-stained amniotic fluid in a vertex presentation may indicate _____.

Labor is a stressor that the fetus normally adapts to readily; yet there are certain instances in which a fetus becomes compromised during this process. A number of maternal interruptions in health put the infant at risk during labor; included are diabetes, hypertension, sickle cell anemia, and bleeding. Certain fetal problems make the labor process more hazardous; these include hemolytic incompatibilities, postmaturity, and growth retardation. Most of the above conditions may be assessed before the labor process begins so that the staff will be prepared if difficulties should arise.

Maternal conditions that may put the infant at risk during labor include _____ , _____ , _____ and _____ .

diabetes; hypertension, sickle cell anemia; bleeding

Fetal problems that occur in utero, making labor a more difficult process, include _____ , _____ , and _____ .

hemolytic incompatibilities; postmaturity; growth retardation

During the actual labor process there are other types of stress that may arise, for example, if labor is induced using drugs such as oxytocin or prostaglandins or if the mother is given medications—either analgesics or anesthetics—to relieve the discomfort.

The *maternal position* in itself may create difficulties for the fetus; for example, if the mother becomes hypotensive due to the pressure of the gravid uterus on the inferior vena cava, blood flow to the fetus is decreased. This means that the mother should never be in a supine position during labor. At other times the mother's position may be such that the pressure of the fetus is on top of the cord, causing cord compression, and the mother should be instructed to change her position.

Difficulties during labor may be created for the fetus if medications are given to _____ or _____ .

induce labor; relieve discomfort

Maternal position in labor may create _____ or _____ .

hypotension; cord compression

It is essential that the fetus be monitored closely throughout labor and delivery to determine its status and response to the labor process. Symptoms of fetal distress indicate that the fetus is compromised and is having difficulty. Clinical monitoring with the fetascope will enable the nurse to identify patterns of distress by close observation. Often during labor the mother and the fetus will have electronic monitoring

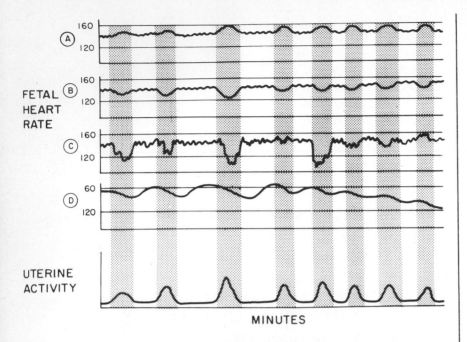

Patterns of fetal heart change associated with uterine contractions. *A* acceleration, *B* early deceleration, *C* variable deceleration, *D* late deceleration. (*From Gynecology and Obstetrics: The Health Care of Women by S. Romney et al. Copyright © McGraw-Hill Book Company 1975. Used with the permission of McGraw-Hill Book Company.*)

recording the contractions and the fetal heart rate, and the nurse will identify patterns of distress from the graph.

Most instances of fetal distress occur because there is an interference in maternal-fetal circulation resulting in a degree of fetal anoxia. The fetus attempts to compensate for this anoxia usually by initial rise in the heart rate. If this attempt is unsuccessful then the heart rate decreases and often acidosis sets in. It is important to ascertain the pattern of the fetal heart rate in relation to the contractions, since this pattern often indicates what type of difficulty is occurring. Dr. Caldeyro-Barcia has identified patterns of fetal heart slowing or deceleration. The three decelerations are termed *early deceleration*, or "type I dip"; *late deceleration*, or "type II dip"; and *variable deceleration*, or "type III dip." The early-deceleration pattern occurs when the fetal heart rate begins to drop at the onset of the contraction and the rate recovers as the contraction ends. This pattern is thought to occur when there is compression of the fetal head and, unless extreme, seems to be well tolerated by the fetus; however, it is important to have the mother examined to rule out a prolapse of the cord. If the decelerations are severe and meconium is present, the delivery should be effected as soon as possible.

Late decelerations are a slowing of the fetal heart rate that begins with the acme and in which the recovery period extends past the end of the contraction. These decelerations are an indication of serious difficulty in the uteroplacental circulation due to insufficiency. If labor is being induced, the drug is stopped immediately and the pattern observed. Many physicians feel that if there are three consecutive late decelerations, fetal blood sampling should be done to determine the degree of fetal anoxia and the delivery should be effected quickly. The mother should be positioned on her left side to enhance circulation to the uterus, and she is given oxygen by mask to increase the amount the fetus is receiving.

Variable decelerations occur when there is a slowing of the heart rate that does not correspond to any phase of the contractions. These decelerations are thought to be the result of cord compression. A vaginal examination is done to assess whether there is a prolapsed cord. The mother's position should be changed and oxygen administered. If the decelerations continue, then delivery should be done as quickly as possible. Studies have indicated that often if there is no prolapse, the cord may be wrapped around the neck of the fetus or may be very short.

Close observations of the fetal heart rate are necessary in order to _____.

> determine the fetal status;

If head compression is occurring, there will be a pattern of _____ Indicated by
_____
_____
_____.

> early decelerations;
> a dropping of the fetal heart rate at the onset of the contraction

If there is insufficient circulation through the placenta, then a pattern of _____ is seen. The heart rate changes by dropping _____
_____.

> late decelerations;
> with the acme
> of the contraction

If the umbilical cord is wrapped around the fetus's neck, then you may see a pattern of _____.
These decreases in the heart rate occur _____
_____.

> variable decelerations;
> independently
> of the phase of the contraction

Fetal blood sampling is done by assessing the pH of the capillaries of the fetal scalp. Normally the pH is lower in the capillaries than in the arterial blood. The critical level that suggests fetal acidosis and probable depression of the neonate has been determined to be a pH of 7.2 or lower. Fetal blood sampling is done after the cervix has dilated enough to make visualization of the fetal scalp possible and the membranes have ruptured. An endoscope is used, and then a small incision is made and the blood is drawn up into a capillary tube that has been heparinized. Problems occurring from this procedure include bleeding from the scalp and infection. Oxygen and carbon dioxide pressures may be assessed, but the pH seems more reliable in determining fetal status.

The perinatal mortality rate has decreased, and many observers feel this result is due to close observation during labor and quick intervention to relieve fetal distress. Although some institutions may find that their primary cesarean section rate is increased, many institutions find that with electronic monitoring, a more accurate assessment of fetal status is possible and fewer cesarean sections are performed.

Other indications of fetal distress are *fetal tachycardia*, which is a fetal heart rate of over 160 beats per minute or a rise in rate of 20 to 30 beats per minute over the basal rate; and *fetal bradycardia*, which is a fetal heart rate of under 120 beats per minute or a persistent slowing.

Tachycardia is the _____ of the fetal heart rate to over _____ beats per minute or an increase of 20 to 30 beats over the _____.

increase;

160;

basal rate

Another nursing observation that might be indicative of fetal distress is the presence of *meconium in the amniotic fluid* when there is a vertex presentation.

When the amniotic fluid is greenish instead of the normal _____ color, it is thought that anoxia, which increases intestinal peristalsis, has caused the fetus to expel the contents of the bowel.

clear

When the fetus is in a vertex presentation and meconium is present in the amniotic fluid, this often is an indication of _____ _____.

fetal

distress

POST-TEST Indicate whether each statement is true or false by circling the appropriate letter. Then turn to page 258 and see how well you have done.

1. Anoxia is a common cause of fetal distress.   T   F

2. A type I dip is more serious for the fetus than a type II dip is.   T   F

3. When a fetal heart rate is monitored when distress is suspected, it should be counted from the onset of a contraction until two minutes after the contraction is over.   T   F

4. A pH of 7.0 from a fetal scalp capillary is considered normal.   T   F

5. Fetal bradycardia means that the fetal heart rate has slowed to 140 beats per minute.   T   F

6. In a vertex presentation, meconium in the amniotic fluid is an indication of fetal distress.   T   F

In the specific areas with which you had difficulty, return to the material and review.

BIBLIOGRAPHY   Hodnett, Ellen, "Fetal Monitoring," *Canadian Nurse*, Vol. 73, No. 3, pp. 44–47, March 1977.

Langhorne, Florence, "The Fetal Monitor: A Friend or Foe?" *Maternal Child Nursing*, Vol. 1, No. 5, pp. 313–314, Sept.–Oct. 1976.

Pritchard, Jack and Paul MacDonald: *Williams Obstetrics*, 15th ed., Appleton-Century-Crofts, New York, 1976.

Tejani, Nergesh A., "The Association of Umbilical Cord Complications and Variable Decelerations with Acid-Base Findings," *Obstetrics and Gynecology*, Vol. 49, No. 2, pp. 159–162, Feb. 1977.

PRETEST ANSWERS   1. Normal   2. Fetal distress   3. A fetal heart rate of over 160 beats per minute   4. A fetal heart rate of under 120 beats per minute   5. Fetal distress

POST-TEST ANSWERS   1. T   2. F   3. T   4. F   5. F   6. T

CHAPTER TWO

PROLAPSE OF THE UMBILICAL CORD

OBJECTIVES   *Define prolapse of the cord.*

Differentiate between apparent and hidden prolapse of the umbilical cord.

Identify three factors that predispose to prolapse of the cord.

Identify nursing intervention when prolapse of the cord complicates the intrapartum period.

GLOSSARY   *Prolapse of the umbilical cord:* Situation in which the umbilical cord is in front of the fetal presenting part after the rupture of membranes

Amniotomy: Rupture of the amniotic sac; usually used in reference to artificial rupture

Knee-chest position: Prone position with the mother resting on her flexed knees and elbows

PRETEST In the spaces provided, fill in the word or words that best complete(s) the statements. Then turn to page 265 and check your answers.

1. Prolapse of the umbilical cord means _____

    _____

    _____

    _____.

2. Prolapse of the cord can be either _____ or _____.

3. Four factors that predispose to prolapse of the cord are _____

    _____, _____, _____, and

    _____.

4. Prolapse of the cord is most dangerous to the _____ since it

    produces _____ and ultimately _____.

5. The first action of the nurse when identifying a prolapse of the cord is to

    _____

    _____.

6. She should then notify the _____ and keep the parents

    _____.

We have thoroughly discussed the observations and nursing intervention pertinent to the care of the mother and fetus during parturition. You are well aware of the necessity for continuous monitoring of the fetal heart rate, uterine contractions, maternal vital signs, and observations of amniotic fluid after amniotomy. Our objectives are, as always, the delivery of a healthy baby to a healthy mother. It therefore is essential that you become familiar with some of the other high-risk situations that can occur during labor and/or delivery and clarify the nursing observations and role in these critical situations.

We have mentioned the necessity for counting the fetal heart rate after procedures such as enema, vaginal examination, and amniotomy. The reason for this is to determine if any signs of *fetal distress* are occurring. The most frequent cause of intrauterine fetal problems at this time is *prolapse of the umbilical cord*.

Prolapse of the umbilical cord occurs following the rupture of the membranes when the umbilical cord falls below the presenting part so that it is between the presenting part and the cervical canal. There is compression of the cord because it is before the presenting part, and each time there is a contraction or as the presenting part moves down into the cervical canal, the degree of compression is increased.

Prolapse of the umbilical cord presents a threat to the life of the fetus because cord compression lasting for any period of time will stop most of the transfer of oxygen between the placenta and the baby. The mother also is suddenly in a high-risk situation, the baby may be lost, and the only possible treatment is major surgery—a cesarean section. Several factors may be the causes of cord prolapse. It may follow when the membranes have prematurely ruptured, when they rupture after an enema is administered, or after a vaginal examination. In short, any condition that may have produced a change in the position of the fetus or which may have served to disturb the integrity of the membranes may lead to prolapse of the cord.

This complication occurs most frequently in breech presentations since the breech does not always fill the pelvis. Similarly, it is found if there are multiple pregnancies or prematurity or if the presenting part is above the ischial spines. That is to say the presenting part is not yet _____.

engaged

Essential at this time is to assess the fetal status by monitoring the fetal heart rate to determine if there is any distress.

When the cord has prolapsed, it sometimes is visible at the vaginal orifice; the situation then is known as an "apparent prolapse." However, should the cord not be visible although prolapsed, the situation

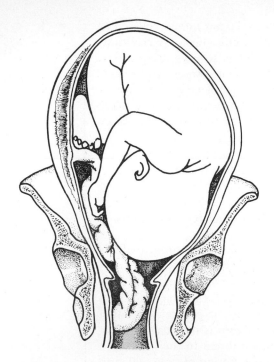

Prolapsed cord.

is termed a "hidden prolapse." Therefore, after rupture of membranes, if the fetal heart rate slows and remains slow, a careful vaginal examination should be performed to see whether or not the cord has prolapsed unseen.

A prolapse of the umbilical cord is most dangerous to the _____, because fetal _____ can occur as a result.

fetus; anoxia (death)

Prolapse of the cord means that, after rupture of membranes, the cord falls before the fetal _____.

presenting part

If a mother with a known multiple pregnancy or breech presentation spontaneously ruptures membranes, the nurse would check the fetal heart rate and observe the perineum for signs of _____.

prolapse

Prolapse of the cord also occurs more frequently in mothers when the presenting part is not yet _____.

engaged

After rupture of membranes, if the fetal heart sustains a slow or irregular rhythm, the mother should be examined to see if there is a _____.

hidden prolapse

⬇

If you are with a mother when prolapse of the cord occurs, it is essential that you slowly change her position to Trendelenberg or knee-chest in order to reverse gravity and, hopefully, remove the pressure of the fetus' presenting part from the cord. This condition does not cause the mother any pain, and she must be carefully told what you are doing and why. It is very difficult for a mother in active labor to be asked to maintain a knee-chest or Trendelenberg position without her complete understanding and cooperation.

You should not leave this mother alone. You should notify the doctor and send for him or her by calling for help with the patient bell. Oxygen is administered to the mother, and the fetal heart rate is monitored continuously.

The infant should be delivered as quickly as possible, usually by cesarean section. The nurse must never attempt to replace the cord in the vagina because additional compression may occur. The nurse should cover the exposed cord with sterile dressings saturated in normal saline solution so that the cord will not dry out.

The nurse should keep the parents informed of what is happening and, when possible, allow them to hear the fetal heartbeat. This crisis— suddenly realizing that they may lose their child—is terrifying for them. They need all the support and understanding that the staff can give.

The following procedures are done quickly: start of intravenous fluids, type and crossmatch of blood, abdominal skin prep, insertion of a Foley catheter, and preparation for the operative procedure. The staff must communicate control of the situation and reassurance to the parents. Should the fetus die, both parents should be told together if possible, for it is at this time that they need the support of one another to cope with this loss.

This also is a difficult time for you, the nurse, who must recognize your feelings and deal with them in order to be effective in support of the parents. You must be sure that you are not losing yourself in nursing tasks as a means of not dealing with your feelings and the needs of the parents.

Should you observe a prolapsed cord at the vaginal orifice, your first action would be to change _____.

It would be changed to _____ or _____ position in order to take _____ off the cord.

The staff can assuage the parents' anxiety somewhat by _____ them about what is happening and by telling them about the _____ of the fetus.

Prolapse of the cord is treated by _____ of the fetus, usually by _____.

	the mother's position
	Trendelenberg; knee-chest;
	pressure
	informing;
	condition
	delivery;
	cesarean section

POST-TEST   Indicate whether each statement is true or false by circling the appropriate letter. Then turn to page 265 and see how well you have done.

1. Prolapse of the umbilical cord causes the mother severe lower abdominal pain.   T   F

2. Prolapse of the umbilical cord always occurs when the membranes rupture and the presenting part is not engaged.   T   F

3. Upon observing prolapse of the umbilical cord, the nurse will put the mother in the Trendelenberg or knee-chest position.   T   F

4. The nurse will refrain from replacing a prolapsed cord in the vagina.   T   F

In the specific areas with which you had difficulty, return to the material and review.

BIBLIOGRAPHY Pritchard, Jack and Paul MacDonald: *Williams Obstetrics*, 15th ed., Appleton-Century-Crofts, New York, 1976.

Romney, Seymour, et al.: *Gynecology and Obstetrics: The Health Care of Women*, McGraw-Hill Book Co., New York, 1975.

Tejani, Nergesh A., "The Association of Umbilical Cord Complications and Variable Decelerations with Acid-Base Findings," *Obstetrics and Gynecology*, Vol. 49, No. 2, pp. 159–162, Feb. 1977.

PRETEST ANSWERS
1. That the umbilical cord is in front of the fetal presenting part after the membranes have ruptured
2. Apparent; hidden   3. Breech presentation; multiparity; prematurity; high station
4. Fetus; anoxia; fetal death   5. Change the mother's position to Trendelenberg or knee-chest
6. Doctor; informed

POST-TEST ANSWERS
1. F   2. F   3. T   4. T

CHAPTER THREE
PREMATURE LABOR

OBJECTIVES   *Define premature labor.*

Identify the risk of premature labor to the mother and to the neonate.

Identify a method of arresting premature labor.

Identify the nursing intervention during premature labor.

GLOSSARY   *Premature labor:* Labor that begins prior to the thirty-sixth week and after the twenty-sixth week of gestation

Perinatal mortality: The rate of death of fetuses and neonates between the twentieth week of gestation and the twenty-eighth day of life compared with 1,000 live births

Perinatal morbidity: Any medical complication occurring during the perinatal period, from the twentieth week of gestation to the twenty-eighth day of life

PRETEST In the spaces provided, fill in the word or words that best complete(s) the statements. Then turn to page 276 and check your answers.

1. Premature labor is labor that begins between the _____ _____ and the _____ week of gestation.

2. Some of the factors that predispose to premature labor are _____ _____ , _____ _____ , _____ _____ , _____ , _____ _____ , _____ , _____ , _____ _____ , or _____ .

3. During premature labor, sedation is _____ .

4. One assesses the fetal status during premature labor by monitoring the fetal heart rate _____ _____ .

Under normal circumstances, the processes of labor generally begin between the thirty-eighth and forty-second weeks of gestation. Labor processes that begin between the *twenty-sixth and thirty-sixth weeks of gestation* are classified as *premature*, and these account for about 50 percent of perinatal mortality since premature onset of labor presents a high-risk situation for the infant.

In the majority of cases, no specific causative factor for the onset of a premature labor can be identified. However, previous interruptions in health or nonhealth states affecting the mother before or throughout the pregnancy are thought to initiate a premature labor. As examples of such nonhealth states we may cite chronic hypertensive vascular disease, acute urinary tract infections, toxemia, abruptio placenta, and/or congenital anomalies. Recent research has shown that smoking during the pregnancy may result not only in lower birth weight in infants but also in prematurity. It also has been noted in recent years that women who are addicted to drugs have a premature labor more often than nonaddicted women do. Other known causes include poor socio-economic conditions, since social factors often influence whether or not the mother receives antepartal care. Finally, it is important to note that about 30 percent of premature labor follows premature rupture of the membranes.

Premature labor creates a crisis situation for the parents. Their thoughts about the many complications and serious problems attributed to prematurity often create a very frightening situation. Often the mother has wished that the pregnancy were over, and now this really may be happening; but the parents' concern then focuses on the welfare of the baby. The parents attempt to determine what action of theirs caused this premature labor, and they may experience guilt feelings that they were responsible for this crisis. It is important to help the parents ventilate their feelings and to provide information so that they are better able to deal with this situation and later will form a positive relationship with the baby. If there is no medical problem that is operating as a stressor, it is helpful for the parents to know that in most instances the cause of premature labor is unknown.

The early onset of labor is one of the leading causes of perinatal mortality and morbidity. The premature infant has a higher incidence of neurological problems and respiratory distress syndrome than a full-term infant has.

Labor that begins after the twenty-sixth week of gestation and before the thirty-sixth week is called _____.

    premature

Some of the known causes of premature labor are placental conditions such as _____, vas-

    abruptio placenta;

cular problems such as _____, maternal conditions

    hypertension;

such as _____, and abuses such as _____

and _____.

    The most pressing concern of the parents is fear for the safety of

_____.

    They also often experience feelings of _____.

toxemia; smoking;

drug addiction

the baby

guilt

    The care and management of the mother begins with an assessment of her status and that of the fetus. If there are indications that the fetus has growth retardation or will be under more stress in utero than once delivered, because of maternal interruptions in health, then the approach is supportive of the labor process and no attempt is made to arrest labor. Often if the gestational dates are not known and there is growth retardation, the situation is confused with premature labor when it is actually term labor. If the mother is examined and is found to have her membranes intact, the cervix is not dilated, and there is no identifiable problem, then an attempt is made to arrest the progress of the premature labor because of the problems of prematurity for the infant. Labor is arrested to gain time for the fetus in utero to attain maturity so that, once born, the adjustment to extrauterine life will be accomplished with ease.

    Some studies have found that bed rest and, possibly, light sedation that would not compromise the infant are effective in stopping premature labor. Previously alcohol was used in an attempt to inhibit the release of oxytocin and stop contractions, but recent studies have indicated that the fetus suffers from the alcohol infusion and may develop adverse symptoms.

    Currently there is an investigation of a drug, terbutaline, which affects the beta receptors of the uterus and inhibits premature labor. The side effects of the medication include an increase in both the maternal and the fetal heart rate. The medication is given intravenously for eight hours and then injected subcutaneously four times a day for three days. The investigators feel that the drug is well tolerated. Other beta receptor drugs, ritodrine and salbutamol, have side effects of tachycardia, nausea and vomiting, dyspnea, and apprehension that are lessened to a degree if the mother is in a lateral recumbent position. The effectiveness of these medications is yet to be determined. Drugs that inhibit prostaglandin synthetase activity seem to halt labor as long as the labor is not in the active phase.

    Attempts to inhibit premature labor may be instituted when

_____

_____ and upon examination it is determined that

there are no fetal or maternal

problems;

_____

_____.

    The medication terbutaline has side effects that are _____

_____.

⟱

there is no cervical dilation

and the membranes are intact

maternal

and fetal tachycardia

    It is to be remembered that any complication during pregnancy requires that the family be given continued support and reassurance. Such is the case when the mother goes into premature labor and delivery.

    Since a premature delivery is likely to produce a high-risk neonate, it is important that the baby's health status be continuously assessed through frequent monitoring of the fetal heart rate. Administration of sedatives and narcotics to the mother at this time is contraindicated since the fetus usually is small and its physiological systems are immature; thus any agent that will produce a physiological depression will produce a serious complication.

    During the second stage of labor, local or regional anesthesia methods such as epidural, caudal, or spinal may be used to decrease the stresses of delivery for the mother. Application of forceps to assist in the delivery also is contraindicated since there is a possibility that the fetal head may be compressed. An episiotomy is done to allow enough room for the baby's head to be delivered, to prevent pressure from the perineal floor on the head and to avoid injury to the baby.

    The cord should be clamped before it stops pulsating so that the blood volume of the baby is decreased and the immature liver is prevented from being forced to try to handle the extra bilirubin level.

    The parents should be kept well informed of the condition and progress of the fetus. Constant monitoring or frequent checks of the fetal heart rate are routine. The mother should be given support and help with breathing and relaxation techniques since analgesia is

_____.

contraindicated

    Susan Lindstrom, a twenty-year-old primigravida, is admitted to labor and delivery. She is 36 weeks gestation according to dates and estimated size of infant. She has a history of contractions beginning five hours before admission and a small amount of fluid leaking. When you check her chart, you find that Susan is having contractions every three to five minutes, the presentation is vertex, station -1, and the membranes have ruptured. The cervix is 4 centimeters dilated. The fetal heart rate is 144 and regular.

When you enter the room you find Susan fighting the contractions; she tenses up and becomes very restless. Bob, the father, has just arrived from work, and he appears to be very worried and lost. Your interaction with this family which would be most helpful in providing reassurance is:

A. Informing them that since Susan seems so uncomfortable with the contractions, you will talk with the doctor and ask him to write an order for a pain-killing medication that should help Susan to relax.

Go to page 272.

B. Informing the couple that since Susan is in very early labor, it may be possible with the use of intravenous medication to stop the process and then when labor starts again the baby will be older and not have so many problems of prematurity.

Go to page 273.

C. Informing the parents that you are going to be with them; determining if Susan is experiencing discomfort in her back and, if so, having Bob apply pressure while explaining what is happening; and allowing them both to hear the fetal heart rate.

Go to page 274.

Your selection of *A* indicates that you have *not* understood one of the primary rules during premature labor: that is that the mother does not receive analgesia during labor because of the extreme susceptibility of the premature infant.

Return to page 269. Review the material and choose another response from page 271.

In your choice of *B* you have not assessed the current situation accurately and you need to integrate this with criteria for the administration of medication to the mother.

Return to page 269. Review the material and choose another response from page 271.

Excellent. Your selection of *C* indicates that you have integrated the material and identified the status of the mother as well as the best way of providing support. You are helping the couple to relax, ask questions, and know that the baby's heart rate is good.

Advance to page 275 and take the post-test.

POST-TEST   Indicate whether each statement is true or false by circling the appropriate letter. Then turn to page 276 and see how well you have done.

1. A labor that begins anytime after the thirty-sixth week of gestation is termed "premature labor."   T   F

2. Women who are drug abusers are more apt to have a premature labor than nonusers are.   T   F

3. Premature labor is a leading cause of perinatal morbidity and mortality.   T   F

4. Since women in premature labor become very anxious and fearful, it is advisable for sedatives to be administered.   T   F

5. Regional anesthesia is the anesthesia of choice when delivery is imminent in a premature labor.   T   F

In the specific areas with which you had difficulty, return to the material and review.

BIBLIOGRAPHY Hauth, John C., et al., "Early Labor Initiation with Oral PGE$_2$ After Premature Rupture of the Membranes at Term," *Obstetrics and Gynecology*, Vol. 49, No. 5, pp. 524–526, May 1977.

Ingemarsson, Ingemar, "Effect of Terbutaline on Premature Labor," *American Journal of Obstetrics and Gynecology*, Vol. 125, No. 4, June 15, 1976.

Pritchard, Jack and Paul MacDonald: *Williams Obstetrics*, 15th ed., Appleton-Century-Crofts, New York, 1976.

PRETEST ANSWERS 1. Twenty-sixth; thirty-sixth   2. Any of the following: acute urinary tract infections; chronic hypertensive disease; toxemia; incompetent cervical os; multiple pregnancy; poor maternal nutrition; drug addiction; congenital abnormalities   3. Minimal   4. More frequently than is done in normal labor

POST-TEST ANSWERS 1. F   2. T   3. T   4. F   5. T

CHAPTER FOUR

PREMATURE RUPTURE OF MEMBRANES

OBJECTIVES *Identify the characteristics of premature rupture of membranes.*

Identify the significance of premature rupture of membranes.

Identify the nursing intervention with the mother who has prematurely ruptured membranes.

GLOSSARY *Amnionitis:* An inflammation of the amnion, usually due to an intrauterine infection following premature rupture of membranes

Premature rupture of membranes: A break or tear in the amnion and chorion prior to the onset of true labor

PRETEST   In the spaces provided, fill in the word or words that best complete(s) the statements. Then turn to page 283 and check your answers.

1. Premature rupture of membranes occurs _____

   _____ .

2. Premature rupture of membranes causes more risk to the fetus than to the mother since it is one of the most frequent causes of

   _____ .

3. Some factors contributing to premature rupture of membranes are

   _____ , _____ ,

   _____ , _____

   _____ , and _____ .

4. The maternal complication following premature rupture of membranes is

   _____ .

Premature rupture of membranes, or rupture of membranes before the onset of true labor, is one of the leading causes of prematurity. Since this is so, if premature rupture of membranes occurs before the thirty-sixth week, a crisis situation is produced for the fetus. The membranes may rupture at term before the uterine contractions begin. The rupture may be *complete*, that is, the amnion and chorion completely rupture, allowing all of the amniotic fluid to escape through the vagina, or *partial*, that is, there may be a small leak or tear in the amnion through which a small portion of amniotic fluid is lost through the vagina.

Studies of prematurely ruptured membranes indicate that near the rupture the membrane is thinner and less elastic. Also there is much controversy about the possibility of enhanced fetal lung maturity because cortisol is released by the mother due to stress when there is rupture of membranes before the thirty-sixth or thirty-seventh week. Some investigators found that there is a decreased incidence of respiratory distress syndrome in premature labor when the membranes rupture prematurely. They attribute this reduction to the cortisol levels. Other researchers do not find any significant decrease in respiratory distress rates.

If a mother calls the obstetrician or clinic to report that clear fluid is escaping from her vagina, and questioning reveals that she is having no contractions, the nurse might suspect that the mother has _____ _____.

premature rupture of membranes

The rupture may be either _____ or _____.

complete; partial

Once the membranes are ruptured, the danger of infection is great for both the mother and the fetus in utero. If the rupture occurs very early, around the thirtieth week of pregnancy, then the mother is usually observed for signs of labor and sepsis and remains in bed. It is hoped that the leak will seal off and the fetus will gain more time in utero. If the rupture occurs later in pregnancy, then the danger of infection and the possible morbidity and mortality problems due to infection of the neonate and the mother mandate that delivery should be effected within 24 hours or less. Unless the mother goes into labor spontaneously within three hours following the rupture, chances are that the delay will be longer than desired. Thus labor is established by the use of oxytocin or prostaglandin E_2, providing that vaginal delivery is possible; otherwise a cesarean section is performed. Some institutions automatically start the mother on antibiotics whether or not she has a temperature elevation, although the medication does not cross the placenta to prevent infection in the infant. The infant is often placed in the suspect

nursery following delivery and may or may not be treated with prophylactic antibiotic therapy.

Problems for both the mother and the fetus once the membranes
rupture include _____ and _____   maternal; fetal
_____. If premature rupture of the membranes occurs very   infection;
early, around the thirtieth week, the regime is _____   bed rest;
and _____   observation of labor or
_____.   sepsis

At term if the membranes have ruptured but no contractions have
started, the choice of action is _____   to initiate labor;
if _____.   a vaginal delivery is possible;

If the mother's temperature rises during labor, she will receive
_____. The infant is observed closely for signs of   antibiotics;
_____.   infection

When a mother is admitted early to the hospital for premature
rupture of membranes, the entire family unit is disrupted. In addition
to the fears for the child who may be born too soon is the fear for the
life of the mother, since pregnancy is not usually associated with hospitalization for anything other than the normal birth of the baby. Obviously, this unforeseen complication introduces additional stressors;
for example, there may be financial difficulty meeting an unexpected
hospital bill, difficulty in getting someone to care for other children at
home, or psychological unpreparedness for separation from the family
unit and fear of the results of this complication.

Old wives' tales may serve to complicate the picture further. It
is felt by many lay people that a more difficult labor results from the
premature loss of amniotic fluid. They speak of a "dry-birth" and feel
that friction in the birth passage is increased, causing increased pain
and difficulty. It must be carefully explained that some additional amniotic fluid is produced and there are other bodily secretions from the
lining of the birth canal which facilitate delivery.

The nurse also must support the family unit by identifying its
strengths and utilizing them to help the family adapt to the introduction
of the new stressor.

In addition to providing and communicating pertinent information,
the nurse will need to recognize that the management of the mother
will be different from the management of a mother with a normal pregnancy. Pelvic exams will, of necessity, be limited to prevent infection,
and bed rest is indicated for the same reason. It is very important that

the nurse assess the labor pattern in order to determine the progress. The mother's reaction and the characteristics of the contraction will help to indicate the mother's status. It is important to keep in mind that the length of labor is often shorter if the baby is premature than if it is full-term.

Food may be withheld in case labor is imminent. The mother must be helped to understand the reason for these measures and for the introduction of intravenous therapy for the purpose of maintaining fluid and electrolyte balance if the mother is to be given nothing by mouth.

When the mother does go into active labor, the nursery should be informed that a high-risk infant will be admitted. The baby is classified in this way because it may show signs of infection due to premature rupture of membranes and/or may be a premature infant (one born between the twenty-sixth and thirty-sixth weeks of gestation). The infant's neurological and respiratory systems are particularly immature and do not function properly, and they may need medical assistance to maintain respirations, temperature, and other bodily functions. The premature infant and its needs will be discussed in Unit VII, Chapter Two.

POST-TEST   Indicate whether each statement is true or false by circling the appropriate letter. Then turn to page 283 and see how well you have done.

1. Premature rupture of membranes occurs after the first stage of labor is completed.   T   F

2. A rupture of membranes is not always complete.   T   F

3. The greatest danger of premature rupture of membranes is to the fetus.   T   F

4. Antibiotics can be given to the mother to prevent infection developing in the fetus.   T   F

In the specific areas with which you had difficulty, return to the material and review.

BIBLIOGRAPHY   Artal, Raul, "The Mechanical Properties of Prematurely and Non-Prematurely Ruptured Membranes," *American Journal of Obstetrics and Gynecology*, Vol. 125, No. 5, p. 658, July 1, 1976.

Hauth, John C., et al., "Early Labor Induction with Oral PGE₂ After Premature Rupture of the Membranes at Term," *Obstetrics and Gynecology*, Vol. 49, No. 5, pp. 524–526, May 1977.

Sell, Elsa Joyce and Thomas Harris, "Association of Premature Rupture of Membranes with Idiopathic Respiratory Distress Syndrome," *Obstetrics and Gynecology*, Vol. 49, No. 2, p. 167, Feb. 1977.

Worthington D., et al., "Fetal Lung Maturity, I. Mode of Onset of Premature Labor," *Obstetrics and Gynecology*, Vol. 49, No. 3, pp. 275–279, March 1977.

PRETEST ANSWERS   1. Before the actual onset of labor   2. Prematurity   3. Multiple pregnancies; polyhydramnios; cephalopelvic disproportion; fetal position; premature cervical dilatation   4. Infection

POST-TEST ANSWERS   1. F   2. T   3. T   4. F

CHAPTER FIVE
PROLONGED LABOR

OBJECTIVES   *Define dystocia.*

Define uterine dysfunction or inertia.

Differentiate between hypotonic and hypertonic uterine inertia.

Identify intervention measures when a labor is complicated by either hypertonic inertia or hypotonic inertia.

Identify nursing intervention when a labor is complicated by uterine inertia.

GLOSSARY   *Active phase of labor:* The part of labor that occurs after 3 centimeters of cervical dilatation

Latent phase of labor: The part of labor that occurs prior to 3 centimeters of cervical dilatation

Cephalopelvic disproportion: The disparity between the size of the fetal head and the size of the maternal bony pelvis

Dysfunction (uterine): An interruption in the uterine forces causing prolongation in any phase or stage of labor

Dystocia: A stopping or slowing of the labor processes

Hypertonic uterine contractions: Intense, painful, but ineffectual contractions of the uterus

Hypotonic uterine contractions: Mild, often irregular contractions that produce little discomfort and are of low intensity

Malposition: Fetal position other than occiput anterior which may cause prolonged labor

Uterine inertia: Uterine dysfunction

PRETEST In the spaces provided, fill in the word or words that best complete(s) the statements. Then turn to page 296 and check your answers.

1. The definition of "dystocia" is _____
   _____.

2. Uterine dysfunction or inertia is _____
   _____
   _____.

3. The three major factors causing prolonged labor, either singly or in combination, are _____
   _____;
   _____ , _____
   _____ , _____
   _____ ; and _____
   _____.

4. Hypotonic dysfunction usually occurs during the _____
   phase of labor or after the cervix has dilated _____ centimeters.

5. Hypotonic uterine inertia responds well to the use of _____.

6. Hypertonic uterine inertia usually occurs during the _____
   phase of labor.

7. Hypertonic uterine inertia is first treated by the use of _____
   _____ to stop contractions and _____ to allow the mother to rest.

8. Fetal distress in hypotonic inertia occurs after _____
   develops.

9. The most severe complication of uterine dysfunction is fetal _____.

Prolonged labor is a common interruption in the health state which is seen during the intrapartum period. This phenomenon is referred to as *dystocia*, meaning the slowing or stopping of the progress of labor. Dystocia can occur in any stage of labor. The stressors producing this interruption are in any of three areas: those of the uterine forces, i.e., the contractions; the passenger, i.e., the fetal size or presentation; and the passage, i.e., the maternal pelvis. Stressors in these areas may operate singly or in combination with others.

Dystocia occurs due to stressors operating in the areas of

_____, _____, and   uterine forces; passenger;

_____.   passage

The beginning phase of labor from 0 to 3 centimeters of cervical dilatation is referred to as the *latent phase*. The criteria for prolongation in this phase for the primigravid woman is labor longer than 20 hours and for the multigravid woman, more than 14 hours. During the *active phase*, from 4 centimeters to full cervical dilatation, the criteria for prolongation of labor is 1.2 centimeters or less of dilatation per hour for the primigravid woman and 1.5 centimeters or less of dilatation per hour for the multigravid woman.

The latent phase of labor is _____   from 0 to 3 centimeters

cervical dilatation.

The active phase of labor is _____   from 4 to 10 centimeters

cervical dilatation.

Dystocia in the latent phase for the primigravid woman is defined

as a period of _____.   20 hours or longer

During the active phase, prolonged labor in the multigravid

woman is cervical dilatation of _____   1.5 centimeters

_____.   or less per hour

In this chapter we are going to discuss prolonged labor that results when the uterine forces are involved. When the normal pattern of uterine contractions is interrupted, this is described as "uterine dysfunction" or "uterine inertia," both terms being synonymous. Often uterine dysfunction occurs as a response to various stressors. Uterine dysfunction appears at different phases in labor with a pattern that is characteristic. During the latent phase the contractions often are intense, regular, painful, and ineffectual. These contractions are *hyper-*

tonic. In the active phase of labor the contractions tend to be irregular and mild and produce little discomfort. These contractions are *hypotonic*.

⬇

When the normal pattern of uterine contractions is interrupted, this is described as _____ or

_____ .

uterine dysfunction;

uterine inertia

When uterine dysfunction occurs during the latent phase the contractions are _____, _____,

_____, and _____.

intense; regular;

painful; ineffectual

These contractions are called _____.

hypertonic

In the active phase of labor, contractions of uterine dysfunction are _____ and _____ and _____

_____ .

mild; irregular; produce

little discomfort

These are called _____.

hypotonic

Stressors that may produce uterine dysfunction include large amounts of analgesia or regional anesthesia given during early labor, overdistension of the uterus such as might occur in a multiple pregnancy, and fear and anxiety about the labor and delivery process. Uterine inertia is an adaption of a protective mechanism in instances of pelvic contraction and fetal malposition. Many times the specific stressor is unknown.

Uterine dysfunction results from known stressors such as

_____ ,

_____ , _____ , _____

_____ , or _____ .

analgesia early in labor;

overdistension; fear; pelvic

contraction; malpresentation

The complications that can arise from prolonged labor are fetal distress occurring early with a hypertonic pattern of labor and occurring later, following uterine infection, with a hypotonic pattern of labor. The mother becomes exhausted and may develop an infection after the rupture of membranes. Uterine infection can be treated with antibiotics, but the fetus does not respond and the fetal mortality rate is high.

In hypertonic labor, fetal distress occurs _____.

early

In hypotonic labor, fetal distress occurs _____

_____ .

following

uterine infection

Maternal complications that occur during prolonged labor are
_____ and _____.

exhaustion; infection

Once hypertonic uterine dysfunction is diagnosed, the treatment is to arrest this pattern of labor by sedating the mother with morphine and a short-acting barbiturate. Following this, usually the mother awakens and a normal pattern of uterine contractions becomes established. If this does not occur, then half the usual dose of oxytocin is tried, and if this is unsuccessful, then a cesarean section is performed.

If the mother in labor develops a pattern of hypotonic uterine dysfunction, then the adequacy of the pelvis is reexamined and the presenting part determined in relationship to the pelvis. Often this is assessed more accurately by x-ray pelvimetry than by vaginal examination. If there is no cephalopelvic disproportion, the contractions are stimulated by the intravenous administration of oxytocin or prostaglandins. (See nursing implications during stimulation by oxytocin, pages 102–103.)

Hypertonic uterine dysfunction is treated with _____ and _____.

morphine; sedation

Once hypotonic uterine dysfunction is diagnosed, before treatment is initiated _____ _____ is necessary.

evaluation of the adequacy of the pelvis

If there is no cephalopelvic disproportion or malpresentation when hypotonic contractions occur, then the treatment is _____.

stimulation by oxytocin

The need for constant nursing intervention, support, and understanding during labor becomes accentuated during a difficult labor and delivery. The parent's anxiety levels are increased by this additional crisis, and they find it difficult to comprehend that labor is not proceeding as it would under normal circumstances. Thus, the parents become fearful and tired and often do not know how to handle the situation. Constant reassurance, support, and understanding on the part of the nurse are most important during this particularly critical period of time.

Specific nursing intervention measures are geared to the maintenance of an environment conducive to relaxation. Frequent sponge baths, repositioning of the patient, soothing backrubs, and frequent changes of linen are nursing activities that contribute to a sense of well-being and comfort.

The staff must maintain strict aseptic technique to prevent development of infection. Also, the mother's status should be assessed through observation of her temperature every two hours. If the mother's temperature rises, antibiotic therapy is initiated.

The fetal heart rate should be monitored carefully, preferably by continuous external or internal monitor. If these devices are not used, assessment should be more frequent than the usual every 15 minutes. Other signs of fetal distress, such as meconium in the amniotic fluid, should be reported to the physician if they develop.

Comfort measures that can be provided for the mother are _____, _____, _____, and _____.

> sponge baths; repositioning; backrubs; change of linen

A means of assessing the mother's possibility of developing an infection is _____.

> checking her temperature

The well-being of the fetus can be identified by the _____ _____ and the _____ _____.

> fetal
> heart rate; color of amniotic
> fluid

Although rest and sleep are important since the mother may be exhausted by the prolonged process, she should not be maintained in isolation; interpersonal relationships are most significant at a time when fears and anxieties may be exacerbated. Explanations as to what is being done and what is to follow should be carefully given to the mother.

Since dehydration may occur as a result of exhaustion and energy expenditure taking place when labor is prolonged, fluids are given intravenously, thus ensuring maintenance of electrolyte balance; 2,000 cubic centimeters or more may be administered within a period of 24 hours.

Therefore the nurse must maintain careful watch for signs of fluid and electrolyte imbalance and report these immediately to the physician.

A prolonged labor may severely exhaust the mother's resources. Imbalances of _____ and _____ may occur. To prevent this, the physician may order _____ intake of fluids. An amount equal to _____ _____ over a period of _____ hours may be administered.

> fluid; electrolyte
> intravenous
> 2,000 cubic
> centimeters; 24

Let us see how this information might be applied to the care of a woman you might meet in the hospital.

Marie and George Galliano called the obstetrician after Marie's membranes ruptured at 5 A.M. The doctor told them to go to the hospital, where he met them and admitted Marie. Upon admission you note that Marie is a Gravida III, Para II, 40 weeks gestation. The presentation is vertex with station −2, cervix 3 centimeters dilated, and membranes ruptured. The fetal heart rate is 136 per minute and regular. At a vaginal examination two hours ago, the findings were the same as those currently, at 9 A.M.: cervix 5 centimeters dilated, station −2. The intensity of the contractions is 2+ and the doctor orders x-ray pelvimetry. While you are preparing Marie for the x-rays, the parents begin to express their fears and concerns that something is wrong.

Choose which response is best in helping them to understand what is happening.

A. This is nothing to worry about. It's just like having a chest x-ray. You don't feel anything, and then it's all over. Go to page 292.

B. Since the progress of your labor has slowed, it is important to make sure that the baby can pass through your pelvis, and these x-rays will give this information. It may be tiresome and uncomfortable on the x-ray table but it does not last long. Go to page 293.

C. It is obvious that something is wrong because the baby is not descending and your cervix has stopped dilating. It may be because the baby is too big to go through, and that is what the x-rays will show. Go to page 294.

Your choice of *A* is poor. You have only heightened the couple's fears, since if you are not willing to discuss the matter, it must be very serious. You also have closed the door to any more discussion.

Return to page 291. Review the material and choose another response.

B is a very good choice. You have informed the parents about what is happening and why things are being done. It is impossible to tell them anything definite, but you have given background information so that they can understand and cope with this stressor in labor. You also have left the conversation open so that they can communicate their fears or questions. Great!

Advance to page 295 and take the post-test.

Your choice of *C* is a very poor one. You have confirmed for the couple that their worst fears are true. You have presumed certain things were true, such as ". . . the baby is too big." Also you have indicated that the parents should know all this is going on. There is nothing in this response which is supportive.

Return to page 291. Review the material and choose another response.

POST-TEST Indicate whether each statement is true or false by circling the appropriate letter. Then turn to page 296 and see how well you have done.

1. Dystocia is a cessation or slowing of the labor process. T F

2. ''Uterine dysfunction'' and ''uterine inertia'' mean the same thing. T F

3. Uterine dysfunction can be caused only by an overdistended uterus or cephalopelvic disproportion. T F

4. The active phase of labor occurs in the first stage of labor, after 3 centimeters of cervical dilatation. T F

5. The latent phase of labor occurs before the cervix has dilated to 3 centimeters. T F

6. Hypertonic inertia is characterized by painless contractions. T F

7. Fetal distress in hypertonic inertia is due to intrauterine infection. T F

8. Hypotonic uterine dysfunction may be caused by fetal malposition. T F

9. Hypotonic inertia occurs in the latent phase of labor. T F

10. An oxytocic is contraindicated when hypotonic uterine inertia is diagnosed. T F

11. If an antibiotic is given to a mother to prevent infection, it also will prevent infection in the fetus. T F

In the specific areas with which you had difficulty, return to the material and review.

BIBLIOGRAPHY Beck, Paul and Max I. Lilling, "Induction of Labor with Intravenous Prostaglandin," *American Journal of Obstetrics and Gynecology*, Vol. 125,
No. 5, pp. 648–652, July 1, 1976.

Cohen, Wayne R., "Influence of the Duration of Second Stage Labor on Perinatal
Outcome and Puerperal Morbidity," *Obstetrics and Gynecology*, Vol. 49,
No. 3, pp. 266–268, March 1977.

Romney, Seymour L., et al.: *Gynecology and Obstetrics: The Health Care of
Women,* McGraw-Hill Book Co., New York, 1975.

**PRETEST
ANSWERS**   1. The slowing or cessation of the progress of labor   2. An interruption in uterine action
prolonging the duration of any stage of labor   3. Uterine contractions of insufficient force and/or
effect; fetal malpresentation, disproportion in size, or congenital malformation of the fetus; disproportion in size or structure of the birth canal   4. Active; 3   5. Oxytocics   6. Latent
7. Morphine sulphate; barbiturates   8. Infection (intrauterine)   9. Death

**POST-TEST
ANSWERS**   1. T   2. T   3. F   4. T   5. T   6. F   7. F   8. T   9. F
10. F   11. F

CHAPTER SIX

MALPOSITIONS AND MALPRESENTATIONS

OBJECTIVES   *Identify the characteristics of the position occiput posterior.*

Identify the patterns of labor when the fetus is in the occiput posterior position.

Identify the three types of breech presentations.

Identify the pattern of labor when there is a breech presentation.

Identify the characteristics of a face presentation.

Identify the characteristics of a brow presentation.

Identify the characteristics of a shoulder presentation.

Identify nursing intervention measures.

GLOSSARY   *Breech extraction:* The procedure in which the fetus, in a breech presentation, is delivered, either completely or partially, by traction applied by the person effecting the delivery. The traction can be applied either manually or through the use of forceps

Breech presentation: The presentation in which the fetus is in a longitudinal lie with the buttocks and/or feet the presenting part

Complete breech: The presentation in which the buttocks and one or both feet present at the internal os, with the thighs flexed on the fetal abdomen and the legs flexed upon the thighs

Footling breech: The presentation in which one or both feet are presenting at the internal os

Frank breech: A buttocks presentation with the fetal legs extended over its anterior torso

PRETEST In the spaces provided, fill in the word or words that best complete(s) the statements. Then turn to page 309 and check your answers.

1. An occiput posterior position is a position in which _____

   _____

   _____ .

2. When the fetus is in an occiput posterior position, during labor the mother

   may experience _____ .

3. The position of the fetus in an occiput posterior may be persistent or

   _____

   _____ .

4. A complete breech presentation is a presentation in which _____

   _____

   _____ .

5. When the fetus is in a breech presentation, the assessment of the fetal heart

   is more frequent than usual because of _____

   _____ .

6. A frank breech is a presentation in which the fetus _____

   _____

   _____ .

7. When the infant is in a face presentation, the fetal head is _____

   _____ .

8. A face presentation often occurs if there is _____

   _____ .

9. A brow presentation is a presentation in which the fetal head is

   _____ .

10. Delivery of a brow presentation is usually by _____

    _____ .

11. When the infant is in a transverse lie, the presenting part is the

    _____ .

12. Delivery when the fetus is in a transverse lie is by _____

    _____ .

The presentation of the fetus and the position that it assumes in utero determine the type of labor and delivery that will follow. The fetal presentation and position are usually adaptations to the existing space within the uterus and the pelvis. If space is decreased because of placenta previa, the fetus often assumes a presentation other than vertex, or if there is pelvic contracture, the fetal head may be extended rather than flexed in an attempt to accommodate to space available. There are instances when a position such as occiput posterior is transitory and becomes occiput anterior during the labor process; at other times another position or presentation may persist, thus altering the pattern of labor. Often medical intervention, such as the use of forceps or abdominal delivery, is necessary in these instances for the health of both the mother and the baby.

Generally, any type of interruption affecting the already emotionally charged events of labor and delivery will exacerbate feelings of anxiety and fear that may be communicated by both mother and father. Thus, skillful identification of emotional components at this time is of the essence. Through constant explanations and reinforcement of any teachings needed, the nurse can do much to assist the parents throughout this most difficult period. It is important, however, that no absolute reassurances be given at this time, since when interruptions are present, the course and events of the labor process cannot be predicted.

When the fetus is in a vertex presentation, the most common position for the occiput is the anterior. In some instances the fetal head does not rotate to that position but rather to the posterior aspect of the maternal pelvis. This position is described as *occiput posterior* and is written "ROP" if the occiput is to the right and posterior. The fetal position is LOP when _____

_____

_____.

| the occiput is on the left posterior side of the maternal pelvis

Frequently when the fetus is in an occiput posterior position, this position will change spontaneously to an anterior position during the labor process. Should this rotation occur, no major problem is incurred by the fetus' having been in the posterior position, and the labor often is lengthened by only a contraction or two.

When the fetus is in an occiput posterior position, this may spontaneously _____

_____.

| rotate to an anterior position

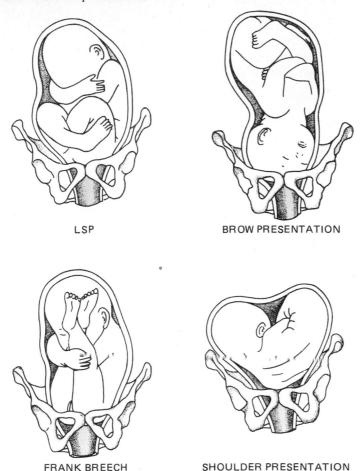

LSP

BROW PRESENTATION

FRANK BREECH

SHOULDER PRESENTATION

Malpositions and malpresentations.

During labor, when the fetus is in a posterior position, the mother often experiences increased back pressure that does not seem to be relieved by relaxation or counterpressure. It is felt that the fetus can be helped to rotate by the force of gravity if the mother is placed in Simm's position, on her side with her top leg across. When the fetus is in the posterior position, the fetal heart is heard toward the midline of the mother, and when abdominal palpation is done, the fetal back cannot be felt.

If there is slight contracture of the maternal pelvis and the occiput is posterior, this position often persists throughout labor. When this occurs, the labor is prolonged because the infant's head must mold to be able to pass through the birth canal. Constant encouragement and reinforcement of the mother are necessary since she often becomes tired quickly because of the discomfort and the prolonged time.

The baby may be delivered in the posterior position, or the physician may rotate the head of the infant manually or by forceps to an anterior position if there is enough room before extraction. It is important that the mother not receive narcotics or general anesthesia, which would depress the baby further, since the infant already is subject to more stress than usual and the time period of delivery often is lengthened. Assessment of the fetal heart rate is very important throughout labor and especially during delivery.

If the posterior position is persistent, this often means that the mother's pelvis is _____.

slightly contracted

Labor takes a longer time when the occiput is posterior than when it is anterior because of _____
_____.

the molding of

the fetal head

Narcotics are not given to the mother since _____
_____
_____
_____.

the baby

is subject to more stress than

usual and is likely to be

depressed

When the fetus is in a longitudinal lie with the buttocks and/or feet closest to the internal os, this is a *breech presentation*. When Leopold's maneuver is done, one can feel the head of the fetus in the fundus and the head is easily moved. If the presenting part is not engaged, the buttocks can be palpated above the symphysis pubis as an irregular soft mass. There are three classifications of breech presentations depending on the position of the feet in relationship to the buttocks. These classifications are as follows:

- *Frank breech:* Where the buttocks alone are the presenting part and the legs are extended across the body

- *Complete breech:* Where the feet and the buttocks together form the presenting part since the legs and thighs of the fetus are flexed

- *Incomplete breech:* Where the feet alone, singly or together, or the knees of the fetus are the lowermost presenting parts

A frank breech occurs when _____
_____.

the buttocks alone

are the presenting part

When the feet or knees of the fetus are the presenting part, this is _____.

an incomplete breech

When the legs and thighs are flexed so that the feet and the buttocks are closest to the internal os, this presentation is _____ _____ .

a

complete breech

Breech presentations are seen more frequently when the fetus is premature or when the mother is a multiparous woman and the uterus is more relaxed than it is in a primiparous woman. Also, if there is placenta previa, the fetus often is in a breech presentation to accommodate to the available space.

During labor, when the fetus is in a breech presentation, the position is determined by the relationship of the sacrum to the maternal pelvis; thus if the sacrum is on the right side of the mother and to the anterior, the position written "RSA." When the presentation is incomplete, often it is described as a "single footling" or a "double footling," and the position is difficult to identify.

If on the chart the position is written "LSP," this note means that _____ _____ _____ _____ .

the sacrum is on the left

of the mother's pelvis and to

the posterior

When the baby is in a breech presentation, then the fetal heart rate is heard in the upper quadrants of the mother's abdomen. The membranes often rupture prematurely or early in the labor; therefore close observation of both the maternal and the fetal status is necessary. Since in both a frank breech and an incomplete breech, the maternal pelvis is not completely filled by the presenting parts, there is a danger of prolapse of the cord. Thus, the fetal heart rate should be monitored every five minutes, and the perineum should be checked frequently to observe for prolapse of the cord.

Careful assessment of the fetus during labor is important because of the possibility of _____ .

prolapse of the cord

Once the membranes are ruptured, the mother's status is determined by frequently checking _____ .

her temperature

Assessment of the fetal head size is important during labor. If there is any question that the head may not pass through the maternal pelvis with ease, x-ray pelvimetry is done. When the fetus is in a breech presentation, the biggest part, the head, is last to be delivered, and should there be cephalopelvic disproportion, the fetal mortality rate is high.

When the fetus is in an incomplete or a frank breech presentation, often the buttocks/feet are seen extending from the vagina before the cervix is fully dilated. The presenting part often appears bruised because these soft tissues have acted as a dilator against the maternal cervix. During labor, if there is meconium in the amniotic fluid, this is not considered to be an indication of fetal distress since there is a lot of pressure on the fetal abdomen when the thighs are flexed, and meconium is expelled.

Delivery of the baby may be spontaneous or assisted. When there is assistance, the procedure is termed "breech extraction." Once the fetus has delivered up to the level of the umbilicus, the oxygen supply is limited because of the compression of the cord. During delivery it is important to have general anesthesia readily available since the head is the last part and the biggest and, if the cervix is not completely dilated or contracts down after the body is delivered, there is danger of the head being caught. General anesthesia allows for relaxation of the cervix, which then can be slipped over the baby's head.

A breech extraction can be a manual procedure in which the physician applies traction and delivers the shoulders one at a time in an anterior-posterior position, then rotates the body to deliver the head by flexion, also in the anterior and posterior planes; or at times the physician may use forceps to deliver the head once the body of the infant is out.

A breech delivery is usually traumatic for the infant, and often the infant needs resuscitative measures immediately. The infant frequently appears to be in shock and needs careful nursing observations. Since the delivery usually involves maneuvering of the fetus, there may be fractures of the clavicle and humerus, injury to the brachial plexus, and, more serious, intracranial hemorrhage following difficult extractions. Added to this is the fact that the infant may be premature, with the inherent problems related to immaturity.

When the fetus is in the position RSA, you would listen for the fetal heart rate in the mother's _____   right upper

_____.   quadrant

Assessment of fetal well-being is done by _____   monitoring

_____   the fetal heart rate every five

_____.   minutes

The mother's perineum is checked frequently for _____   presence

_____.   of the cord (prolapse)

X-ray pelvimetry may be done so that _____

_____.

The presence of meconium in the amniotic fluid means that

_____

_____.

A breech extraction is a procedure in which _____

_____

_____.

Immediately following the delivery of the baby, there often is need for _____.

The infant should be observed for signs of _____,

_____, _____

_____, and _____.

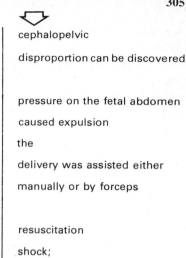

cephalopelvic

disproportion can be discovered

pressure on the fetal abdomen

caused expulsion

the

delivery was assisted either

manually or by forceps

resuscitation

shock;

fractures; injury to the brachial

plexus; intracranial hemorrhage

Nursing assessment of the family during labor includes determining their understanding and fears about a breech delivery. There is an abundance of old wives' tales about breech deliveries which instill fears and uncertainties that may add greatly to the mother's difficulty during labor. Clarification of misinformation is important, and then constant information on the mother's progress will help the family to relax. Often when the baby's feet or buttocks protrude so that they are within the mother's line of vision, she becomes overwhelmed and has difficulty following directions and participating in the delivery. Good preparation early in labor may help to alleviate this. The nurse must constantly encourage and guide the family to assist them in adapting successfully. Following delivery, any treatment or measures used on the baby should be clearly explained to the parents. They should see and hold the infant as soon as possible. If the baby is premature, it usually is taken to the nursery quickly, and the parents have only a moment to meet this new member of their family.

When the fetus is in a longitudinal lie and the fetal head is extended fully, this is a *face presentation*, with the chin or mentum as the presenting part. Face presentations occur if there is some pelvic contracture at the inlet and if the baby is large. The adequacy of the pelvis is assessed by x-ray and, if necessary, a cesarean section is done. If the fetus has the face presenting, then upon abdominal palpation the cephalic prominence is felt on the same side as the fetal back because of the extension of the head. The back is turned toward the maternal spine; thus the fetal heart is heard through the thorax of the baby. The mechanism of the fetal cardinal movement is altered so that with descent there is extension of the fetal head; this is followed by internal rotation, and delivery is by flexion. Before normal delivery can take place, the chin or mentum must rotate so that it is directly under the symphysis pubis. The labor often is longer than in a vertex presentation, and the face of the infant is edematous and often ecchymotic because of the pressure during delivery.

When the fetus has the face presenting, the presenting part is the

_____ or _____.   chin; mentum

Evaluation of the pelvis and fetal head is important so that

_____ can be ruled out.   cephalopelvic disproportion

Following this type of delivery, the infant's face usually appears

_____ and _____.   edematous; ecchymotic

The fetus is in a *brow presentation* when the fetal head, instead of being flexed, is partially extended so that the brow of the infant is closest to the internal os. Diagnosis is made by vaginal examination. A brow presentation is seen when the infant is premature or when there is contracture of the inlet of the pelvis. If the infant is small, then often a normal spontaneous delivery will follow a prolonged labor since the head usually must undergo a degree of molding for this broadest diameter of the head to pass through the maternal pelvis. Careful evaluation of the pelvis and the size of the infant is necessary since if the brow presentation persists a cesarean section usually is indicated when the infant is of normal term size.

A brow presentation occurs when _____   the brow of

_____   the fetus is the part closest to

_____.   the internal os

Difficulty occurs when the fetus is in a brow presentation

because _____   the brow is the broadest

_____.   diameter of the head

Usual delivery at term is by _____.   cesarean section

When the fetus is in a *transverse lie*, then the presenting part is the *shoulder*. A shoulder presentation can be determined by Leopold's maneuver or by vaginal examination. The infant may be found in a transverse lie when the mother is a grand multiparous woman, when placenta previa occurs, or when there is pelvic contracture. Vaginal delivery is impossible in most instances except with the second premature twin. Thus, once a transverse lie is diagnosed, the mother will

be scheduled for an elective cesarean section because the labor contractions are detrimental to the fetus' circulation and may cause uterine
rupture.

When the infant has a shoulder presentation, then the lie is
_____.

transverse

Delivery of an infant in this presentation is by _____

cesarean

_____.

section

POST-TEST Indicate whether each statement is true or false by circling the appropriate letter. Then turn to page 309 and see how well you have done.

1. When the fetus is in an occiput posterior position, there may be spontaneous rotation to an anterior position. T F

2. If the fetus is in an ROP position, the mother will complain of severe abdominal pain. T F

3. In a breech presentation, the delivery always will be by cesarean section. T F

4. In a full breech presentation, the buttocks and feet are presenting. T F

5. Meconium-stained amniotic fluid is a sign of fetal distress in a breech presentation. T F

6. In an incomplete breech, the buttocks and one or both feet are presenting. T F

7. A complication of breech presentation might be prolapse of the umbilical cord. T F

8. In a face presentation, the fetal head is fully extended. T F

9. In a brow presentation, the fetal head is fully extended. T F

10. If the doctor tells you that the shoulder of the fetus is presenting, you can expect a long labor but a vaginal delivery. T F

In the specific areas with which you had difficulty, return to the material and review.

BIBLIOGRAPHY   Hibbard, Lester T., "Changing Trends in Cesarean Section," *American Journal of Obstetrics and Gynecology*, Vol. 125, No. 6, p. 798, July 15, 1976.

Pritchard, Jack and Paul MacDonald: *Williams Obstetrics*, 15th ed., *Appleton-Century-Crofts*, New York, 1976.

Walter, David F., "Patterns of Management with Breech Presentation," *American Journal of Obstetrics and Gynecology*, Vol. 125, No. 6, p. 733, July 15, 1976.

PRETEST ANSWERS   1. The occiput of the fetus is toward the back of the mother's pelvis   2. More back discomfort   3. May rotate spontaneously to an anterior position   4. Both the feet and the buttocks are presenting   5. The possibility of prolapsed cord   6. Has the legs extended over the body, and the sacrum is the presenting part   7. Fully extended   8. Contracture of the pelvis   9. Partially extended   10. Cesarean section   11. Shoulder   12. Cesarean section

POST-TEST ANSWERS   1. T   2. F   3. F   4. T   5. F   6. F   7. T   8. T   9. F   10. F

CHAPTER SEVEN

OBSTETRICAL ANESTHESIA AND ANALGESIA

OBJECTIVES   *Identify types of analgesia used during labor.*

Identify the two types of anesthesia.

Identify the types of regional anesthesia.

Identify the nursing intervention when the mother receives anesthesia and/or analgesia.

GLOSSARY   *Twilight sleep:* A type of analgesia achieved by the combination of morphine and scopolamine

General anesthesia: A type of anesthesia in which sedation of the person occurs and the whole body is anesthetized

Regional anesthesia: Conduction anesthesia that decreases the sensitivity of or anesthetizes only a specific area of the body

Pudendal block: A type of regional anesthesia achieved by placing the agent into the pudendal nerves, desensitizing the vulva and perineum

Caudal anesthesia: A type of regional anesthesia achieved by injecting the agent into the caudal canal so that the pelvic area is desensitized

Epidural anesthesia: A regional anesthesia achieved by injecting the anesthetic agent into the spinal canal outside the dura

Spinal anesthesia: A regional anesthesia achieved by injecting the anesthetic agent into the dura

PRETEST In the spaces provided, fill in the word or words that best complete(s) the statements. Then turn to page 319 and check your answers.

1. When giving analgesia or anesthesia to the mother during labor, it is important to consider the welfare of _____ _____.

2. If after delivery the infant is depressed from the administration of Demerol, the medication that can counteract the effect is _____ _____.

3. Barbiturates rarely are given to the mother during labor because _____ _____ _____.

4. Twilight sleep is accomplished by the combination of _____ and _____.

5. Anesthesia is of two types: _____ and _____.

6. When the mother receives general anesthesia, the danger of aspiration is decreased by _____ _____.

7. The mother can administer anesthesia to herself with a _____ _____.

8. Nitrous oxide with oxygen provides _____ _____.

9. A pudendal block anesthesizes _____ _____.

10. Caudal anesthesia results when the anesthetic is injected into the _____.

11. A saddle block is a _____ _____.

Anesthesia and analgesia are important agents that are used to promote the welfare of both the mother and the baby during labor and delivery. At times they are used because of the mother's need, and at other times they are necessary because some type of interruption in the processes of labor and delivery indicates the need for operative obstetrics. At all times both the infant and the mother must be considered.

The use of barbiturates during active labor is contraindicated because the baby will be depressed from the medication at birth and there is no means available to counteract the effects. In the first volume of this series, the use of Demerol in combination with the mild tranquilizers was discussed as a means of assisting the mother to cope with the discomforts of the contractions. The medications should be past their peak of action before the actual delivery of the infant. At times, the rate of labor is difficult to assess. For example, the mother who was examined and was found to be 5 centimeters dilated may progress rapidly to full dilatation shortly after the administration of Demerol, and the baby will be depressed at birth. There are narcotic antagonists (Nalline or Lorfan) that can be administered either to the mother immediately prior to delivery or to the infant following delivery which will counteract the effect of the Demerol and relieve the depression of the infant. It is important that these narcotic antagonists, Nalline and Lorfan, not be given when the infant's depression is due to other factors, since these drugs themselves can cause respiratory depression. Narcan is a narcotic antagonist that is effective in reversing respiratory depression within two minutes and has the advantage of not producing any respiratory depression if a narcotic is not responsible for depressed respiratory function.

In active labor, the drugs that rarely are used are

_____.

barbiturates

When one is giving Demerol and a tranquilizer to the mother in labor, it is important to know _____

_____ and the mother's _____.

the time of their peak action; progress in labor

If at birth the baby is depressed due to narcotics, then

_____

_____.

a narcotic antagonist is administered

ANALGESIA

A number of years ago, "twilight sleep" was popular for mothers who were very anxious about the labor and delivery process and did not wish to be alert and aware during this time. It is not used as frequently today because of the side effects. Twilight sleep is achieved by the combination of morphine with scopolamine. These medications not only sedate the mother but also often cause her to forget her labor because scopolamine has an amnesic effect. A similar amnesic effect is achieved by using Demerol instead of morphine with scopolamine. One of the side effects that may develop is that the mother loses contact with reality, attempts to climb out of bed, and becomes very restless. The mother also may verbally assault those about her, so the father must be prepared for this occurrence. If the mother is very heavily sedated during labor, the nurse must rely on personal observations of the labor progress and not on the reactions of the mother. Also, preparations to resuscitate the baby following delivery are necessary because respiratory depression often occurs.

Twilight sleep results from the use of _____ _____.

morphine and scopolamine

As well as sedating the mother, twilight sleep has the effect of _____.

amnesia

A side effect of this medication is _____.

restlessness

GENERAL ANESTHESIA

Anesthesia may be one of the two types, *general* or *regional*. General anesthesia usually is used for a difficult operative procedure using forceps or a cesarean section. Preparation of the mother is difficult. Usually the mother has a full stomach because of the slowed peristalsis, even if she has had nothing by mouth during labor. There is a danger of aspiration pneumonia should the mother regurgitate during anesthesia administration. If the gastric contents are aspirated, the high acidity destroys the lung tissue and there is a high fatality rate. Precautions include administering an antacid such as milk of magnesia to reduce the acidity and having the mother fast if possible for 12 hours before receiving the anesthesia. It is very important that the mother be intubated with an endotracheal tube so that this danger of aspiration is reduced.

There is a trend in anesthesia away from the use of explosive gases such as Cyclopropane because of the grave danger they present.

Frequently a combination of three medications is used to give good anesthesia, muscle relaxation, and sedation for operative procedures. Limited amounts of sodium pentothal, a general anesthetic, are given intravenously. Only slight depression of the infant occurs with the use of this barbiturate because of the small amounts administered and the fact that the baby is delivered quickly, within three to five minutes following administration. A muscle relaxant, succinylcholine chloride, produces temporary paralysis of the muscles of the mother, including the respiratory ones, so that assisted ventilation is a must. This drug does not cross over and affect the fetus. The mother usually stays in a state of light anesthesia by inhaling a combination of nitrous oxide and oxygen. The mother must receive at least 20 percent oxygen in this combination.

A general anesthesia can be achieved by the combination of
_____, _____
_____, _____,
and _____.

> sodium pentothal; succinyl-
> choline chloride; nitrous oxide;
> oxygen

Intravenous thiopental is a rapidly acting barbiturate producing good relaxation of the uterus and yet little problem of postpartum hemorrhage or vomiting. It is not an effective analgesic, so is often given in combination with nitrous oxide and a muscle relaxant.

Sometimes the mother administers the anesthesia agent herself, as in the case of a *Penthrane whistle*. This is a bracelet that fits on the mother's arm and has a mask containing the anesthetic agent Penthrane. The mother holds this over her face until she breathes enough anesthesia to put her out. At this time her arm falls away from her face, preventing her from receiving too much anesthesia. It is extremely important that the nurse not hold this mask for the mother.

A Penthrane whistle allows the mother to _____
_____.

> administer
> anesthesia to herself

During delivery nitrous oxide can be used alone with oxygen to relieve the discomfort of contractions. Nitrous oxide, although not a true anesthetic, does relieve the discomfort and lightly sedates the mother. Occasionally the mother may become slightly "high" and disoriented for a brief period following administration of nitrous oxide.

Nitrous oxide with oxygen will produce _____
_____and _____.

> light
> analgesia; sedation

Precautions should be taken so that the staff does not suffer effects of these agents. The delivery rooms should be well ventilated, since some of the gas escapes. There have also been studies indicating that women who work in areas where anesthesia is administered have a high abortion and malformed offspring incidence.

REGIONAL ANESTHESIA

Regional anesthesia, also called "conduction anesthesia," is the blocking of an area of the sensory nerve impulses (autonomic system) to relieve discomfort. The anesthetic agent used is usually Xylocaine (lidocaine). During delivery the perineum is infiltrated with the anesthetic agent. Care is taken that introduction of the anesthesia into the vascular system is avoided. This is termed a *local block*. A *pudendal block* is achieved by injection of the medication into the pudendal nerves near the ischial spines. The needle is inserted through either the vagina or the perineum, and extreme care is taken not to inject the medication into the baby's head. This provides anesthesia of the perineum and vulva.

Regional anesthesia may be used during labor to relieve the mother's discomfort. The cervix must be at least 4 to 5 centimeters dilated before this is employed, or the anesthesia will stop the progress of labor. *Paracervical anesthesia* produces anesthesia of the cervix. This is a difficult type of anesthesia to administer since it must be placed accurately on both sides near the base of the broad ligament. Sometimes it is effective, but occasionally only one side is effectively anesthetized. The medication is injected through a polyethylene catheter which is left in place for the effect to be continuous. If a large amount of anesthesia is used during labor, as a result the fetus may have a decreased heart rate.

Regional anesthesia can be used to desensitize a broader area when the anesthetic agent is injected into different parts of the spinal canal to produce anesthesia of the lower extremities in three forms: caudal, epidural, and spinal. *Caudal anesthesia* is accomplished when the anesthetic agent is injected into the caudal canal within the sacrum; when a polyethylene catheter is inserted the administration can be continuous. This medication anesthetizes the pelvic area. Not all women have a caudal canal; therefore its presence must be determined before administration is considered. The anesthetic agent is heavier than the spinal fluid and therefore settles at the bottom of the spinal canal when the mother is in semi-Fowler's position. Should the mother lie down, the agent will travel up the canal and anesthetize the body at a higher level. This includes the respiratory muscles. An important nursing aspect of caudal anesthesia is that a side effect of the medication is hypotension, which is dangerous to both the mother and the infant; thus frequent assessment of the mother's blood pressure is necessary, and a hypertensive agent should be readily available to be administered intravenously to counteract the effect. This means that the mother should have an intravenous infusion running. The second stage of labor usually is prolonged so low forceps are used to deliver the baby.

Paracervical anesthesia can be produced by _____   anesthetizing

_____.

    For this to be a continuous anesthesia, _____

_____

_____.

    The fetus may show an effect by having _____

_____.

    Caudal anesthesia occurs when the anesthetic is injected into

_____.

    The mother must be kept in a _____
position.

    A major side effect of Xylocaine is _____.

An *epidural anesthetic* is administered generally in the lumbar region, and the anesthetic agent is injected into the spinal canal outside of the dura, while a *spinal* differs by having the medication injected into the dura. In labor a spinal also may be termed a "saddle block" since the area that is anesthetized is the lower part of the body. The precautions necessary are that the mother must not be flat and the blood pressure must be observed carefully. If the delivery is by cesarean section, then the spinal or epidural is administered at a higher level, usually in the lower thoracic area. During recovery from a spinal, however, the mother should remain flat since some of the cerebrospinal fluid is lost and the mother will experience severe headaches if she sits up.

    It is important to prepare the mother before she receives a regional anesthetic by telling her that she will lose sensation of her lower extremities and will have difficulty moving her legs. Sometimes mothers experience uncontrollable shaking of the legs that disappears within a short period of time. Also, the loss of bladder sensation means that the nurse must closely monitor the mother's voiding and possibly catheterize her when the need arises. If epinephrine is added to the lidocaine, there is often a diminution of uterine activity, thus slowing the progress.

    Whenever Procaine or lidocaine is used, there is a possibility of anaphylactic shock occurring in persons who are allergic to the medication. A careful history of drug allergy must be taken, and the mother must be observed closely for any untoward reactions. If lidocaine is injected accidentally into the maternal vessels, the mother may experience vertigo, tinnitus, heart palpitations, and a strange metallic taste. At the same time she may become excited or confused.

    An epidural is administered into _____

_____.

---

the paracervical nerves

medication is

injected through a polyethylene

catheter

a decreased

heart rate

the caudal canal

semi-Fowler's

hypotension

the space

outside the dura

A saddle block is the same as a _____.   lumbar spinal

The position of the mother who has a continuous epidural being administered should be _____.   semi-Fowler's

When the mother is to have a cesarean section, the epidural anesthetic is administered in the _____.   thoracic area

Lidocaine can produce _____.   anaphylactic shock

HYPNOSIS

Hypnosis has been used successfully in labor. Although about only half of pregnant women are considered good candidates, if preparation time is available this is a very satisfactory method without side effects.

ACUPUNCTURE

As yet there has been little use of acupuncture in this country. Several studies indicate that the use of electroacupuncture, in which the acupuncture needles are connected to electric current, has been very effective in relieving discomfort. They predict that this method will be very popular. Again, this method eliminates unpleasant and serious side effects and may turn out to be very useful indeed.

POST-TEST Indicate whether each statement is true or false by circling the appropriate letter. Then turn to page 319 and see how well you have done.

1. The use of anesthesia and analgesia during labor and delivery can promote the welfare of both the mother and the infant.   T   F

2. Barbiturates rarely are used during active labor.   T   F

3. Demerol and Vistaril in combination cause no respiratory depression of the infant.   T   F

4. It is important not to use analgesia or anesthesia too early in the labor process.   T   F

5. Twilight sleep provides amnesia for the mother.   T   F

6. Succinylcholine chloride produces muscle paralysis.   T   F

7. The nurse should support the mother and help her hold the Penthrane whistle so that the discomfort will be relieved.   T   F

8. A local block is an anesthetic that is injected into the perineum.   T   F

9. When the mother receives an epidural, hypotension is a major side effect.   T   F

10. There is a danger of anaphylactic shock when lidocaine is used.   T   F

In the specific areas with which you had difficulty, return to the material and review.

BIBLIOGRAPHY Goodlin, Robert C., et al., "Post-Paracervical Block Bradycardia: Its Prediction And Preventability," *American Journal of Obstetrics and Gynecology*, Vol. 125, No. 5, p. 665, July 1, 1976.

Grad, Rae Krohn and Jack Woodsie, "Obstetrical Analgesics and Anesthesia," *American Journal of Nursing*, Vol. 77, No. 2, pp. 242–245, Feb. 1977.

Matadil, Lennox and Luis A. Cibils, "The Effect of Epidural Anesthesia on Uterine Activity and Blood Pressure," *American Journal of Obstetrics and Gynecology*, Vol. 125, No. 6, p. 846, July 15, 1976.

PRETEST ANSWERS   1. Both the mother and the infant   2. Nalline or Lorfan   3. They cause irreversible respiratory depression of the infant at birth   4. Scopolamine; morphine   5. General; regional   6. Intubation with an endotracheal tube   7. Penthrane whistle   8. Light analgesia and sedation   9. The perineum and vulva   10. Caudal canal   11. Spinal given in the lumbar area

POST-TEST ANSWERS   1. T   2. T   3. F   4. T   5. T   6. T   7. F   8. T   9. T   10. T

CHAPTER EIGHT

OPERATIVE OBSTETRICS

GLOSSARY   *Cesarean section:* An operative procedure by which the uterus is entered through an abdominal incision so that the products of conception can be removed

Induction of labor: The instituting of labor, by chemical means, after the period of viability

Obstetric forceps: Instruments used to assist the person effecting the vaginal delivery during the second stage of labor

Perineal laceration: An uncontrolled tear of the perineal body during the second stage of labor

Podalic version: An internal procedure of manually turning the fetus from any undesirable position into a breech presentation

Stimulation of labor: The increasing of the strength and effect of uterine contractions during the first stage of labor by chemical means

PRETEST In the spaces provided, fill in the word or words that best complete(s) the statements. Then turn to page 336 and check your answers.

1. Stimulation of labor is a procedure in which _____

   _____

   _____.

2. Induction of labor differs from stimulation in the following way:

   _____

   _____.

3. Forceps are _____

   _____

   _____

4. Give four maternal and three fetal indications for the use of forceps to effect a delivery. Maternal: _____,

   _____, _____, and _____

   _____. Fetal: _____,

   _____, and _____.

5. A cesarean section is _____

   _____

   _____

6. Describe a classicial section and a low-segment section. Classical:

   _____

   _____. Low-segment: _____

   _____

   _____

7. Give five maternal and two fetal indications for effecting a cesarean section delivery. Maternal: _____, _____

   _____, _____, _____

   _____, and _____

   Fetal: _____ and _____.

8. Podalic version is _____

   _____

   _____.

9. What is the difference between a first-degree, second-degree, third-degree, and fourth-degree perineal laceration? First-degree: _____

_____

_____

Second-degree: _____

_____

_____ Third-degree: _____

_____

Fourth-degree: _____

_____.

If the necessity for operative intervention arises, this event often creates a crisis for the family. When a prepared mother learns that forceps, cesarean section, induction of labor, or stimulation of labor is required, she often feels let down or inept. The nurse should recognize the psychological effect of medical intervention and should be prepared to support the family.

Some expectant mothers want complete freedom from discomfort through heavy sedation and analgesia during the entire labor period. An increasing number of families, however, have had some type of preparation for exposure to the labor process and come to the hospital determined to participate fully in the event.

INDUCTION AND STIMULATION OF LABOR

Induction of labor means that labor is initiated by the use of chemical agents after the period of viability. The drugs most commonly used are an oxytocin and prostaglandin E_2.

There are certain high-risk situations for the mother or the baby in which induction of labor is necessary. These include the diabetic mother, the preeclamptic mother, or the mother who has premature rupture of membranes.

Research has indicated that one can determine how the mother will respond to the induction of labor and whether she will respond to trials of induction or be a better candidate for an elective cesarean section. The mother's status is determined by a vaginal examination. Bishop has outlined certain factors that are used to make the prediction; these factors include the station of the fetal head, the dilatation of the cervix, the length of the cervix measured in centimeters, the consistency of the cervix (firm to soft), and the position of the cervix (posterior to anterior). The most significant of these factors in determining response to induction was found to be the dilatation of the cervix. Administering prostaglandin E_2 extra-amniotically through the cervix by means of a catheter has been successful in improving the status of the cervix and thus making induction possible.

The use of oral prostaglandin E_2 for elective induction is recommended in multiparous women. It is important to note that uterine sensitivity alters during the different phases of labor, and once active labor is established the medication is stopped. Close monitoring of the mother and the fetus is essential. The beginning dosage of prostaglandin E_2 is 0.5 milligrams repeated in one and a half hours if the mother is still in the latent phase. If any hypercontractility occurs, the medication is stopped immediately and is continued, two hours later, only if the contractions have been normal. Nausea, vomiting, and diarrhea—common side effects of prostaglandin E_2—are minimal or low with the oral dose.

In both procedures the baby and placenta are removed manually. Immediate assessment of the baby is necessary, and resuscitative measures are instituted when indicated. The baby may be depressed from the anesthesia and/or from the factors precipitating the need for the cesarean section.

The cesarean section that is done through a horizontal incision into the least contractile zone of the uterus is called a _____ technique.

low-segment

The technique that requires a vertical incision into the body of the uterus is called a _____ section.

classical

Elective sections may be done in the case of a _____ section or in _____.

previous; cephalopelvic disproportion

An emergency section may be initiated in cases of placental problems such as _____ or _____.

placenta previa; abruptio placenta

Preoperative preparation consists of an abdominal and perineal shave and insertion of a Foley catheter. Anesthesia used during the operation is regional (epidural or spinal) or general anesthesia. The operating suite must have the equipment necessary for the care of a high-risk neonate, and a pediatrician should be available.

Postoperative care is geared to assisting the maternal systems to adjust to a nonpregnant state and recover from major abdominal surgery. Vital signs are monitored frequently until stable, and the lochia observed closely so that the blood loss can be assessed. It is important to recognize that the lochia is less than that in a vaginal delivery because when the placenta is removed, the rest of the decidua is removed manually. Intake and output are measured, and the mother gradually begins to take oral diet. Turning the mother, deep breathing and coughing and postoperative exercises are preventive and promotive measures. Assessment of involution of the uterus by palpation of the fundus is possible.

Often if the cesarean section was an emergency procedure, the mother may feel depressed about not having had a vaginal delivery. Helpful for the nurse to allow her to verbalize these feelings. If the mother had general anesthesia, it is usually on the following day she meets her new infant. The nurse can be supportive at this time, recognizing that the mother tires easily and may need assistance in holding.

Induction means _____.

the initiation of labor

Stimulation of labor means that ineffective uterine contractions during labor are made more effective by the use of the chemicals oxytocin or prostaglandin. Stimulation of labor often is necessary when there is hypotonic uterine dysfunction.

The difference between an induced labor and a stimulated labor is that when we speak of "induction" the labor has not yet _____ while "stimulation" means that there is an _____ labor.

begun; ineffective

The drugs used for both of these procedures are _____ and _____.

oxytocin; prostaglandin

Pitocin usually is administered by intravenous infusion or by tablets absorbed in the peribuccal spaces. Oxytocic drugs have a powerful effect on the uterine muscles, so the dosage during labor must be closely controlled. Close observation of mother and fetus is needed so that serious complications that can arise with the use of oxytocics are detected. Every contraction must be monitored so that the occurrence of *tetanic contractions* may be detected; these are contractions in which the uterus remains contracted for 90 seconds or more, constricting the umbilical flow and causing fetal anoxia. Should tetanic contractions or incomplete uterine relaxation occur, administration of the drug must be stopped immediately, the fetal heart rate assessed, and the doctor notified. As well as continuously monitoring the contractions, the nurse must check the fetal heart rate for bradycardia and the mother's blood pressure for hypertension every 15 minutes. Should these complications occur, the nurse should stop the medication and consult with the doctor.

A tetanic contraction is one that lasts over _____ seconds.

90

The danger of a tetanic contraction is _____.

fetal anoxia

Another side effect of an oxytocic is fetal _____.

bradycardia

The mother's _____ must be monitored every 15 minutes.

blood pressure

FORCEPS DELIVERY

Obstetric forceps, used to assist the physician in delivering the fetal head, were first introduced in the late 1700s although actually invented 200 years earlier. There are many different kinds of forceps. They have

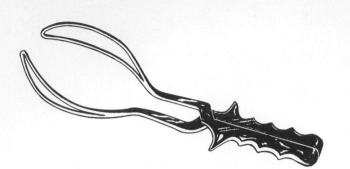

Simpson's forceps.

right and left blades designed to fit the head of the fetus as well as the axis of the maternal pelvis. Forceps are used as an extension of the physician's hands, enabling him or her to reach the fetal head, apply traction, and in some instances, rotate the head to a more favorable position so that delivery can be effected with more ease.

Some of the *maternal indications* for the use of forceps are exhaustion, heart disease, toxemia, or premature separation of the placenta. *Fetal indications* are prolapsed umbilical cord, malposition, and fetal distress.

The proper use of forceps contributes to the safety of both mother and baby by effecting a quick delivery when indicated. Forceps are applied after full cervical dilatation, and traction is applied with the uterine contraction. Forceps deliveries are classified according to the level of descent of the fetal head. *Low, or outlet, forceps* are applied when the fetal head is on the perineum; they are used most frequently. *Mid forceps* are used when the fetal head is at the level of the ischial spines, a more difficult type of delivery. *High forceps* used to be used when the fetal head was above the ischial spines but are no longer used because of the high risk of complications. This technique has been replaced by delivery through cesarean section.

The maternal complications that are indications for the use of

forceps are _____, _____, _____

_____, and _____

_____.

     exhaustion; toxemia; heart

     disease; premature separation

     of placenta

The fetal complications that call for forceps intervention are

_____,

_____, and _____.

     prolapsed umbilical cord;

     malposition; fetal distress

Maternal complications that may arise from the use of forceps are lacerations of the perineum, vagina, and cervix; trauma to the bladder; and hemorrhage. Fetal complications include temporary forceps marks

---

and transitory facial paralysis. A more serious fetal complication that occasionally occurs is intracranial hemorrhage.

If a forceps delivery is anticipated, as in instances of maternal cardiac conditions, the nurse can explain the procedure to the family and clarify any misconceptions. When forceps delivery is an emergency procedure, the nurse often interprets the need for the procedure and explains what is involved. Following the procedure, a nursing assessment of the mother and baby is necessary so that their status can be determined.

Maternal complications following forceps delivery are

_____

_____; _____

_____; and _____.

Common fetal complications are _____

_____ and _____

_____.

A more serious possible fetal complication is _____

_____.

     lacerations of the perineum,

     vagina, and cervix; trauma to

     the bladder; hemorrhage

     temporary

     forceps marks; transitory facial

     paralysis

     intracranial

     hemorrhage

DELIVERY BY CESAREAN SECTION

Cesarean section is the delivery of the fetus through an abdominal incision into the uterus. The surgery can either be elective, as in the case of known cephalopelvic disproportion or previous cesarean section, or emergency, as in the case of severe toxemia, placenta previa, abruptio placenta, fetal distress, or breech presentation.

The psychological preparation of the mother and father is most important. If the surgery is elective, the parents will have time to explore their feelings and make plans for a longer recuperative period and hospital stay. If the operation is of an emergency nature, it often is impossible to give more than brief information and there is little or no time for discussion. If you care for the mother after the surgery, you should know how much preparation she has had so that you will be better able to identify her needs.

Two operative techniques are commonly used in cesarean section: low-segment and classical. In both operative procedures, the initial abdominal incision most often is a vertical midline one. The technique of choice is the low-segment technique. In this technique, the uterus is entered through a horizontal incision into the least contractile portion, the lower segment of the uterus. In a classical section, the uterus is entered directly through the body of the uterus by a vertical incision.

PODALIC VERSION

Internal podalic version involves the turning of the fetus in utero from another presentation to a breech presentation. The physician places one hand inside the uterus, grasps the feet, and performs a breech extraction. This technique is not commonly done but may be used to deliver the second twin who is high up in the uterus, the fetus who is in a transverse lie when the membranes are intact, and the fetus with a prolapsed cord and unengaged head. This is a method of expediting delivery. In all instances the cervix must be fully dilated. Intact membranes provide a larger uterine environment in which to maneuver the baby, so the physician can place a hand inside and just rupture the membranes when grasping the feet of the infant. General anesthesia is important for good relaxation. Careful observation of both the mother and the baby is important following this procedure. The maternal complications that follow include uterine rupture and postpartum hemorrhage. Fetal problems seen include hypoxia, head injuries, and fractures.

"Internal podalic version" means _____ _____.

turning the fetus

in utero to breech presentation

Before this procedure is carried out, the cervix _____ _____.

must

be fully dilated

Nursing observations of the mother following this operation should be geared toward signs of _____ and _____.

uterine rupture;

hemorrhage

The baby should be observed for signs of _____ , _____ , and _____ .

hypoxia;

head injuries; fractures

PERINEAL LACERATIONS

Lacerations of the perineum are tears that occur at the time of delivery of the head or shoulders. They are seen more frequently in multiparous women when no episiotomy is performed than in primigravid women who have had an episiotomy at delivery. When the delivery is precipitous, the perineum does not have time to become stretched and thinned, and lacerations may occur. Other instances in which lacerations are apt to occur are a difficult forceps delivery, a persistent occiput posterior that presents a larger diameter, a breech delivery, and a delivery in which the mother is placed in an exaggerated lithotomy position so that the perineum is under tension. If the outlet is narrow, then the head is forced toward the rectum as it is delivered. This puts extra strain on the perineum and can cause lacerations. If an episiotomy is performed, there are times when it extends and lacerations occur. Perineal lacerations are classified according to the degree to which they extend; the tissues involved determine this extent.

- A *first-degree laceration* involves the fourchet, the mucus membrane of the vagina, and the skin of the perineum.

- A *second-degree laceration* involves those tissues in the first-degree laceration and the muscles of the perineum.

- A *third-degree laceration* involves those tissues in the second-degree laceration and the rectal sphincter.

- A *fourth-degree laceration* involves those tissues in the third-degree laceration and the anterior wall of the rectum.

Lacerations are easily repaired by suturing, and healing usually takes place with no residual effects.

Let us identify the areas involved in each type of laceration.

A first-degree laceration involves only the _____,   fourchet;

_____ of the perineal body, and vaginal _____.   skin; mucosa

In a second-degree laceration, the laceration also includes the

_____ of the perineum.   muscles

A third-degree laceration also includes the _____   rectal

_____.   sphincter

A fourth-degree laceration is one that extends into the _____.   rectum

The nurse on the postpartum unit must be aware of the type of episiotomy and/or laceration sustained by the mother in order to identify the needs of the mother and thus recognize appropriate nursing intervention. Perineal care is extremely important.

When the perineum is checked every morning, the lacerations should be observed for signs of inflammation, swelling, infection, or hematomas. Mothers who have a first-degree laceration complain of pain, especially as they sit. It is helpful to teach them to tighten their gluteal muscles as they sit. If a sitz bath or heat lamp is ordered, these increase the circulation and healing is promoted. When the muscles of the perineum are involved, the pain that the mother experiences is more pronounced when she walks, when she attempts to void, and especially when she defecates. Often these mothers require analgesics and topical sprays and ointments, which are soothing and tend to reduce any edema present. Stool softeners, which aid in reducing some of the discomfort when the mother has a bowel movement, often are given. When the mother has a third- or fourth-degree laceration, it is important

Induction means _____.

the initiation of labor

Stimulation of labor means that ineffective uterine contractions during labor are made more effective by the use of the chemicals oxytocin or prostaglandin. Stimulation of labor often is necessary when there is hypotonic uterine dysfunction.

The difference between an induced labor and a stimulated labor is that when we speak of "induction" the labor has not yet _____ while "stimulation" means that there is an _____ labor.

begun; ineffective

The drugs used for both of these procedures are _____ and _____.

oxytocin;

prostaglandin

Pitocin usually is administered by intravenous infusion or by tablets absorbed in the peribuccal spaces. Oxytocic drugs have a powerful effect on the uterine muscles, so the dosage during labor must be closely controlled. Close observation of mother and fetus is needed so that serious complications that can arise with the use of oxytocics are detected. Every contraction must be monitored so that the occurrence of *tetanic contractions* may be detected; these are contractions in which the uterus remains contracted for 90 seconds or more, constricting the umbilical flow and causing fetal anoxia. Should tetanic contractions or incomplete uterine relaxation occur, administration of the drug must be stopped immediately, the fetal heart rate assessed, and the doctor notified. As well as continuously monitoring the contractions, the nurse must check the fetal heart rate for bradycardia and the mother's blood pressure for hypertension every 15 minutes. Should these complications occur, the nurse should stop the medication and consult with the doctor.

A tetanic contraction is one that lasts over _____ seconds.

90

The danger of a tetanic contraction is _____.

fetal anoxia

Another side effect of an oxytocic is fetal _____.

bradycardia

The mother's _____ must be monitored every 15 minutes.

blood pressure

FORCEPS DELIVERY

Obstetric forceps, used to assist the physician in delivering the fetal head, were first introduced in the late 1700s although actually invented 200 years earlier. There are many different kinds of forceps. They have

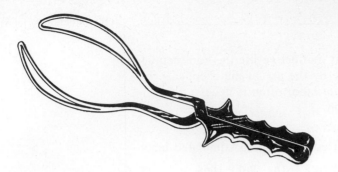

Simpson's forceps.

right and left blades designed to fit the head of the fetus as well as the axis of the maternal pelvis. Forceps are used as an extension of the physician's hands, enabling him or her to reach the fetal head, apply traction, and in some instances, rotate the head to a more favorable position so that delivery can be effected with more ease.

Some of the *maternal indications* for the use of forceps are exhaustion, heart disease, toxemia, or premature separation of the placenta. *Fetal indications* are prolapsed umbilical cord, malposition, and fetal distress.

The proper use of forceps contributes to the safety of both mother and baby by effecting a quick delivery when indicated. Forceps are applied after full cervical dilatation, and traction is applied with the uterine contraction. Forceps deliveries are classified according to the level of descent of the fetal head. *Low, or outlet, forceps* are applied when the fetal head is on the perineum; they are used most frequently. *Mid forceps* are used when the fetal head is at the level of the ischial spines, a more difficult type of delivery. *High forceps* used to be used when the fetal head was above the ischial spines but are no longer used because of the high risk of complications. This technique has been replaced by delivery through cesarean section.

The maternal complications that are indications for the use of forceps are _____, _____, _____ _____, and _____ _____.

exhaustion; toxemia; heart disease; premature separation of placenta

The fetal complications that call for forceps intervention are _____, _____, and _____.

prolapsed umbilical cord; malposition; fetal distress

Maternal complications that may arise from the use of forceps are lacerations of the perineum, vagina, and cervix; trauma to the bladder; and hemorrhage. Fetal complications include temporary forceps marks and transitory facial paralysis. A more serious fetal complication that occasionally occurs is intracranial hemorrhage.

If a forceps delivery is anticipated, as in instances of maternal cardiac conditions, the nurse can explain the procedure to the family and clarify any misconceptions. When forceps delivery is an emergency procedure, the nurse often interprets the need for the procedure and explains what is involved. Following the procedure, a nursing assessment of the mother and baby is necessary so that their status can be determined.

Maternal complications following forceps delivery are
_____
_____ ; _____
_____ ; and _____ .

Common fetal complications are _____
_____ and _____
_____ .

A more serious possible fetal complication is _____
_____ .

lacerations of the perineum, vagina, and cervix; trauma to the bladder; hemorrhage

temporary forceps marks; transitory facial paralysis

intracranial hemorrhage

DELIVERY BY CESAREAN SECTION

Cesarean section is the delivery of the fetus through an abdominal incision into the uterus. The surgery can either be elective, as in the case of known cephalopelvic disproportion or previous cesarean section, or emergency, as in the case of severe toxemia, placenta previa, abruptio placenta, fetal distress, or breech presentation.

The psychological preparation of the mother and father is most important. If the surgery is elective, the parents will have time to explore their feelings and make plans for a longer recuperative period and hospital stay. If the operation is of an emergency nature, it often is impossible to give more than brief information and there is little or no time for discussion. If you care for the mother after the surgery, you should know how much preparation she has had so that you will be better able to identify her needs.

Two operative techniques are commonly used in cesarean section: low-segment and classical. In both operative procedures, the initial abdominal incision most often is a vertical midline one. The technique of choice is the low-segment technique. In this technique, the uterus is entered through a horizontal incision into the least contractile portion, the lower segment of the uterus. In a classical section, the uterus is entered directly through the body of the uterus by a vertical incision.

In both procedures the baby and placenta are removed manually. Immediate assessment of the baby is necessary, and resuscitative measures are instituted when indicated. The baby may be depressed from the anesthesia and/or from the factors precipitating the need for the cesarean section.

The cesarean section that is done through a horizontal incision into the least contractile zone of the uterus is called a _____ technique.

low-segment

The technique that requires a vertical incision into the body of the uterus is called a _____ section.

classical

Elective sections may be done in the case of a _____ section or in _____.

previous;

cephalopelvic disproportion

An emergency section may be initiated in cases of placental problems such as _____ or _____.

placenta previa;

abruptio placenta

Preoperative preparation consists of an abdominal and perineal shave and insertion of a Foley catheter. Anesthesia used during the operation is regional (epidural or spinal) or general anesthesia. The operating suite must have the equipment necessary for the care of a high-risk neonate, and a pediatrician should be available.

Postoperative care is geared to assisting the maternal systems to adjust to a nonpregnant state and recover from major abdominal surgery. Vital signs are monitored frequently until stable, and the lochia is observed closely so that the blood loss can be assessed. It is important to recognize that the lochia is less than that in a vaginal delivery because when the placenta is removed, the rest of the decidua is removed manually. Intake and output are measured, and the mother gradually begins to take oral diet. Turning the mother, deep breathing and coughing, and postoperative exercises are preventive and promotive measures. Assessment of involution of the uterus by palpation of the fundus is not possible.

Often if the cesarean section was an emergency procedure, the mother may feel depressed about not having had a vaginal delivery. It is helpful for the nurse to allow her to verbalize these feelings.

If the mother had general anesthesia, it is usually on the following day that she meets her new infant. The nurse can be supportive at this time, recognizing that the mother tires easily and may need assistance with feeding.

PODALIC VERSION

Internal podalic version involves the turning of the fetus in utero from another presentation to a breech presentation. The physician places one hand inside the uterus, grasps the feet, and performs a breech extraction. This technique is not commonly done but may be used to deliver the second twin who is high up in the uterus, the fetus who is in a transverse lie when the membranes are intact, and the fetus with a prolapsed cord and unengaged head. This is a method of expediting delivery. In all instances the cervix must be fully dilated. Intact membranes provide a larger uterine environment in which to maneuver the baby, so the physician can place a hand inside and just rupture the membranes when grasping the feet of the infant. General anesthesia is important for good relaxation. Careful observation of both the mother and the baby is important following this procedure. The maternal complications that follow include uterine rupture and postpartum hemorrhage. Fetal problems seen include hypoxia, head injuries, and fractures.

"Internal podalic version" means _____ _____.

> turning the fetus
> in utero to breech presentation

Before this procedure is carried out, the cervix _____ ___ _____ _____.

> must
> be fully dilated

Nursing observations of the mother following this operation should be geared toward signs of _____ and _____.

> uterine rupture;
> hemorrhage

The baby should be observed for signs of _____ , _____ , and _____.

> hypoxia;
> head injuries; fractures

PERINEAL LACERATIONS

Lacerations of the perineum are tears that occur at the time of delivery of the head or shoulders. They are seen more frequently in multiparous women when no episiotomy is performed than in primigravid women who have had an episiotomy at delivery. When the delivery is precipitous, the perineum does not have time to become stretched and thinned, and lacerations may occur. Other instances in which lacerations are apt to occur are a difficult forceps delivery, a persistent occiput posterior that presents a larger diameter, a breech delivery, and a delivery in which the mother is placed in an exaggerated lithotomy position so that the perineum is under tension. If the outlet is narrow, then the head is forced toward the rectum as it is delivered. This puts extra strain on the perineum and can cause lacerations. If an episiotomy is performed, there are times when it extends and lacerations occur. Perineal lacerations are classified according to the degree to which they extend; the tissues involved determine this extent.

- A *first-degree laceration* involves the fourchet, the mucus membrane of the vagina, and the skin of the perineum.

- A *second-degree laceration* involves those tissues in the first-degree laceration and the muscles of the perineum.

- A *third-degree laceration* involves those tissues in the second-degree laceration and the rectal sphincter.

- A *fourth-degree laceration* involves those tissues in the third-degree laceration and the anterior wall of the rectum.

Lacerations are easily repaired by suturing, and healing usually takes place with no residual effects.

Let us identify the areas involved in each type of laceration.

A first-degree laceration involves only the _____,   fourchet;

_____ of the perineal body, and vaginal _____.   skin; mucosa

In a second-degree laceration, the laceration also includes the

_____ of the perineum.   muscles

A third-degree laceration also includes the _____   rectal

_____.   sphincter

A fourth-degree laceration is one that extends into the _____. rectum

The nurse on the postpartum unit must be aware of the type of episiotomy and/or laceration sustained by the mother in order to identify the needs of the mother and thus recognize appropriate nursing intervention. Perineal care is extremely important.

When the perineum is checked every morning, the lacerations should be observed for signs of inflammation, swelling, infection, or hematomas. Mothers who have a first-degree laceration complain of pain, especially as they sit. It is helpful to teach them to tighten their gluteal muscles as they sit. If a sitz bath or heat lamp is ordered, these increase the circulation and healing is promoted. When the muscles of the perineum are involved, the pain that the mother experiences is more pronounced when she walks, when she attempts to void, and especially when she defecates. Often these mothers require analgesics and topical sprays and ointments, which are soothing and tend to reduce any edema present. Stool softeners, which aid in reducing some of the discomfort when the mother has a bowel movement, often are given. When the mother has a third- or fourth-degree laceration, it is important to assess her output. Usually, by the third or fourth postpartum day, the mother is more comfortable and is able to walk and sit straight.

Treatments that increase the circulation in the perineum are _____ and _____.

sitz bath; heat lamp

It is important to observe the mother's patterns of _____ and _____.

voiding;

defecation

Observation of the laceration includes checking for the presence of _____ , _____ , _____ , or _____.

edema; inflammation; infection;

hematomas

Ruth Jones is in the intensive care area of the obstetrical unit following an emergency low-segment cesarean section that was performed because of severe fetal distress. The baby had an Apgar of 5/8 and seems to be doing well in the special nursery. You are assigned to look after Ruth the morning after the operation. When you go into the room, you find her dozing. As you begin to check her vital signs, she arouses and, with a puzzled expression, asks how the baby is and what time it is. When you answer Ruth's questions, you then ask how she is feeling. She tells you that she is feeling uncomfortable and is concerned that the cesarean section had to be performed because she had gone to childbirth classes and wanted to be awake at delivery. Your response to Ruth's comment would be which of the following?

A.   "Well, It was very lucky that the cesarean section was performed because the baby's life was saved."

Go to page 333.

B.   "I know you are uncomfortable now, so let me go and get the medication for pain and then you can relax and have nothing to worry about."

Go to page 334.

C.   "You must feel very disappointed not to have gone through delivery as you expected. There was nothing you could do to prevent this from happening. It is very difficult when an emergency situation arises over which you have no control."

Go to page 332.

Your choice of *C* is good because you have allowed the mother to express her feelings about the delivery. You were supportive and reassuring. Many women who deliver by cesarean section have feelings of inadequacy as women, and if the nurse provides adequate support and reassurance, the mother is able to handle these feelings.

Advance to page 335 and take the post-test.

Your choice of *A* is *not* good because you are not allowing the mother to relive the experience of labor and delivery and express the feelings she may have.

Return to page 327. Review the material and choose another response.

Your choice of *B* is not the best, although you have identified that the mother is uncomfortable; however, that is not the complete assessment.

Return to page 327. Review the material and choose another response.

POST-TEST   Indicate whether each statement is true or false by circling the appropriate letter. Then turn to page 336 and see how well you have done.

1. Induction of labor means to give a drug to make the labor stronger.   T   F

2. Pitocin is used to induce and stimulate labor.   T   F

3. Pitocin should be discontinued if there is a tetanic contraction, and the nurse can discontinue it without a doctor's order.   T   F

4. Forceps delivery is indicated in instances of maternal exhaustion and fetal distress.   T   F

5. Postpartum hemorrhage is not a complication related to the use of obstetrical forceps.   T   F

6. When a cesarean section is an elective procedure, it is usually a low-segment operation.   T   F

7. The mother who has had a cesarean section will have more lochia than a mother who has delivered vaginally.   T   F

8. When a podalic version is indicated, it can be done any time after the cervix has dilated to 8 centimeters.   T   F

9. A second-degree perineal laceration involves the fourchet, skin, muscle, and rectal sphincter.   T   F

10. The mother with an extensive laceration and repair may have difficulty voiding and defecating.   T   F

In the specific areas with which you had difficulty, return to the material and review.

BIBLIOGRAPHY   Burke, Michael F. and Pamela Buck, ''Forceps Delivery,'' *Nursing Times*, Vol. 73,
                    No. 13, pp. 454–456, March 31, 1977.

                    Harrison, Robert F., et al., ''Assessment of Factors Constituting an Inducibility
                    Profile,'' *Obstetrics and Gynecology*, Vol. 49, No. 3, pp. 270–274, March
                    1977.

                    Pritchard Jack and Paul MacDonald: *Williams Obstetrics*, 15th ed., Appleton-
                    Century-Crofts, New York, 1976.

                    Visscher, Robert D., et al., ''Guidelines for the Elective Induction of Labor with
                    Oral Prostaglandin E_2,'' *Obstetrics and Gynecology*, Vol. 49, No. 1, p. 18,
                    Jan. 1977.

**PRETEST
ANSWERS**

1.   Labor has begun and drugs are used to increase the effectiveness of the contractions   2.   Labor has not yet begun and chemical agents are used to start labor   3.   Instruments used to aid in extracting a fetus vaginally during the second stage of labor   4.   Maternal: heart disease, toxemia, abruptio placenta, and placenta previa; fetal: prolapsed cord, distress, and malposition   5.   An operative procedure in which a fetus is delivered through an abdominal incision   6.   Classical: vertical incision through the body of the uterus; low-segment: horizontal incision through the lower uterine segment   7.   Maternal: previous section, cephalopelvic disproportion, toxemia, placenta previa, and abruptio placenta; fetal: distress and malposition   8.   The turning in utero of a fetal position into a breech presentation   9.   First-degree: laceration of the fourchet, skin, and mucus membranes of the vagina; second-degree: a first-degree laceration plus the muscles of the perineal body; third-degree: a second-degree laceration plus the rectal sphincter; fourth-degree: a third-degree laceration that includes the rectum

**POST-TEST
ANSWERS**

1. F   2. T   3. T   4. T   5. F   6. T   7. F   8. F   9. F
10. T

CHAPTER NINE

UTERINE RUPTURE AND AMNIOTIC FLUID EMBOLISM

OBJECTIVES *Identify the two types of uterine rupture.*

Identify the signs and symptoms of uterine rupture.

Identify the nursing intervention when uterine rupture occurs.

Identify the characteristics of an amniotic fluid embolism.

GLOSSARY *Rupture of the uterus:* Complete renting or partial tearing of the uterus
Amniotic fluid embolism: Amniotic fluid containing fetal cells, lanugo, vernix caseosa, and sometimes meconium which gains entrance into the maternal circulatory system via placental or cervical venous sinuses

PRETEST In the spaces provided, fill in the word or words that best complete(s) the statements. Then turn to page 343 and check your answers.

1. Rupture of the uterus occurs most frequently in the following situations:

    a. _____,

    b. _____, c. _____,

    d. _____.

2. Rupture of the uterus can be either _____ or _____.

3. When the rupture occurs, the mother will complain of _____

    _____ during _____.

4. The treatment for rupture of the uterus is _____.

5. An amniotic fluid embolism occurs after _____

    _____ and usually causes maternal _____.

6. Symptoms of amniotic fluid embolism are _____,

    _____, _____, and _____.

Rupture of the uterus is a serious complication that fortunately is a rare occurrence. There is a very high rate of fetal loss associated with this interruption, and the maternal mortality rate is significant. Rupture of the uterus occurs most frequently when there has been previous uterine surgery, or trauma from an abortion or intrauterine device. It also may occur in mothers of great parity, and the risk of such an occurrence is greatly increased by giving these mothers oxytocics during labor. Other important factors responsible for rupture of the uterus are internal podalic version, fundal pressure, and difficult forceps or breech delivery. Cephalopelvic disproportion often is associated with spontaneous rupture.

When rupture of the uterus follows a previous classical cesarean section, it is most likely to occur in the last part of pregnancy; when it follows low-segment cesarean section, it is most likely to occur during labor. The signs and symptoms are the same for rupture before labor and during it.

Rupture of the uterus occurs most frequently following _____.

uterine surgery

Oxytocics should not be used in labor with _____ _____.

mothers of great parity

When there is a spontaneous rupture of the uterus, often there exists _____.

cephalopelvic disproportion

When there is rupture of the uterus following low-segment cesarean section, the rupture usually occurs _____.

during labor

Rupture of the uterus may be *complete*, in which case the contents of the uterus spill into the abdominal cavity, or *incomplete*, with the contents retained by the uterine peritoneum or broad ligament. When the rupture occurs during a contraction, the mother experiences intense, sharp, shooting pain and may feel that something has "torn inside." Following this the contractions stop and the mother becomes more comfortable. Some slight vaginal hemorrhage may be observed. When the abdomen is palpated, the fetus is felt beside the round firm uterus. Fetal death, due to interference with circulation at the placental site as the uterus contracts, usually follows. Maternal shock follows quickly upon complete rupture.

The signs and symptoms accompanying incomplete rupture are not dramatic and may be more difficult to discern since the contractions may continue, thus delaying diagnosis and increasing the risk to the mother and baby. Signs of fetal distress are often the first indication of rupture.

A complete rupture of the uterus means that _____ the

_____ contents are spilled into the

_____ . abdominal cavity

When the rupture of the uterus is incomplete _____ the

_____ contents remain in the uterine

_____ . cavity

During the incomplete rupture, the signs and symptoms are

_____ less pronounced and difficult

_____ . to recognize

Ziegel and Van Blarcom have described premonitory signs of rupture when there is cephalopelvic disproportion: the nurse can observe a ridge or "ballooning out" of the uterus just above the symphysis pubis as the lower segment thins out and a contractile ring moves up toward the body of the uterus. Also at this time the mother experiences pain in the lower segment, and tetanic contractions may develop. Should these signs be present, immediate notification of the physician is important so that steps can be taken to prevent the rupture.[1]

The treatment includes removal of the fetus by abdominal incision (laparotomy), and usually a hysterectomy is necessary. Replacement of blood, fluids, and electrolytes is important.

The usual treatment is _____ removal of the fetus

_____ and _____ . abdominally; hysterectomy

Nursing care should be geared to close observation of mothers, especially those with a contributing history, so that any of the signs and symptoms that may occur during labor are readily identified and reported. Since there is an emergency situation, the family needs much support and as much information as possible so that family members can begin to cope. Often the baby dies before there is a possibility of saving it by surgery. The family needs help in dealing with this loss, and the mother, if she has had a hysterectomy, may also have feelings of loss of femininity and grief about never being able to have children again.

Nursing is geared to _____ close observation;

and _____ and _____ . providing information; support

An *amniotic fluid embolism* is the introduction of amniotic fluid that usually contains particles of fetal skin, vernix caseosa, and hair and sometimes contains meconium into the maternal circulation. An amniotic fluid embolism can occur during an amniocentesis, during labor or delivery once membranes have been ruptured, and in instances of uterine rupture. This material enters the venous sinuses of the placental site or the cervix and travels to the lungs. An amniotic fluid embolism is fatal in most instances. There are signs of pulmonary involvement, dyspnea, pulmonary edema, cyanosis, and shock with intravascular coagulation and hemorrhage. Death usually follows rapidly. Treatment of the shock and hemorrhage by transfusion and assistance with ventilation may be attempted. Amniotic fluid embolism tends to be found in multigravid women who have fast labors with severe contractions. Fortunately amniotic fluid embolism is a rare occurrence.

An amniotic fluid embolism occurs when _____ _____ _____ _____.

amniotic fluid containing skin, hair, and vernix enters the maternal circulation

The prognosis for the mother with an amniotic fluid embolism is _____.

grave

Signs and symptoms that indicate an amniotic embolism are _____, _____, _____ _____, and _____.

dyspnea; cyanosis; pulmonary edema; shock with hemorrhage

POST-TEST Indicate whether each statement is true or false by circling the appropriate letter. Then turn to page 343 and see how well you have done.

1. Rupture of the uterus usually causes fetal death.   T   F

2. Rupture of the uterus always is complete.   T   F

3. Amniotic fluid embolism occurs less frequently prior to rupture of membranes.   T   F

4. The mother with amniotic fluid embolism will exhibit signs of pulmonary embolism.   T   F

5. Prompt treatment in amniotic fluid embolism usually makes for a favorable prognosis.   T   F

In the specific areas with which you had difficulty, return to the material and review.

REFERENCES   1. Ziegel, Erna and Carolyn Van Blarcom: *Obstetric Nursing*, 6th ed., The Macmillan Co., New York, 1972, p. 436.

BIBLIOGRAPHY   Douglas, C. P., "Rupture of the Uterus," *Nursing Times*, Vol. 73, No. 2, pp. 240–241, Feb. 1977.

Romney, Seymour L., et al.: *Gynecology and Obstetrics: The Health Care of Women*, McGraw-Hill, New York, 1975.

PRETEST ANSWERS   1. a. Weakened cesarean section scar; b. disproportion; c. great parity; d. injudicious use of oxytocics   2. Incomplete; complete   3. Severe cutting pain; a contraction   4. Laparotomy (hysterectomy)   5. Rupture of membranes; death   6. Dyspnea; cyanosis; pulmonary edema; shock

POST-TEST ANSWERS   1. T   2. F   3. T   4. T   5. F

CHAPTER TEN

RESUSCITATION OF THE NEONATE

OBJECTIVES   *Identify factors that predispose to the development of neonatal asphyxia.*

Identify the differences between asphyxia livida and asphyxia pallida.

Identify the treatment for the above.

Identify nursing intervention when the fetus or neonate is in jeopardy.

GLOSSARY   *Apnea:* Cessation of respirations
Asphyxia neonatorum: Asphyxia, occurring shortly following delivery, in which
the infant is apneic, hypoxic, and acidotic
Asphyxia livida: Neonatal apnea characterized by deepening cyanosis
Asphyxia pallida: Neonatal apnea characterized by pallor and a shocklike
condition

PRETEST In the spaces provided, fill in the word or words that best complete(s) the statements. Then turn to page 352 and check your answers.

1. When the infant is delivered by _____,
   asphyxia is more common than when it is delivered vaginally.

2. Asphyxia livida occurs immediately after birth and presents as _____
   _____.

3. Symptoms of asphyxia pallida are _____, _____
   _____, _____
   _____, and _____.

4. When a newborn shows evidence of respiratory problems, the initial action
   of the nurse is to _____.

5. The steps involved in resuscitating the neonate with asphyxia pallida are
   _____, _____
   _____, and _____
   _____.

There are times when it is possible to predict that the baby will be depressed and will need measures instituted immediately after delivery to initiate and maintain respiratory function. This situation follows intrauterine episodes of hypoxia indicated by changes in fetal heart rate; the changes in fetal heart rate signal distress. If fetal blood sampling is done, and acidosis with low pO_2 and high pCO_2, indicating a degree of hypoxia, is present, this result would alert the staff to the need for resuscitation measures immediately following delivery. There also are certain labor and delivery situations—placenta previa, abruptio placenta, maternal diabetes, postmaturity, prolapsed cord, prematurity, toxemia, or cesarean section—which may cause the fetus to undergo a degree of hypoxia. In the above instances the delivery room staff must be alert to the possibility of a depressed infant and ready to begin measures to resuscitate the infant immediately. There also are situations in which labor and delivery are uncomplicated but the infant has undergone anoxia before birth and is in need of intervention for resuscitation.

It is possible to predict that a degree of neonatal hypoxia will be present at birth when _____ and _____ indicate fetal distress.

the fetal heart rate;

fetal blood gases

Those conditions that predispose to fetal hypoxia are _____

placenta

_____, _____,

previa; abruptio placenta;

_____, _____,

prematurity; postmaturity;

_____, _____, _____

prolapsed cord; toxemia; cesarean

_____, and _____.

section; diabetes

The neonate should be observed constantly for signs of respiratory distress while he is in the delivery room and for several hours after he is removed to the newborn nursery. One method of evaluating the newborn is the scoring system developed by Dr. Virginia Apgar. Remember that the five categories of newborn responses scored are _____, _____,

heart rate; color;

_____, _____,

respiratory effort; muscle tone;

and _____.

reflex ability

If the respiratory system is functioning well and there are no congenital anomalies, the infant will have a high Apgar (over 7). It is important to be aware of signs of immediate neonatal respiratory problems and to initiate appropriate intervention without delay.

The first, and most important, action in regard to the newborn is to clear the nasopharynx and observe the baby's respiratory efforts. If the infant does not cry within 30 seconds after birth, it is said to have neonatal respiratory distress or asphyxia neonatorum as a result of a central nervous system injury or depression before birth.

Hypoxia, often associated with acidosis, brain hemorrhage, or maternal oversedation causing fetal narcosis, is considered to be the main cause of asphyxia of the newborn. The resulting apnea may be of very short duration or may be prolonged, sometimes to death. Asphyxia neonatorum has been divided into two types characterized by their different clinical symptoms, and there are specific treatments for each.

Asphyxia livida is characterized by apnea with progressive facial and body cyanosis. The infant's muscle tone is good, and the umbilical blood vessels are full. *Asphyxia pallida* also is characterized by apnea but with skin pallor, poor muscle tone, empty umbilical blood vessels, and the infant appearing to be in shock.

When the neonate has asphyxia livida, it appears _____ and _____ and has _____.

> apneic;
> cyanotic; good muscle tone

On the other hand, the neonate who has asphyxia pallida appears _____ and _____ and has _____ and ___ _____ _____. This infant appears to be in _____.

> apneic; very pale;
> empty cord vessels; poor
> muscle tone; shock

When the infant has asphyxia livida, the intervention method usually is gentle stimulation through tapping of the soles of the infant's feet and rubbing of the back. While the infant is receiving this stimulation, oxygen is administered, often by mask.

If the infant has asphyxia pallida, then immediate measures are initiated. Suctioning of the nasopharynx is done gently so as not to injure the nasopharynx or cause further spasm of the pharynx. Many factors need simultaneous attention. You must keep the infant warm by quickly drying the head and body, to prevent evaporation from causing further decrease of temperature. If the infant is anoxic, the fat and glycogen stores are unable to be metabolized for heat. After suctioning of the nose and nasopharynx, artificial ventilation is attempted by extension of the head to a sniffing position and use of either mouth-to-mouth resuscitation or a positive-pressure mask. Oxygen-enriched air is administered. It is important to check for lung sounds that indicate expansion and airflow. Often this stimulation is enough to start spontaneous respirations. If it is unsuccessful, a laryngoscope is inserted to visualize the trachea below the epiglottis, and an endotracheal tube is inserted. Often deep suction on the endotracheal tube will dislodge

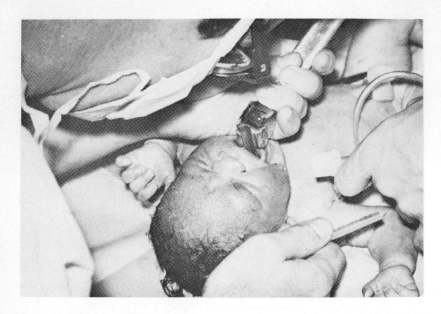

Use of the laryngoscope to insert an endotracheal tube under direct vision. *(From Williams Obstetrics, 15th ed., by Jack Pritchard and Paul Mac-Donald. Copyright © 1976, Appleton-Century-Crofts. Used with permission of Appleton-Century Crofts.)*

foreign debris such as mucus, meconium, or blood that has been aspirated. Then ventilation is begun with the endotracheal tube in place, usually by the operator filling his or her mouth with oxygen from a line and blowing gentle puffs into the tube of not more than 30 centimeters of water pressure. This is done about 30 times a minute. If the heartbeat is absent or below 60 then external cardiac massage is initiated, with the operator's middle and index finger over the middle third of the sternum. The sternum is depressed only 1 to 2 centimeters. The rate is four cardiac beats to one breath. While the lungs are being filled, cardiac massage stops, thereby preventing rupture of the lungs.

When the infant is apneic, there is a rapidly increasing acidosis that adds further to the depression of the respirations. This can be corrected by the administration of sodium bicarbonate, usually given through the umbilical vein. There is some concern about using this vein because of the danger of thrombosis, infection, and air embolism. Suggestions for using the extremities for intravenous medication and fluid have been made, but the problem is that those veins are small and it is difficult to maintain a flow because of infiltration. It is important to administer the sodium bicarbonate in small doses or mixed with glucose so that the hypertonic solution of the sodium bicarbonate itself does not cause damage to the central nervous system. Intracardiac injections of epinephrine are rarely used. Usually the infant responds to these measures. At other times the infant may need artificial ventilation for a long period. The infant is moved to an intensive care area.

Before artificial ventilation is begun it is important to

‗‗‗
‗‗‗‗‗‗‗‗‗‗‗‗‗‗‗‗‗‗‗‗‗‗‗‗‗‗‗‗.

Drying the infant off prevents heat loss through ‗‗‗‗‗‗‗‗‗‗‗.

Often the trachea will be blocked by foreign debris such as
‗‗‗‗‗‗‗‗‗‗, ‗‗‗‗‗‗‗‗‗‗‗‗, and ‗‗‗‗‗‗‗‗‗‗‗‗.

Artificial ventilation is done at the rate of ‗‗‗‗‗‗‗‗‗‗‗‗
‗‗‗‗‗‗‗‗‗‗‗. If the cardiac rate is less than ‗‗‗‗‗‗‗‗‗‗
‗‗‗‗‗‗‗‗‗‗‗‗‗‗‗‗‗‗‗‗‗‗‗‗‗ then external massage is done.

Treatment for the neonate with asphyxia livida is ‗‗‗‗‗‗‗‗‗‗‗‗
and ‗‗‗‗‗‗‗‗‗‗‗‗.

Intervention measures used with the neonate who has asphyxia
pallida include ‗‗‗‗‗‗‗‗‗‗‗‗‗, ‗‗‗‗‗‗‗‗‗‗‗‗‗‗‗‗
‗‗‗‗‗‗‗‗‗‗‗‗‗‗‗‗‗‗‗‗‗‗‗‗‗‗‗‗‗‗‗‗‗‗,
and ‗‗‗‗‗‗‗‗‗‗‗‗‗‗‗‗‗‗‗‗‗‗‗‗.

suction the nose and
nasopharynx
evaporation
mucus; blood; meconium
30 per
minute; 60
beats per minute
stimulation;
oxygen
suction; assisted
ventilation with oxygen;
sodium bicarbonate

Since neonatal resuscitation is the responsibility of the best-prepared person in the delivery room, it is essential that all nurses, doctors,
and anesthetists be well-trained in this technique.

Chemical stimulants have been found to be ineffective in restoring
and promoting respiratory function. However, if the mother has been
sedated with narcotics late in labor, narcotic antagonists such as Lorfan
or Nalline may be administered to the neonate via the umbilical vein.

Once the baby is able to sustain the respiratory function inde-
pendently and has been moved to the nursery, careful observation must
be continuous because the insult of the asphyxia may have seriously
decreased the effectiveness of the infant's adaptive mechanisms. The
nurse must be alert to signs of further respiratory difficulties.

Asphyxia neonatorum or ‗‗‗‗‗‗‗‗‗‗‗‗‗‗‗‗‗‗‗‗‗‗
‗‗‗‗‗‗‗‗‗‗‗‗‗‗‗‗‗‗‗‗ is said to occur if there have been no
respiratory efforts by ‗‗‗‗‗‗‗‗ seconds after birth.

It is thought to be caused by intrauterine ‗‗‗‗‗‗‗‗‗‗‗‗‗‗
‗‗‗‗‗‗‗‗‗‗‗‗‗‗‗‗‗‗‗‗‗‗‗‗‗ injury or depression.

If the asphyxia is caused by narcotism of the mother, the
newborn may be treated with ‗‗‗‗‗‗‗‗‗‗‗‗ antagonists
injected into the umbilical ‗‗‗‗‗‗‗‗‗‗‗‗‗‗‗.

neonatal respiratory
distress;
30
central
nervous system
narcotic;
vein

When being stimulated, the baby should be handled _____   gently;
and should be kept _____.   warm

In the newborn nursery, the baby who has suffered respiratory
distress should be _____.   watched carefully

When resuscitation measures are initiated in the delivery room,
often there are many people crowded about the infant. The parents'
fears for the well-being of the baby become paramount, and it is important for the nurse and the staff to interpret to them the measures
that are being employed with the infant and the reasons why these are
necessary during this crisis situation. The explanations can be simple,
such as, "The baby is having difficulty breathing and needs help and
some oxygen." Usually as soon as the infant begins respiration on its
own, it emits a cry, and this begins to reassure the parents that the
infant is alive. Explanations about the follow-up care in the special
nursery include information that it is important to keep a close watch
over the infant to make sure that everything is all right. Parents can
deal with the truth, and it is important to be honest with them so that
they do not begin to fantasize about the infant's condition.

POST-TEST   Indicate whether each statement is true or false by circling the appropriate letter. Then turn to page 352 and see how well you have done.

1. Neonatal respiratory distress is defined as no respiratory efforts for five seconds or more.   T   F

2. Asphyxia neonatorum is thought to be a result of central nervous system injury or depression.   T   F

3. If the baby does not breathe spontaneously, a respiratory stimulant should be administered after the nasopharynx is cleared.   T   F

4. After the airway is cleared, when the infant is suffering from asphyxia pallida, oxygen should be administered under positive pressure.   T   F

5. It also is important to keep the infant at a stable 95° temperature to decrease metabolism until respirations are restored.   T   F

6. A newborn in respiratory distress should be resuscitated by the best-prepared person.   T   F

In the specific areas with which you had difficulty, return to the material and review.

BIBLIOGRAPHY   Auld, Peter, "Resuscitation of the Newborn Infant," *American Journal of Nursing*, Vol. 74, No. 1, pp. 68–70, Jan. 1974.

Evans, Marian, "Adaptation of the Infant at Birth and Intervention Techniques for Distressed Neonate," *Journal of Nurse-Midwifery*, Vol. XX, No. 4, pp. 18–28, Winter 1975.

Pritchard, Jack and Paul MacDonald: *Williams Obstetrics*, 15th ed., Appleton-Century-Crofts, New York, 1976.

Roberts, Florence Bright: *Perinatal Nursing*, McGraw-Hill Book Co., NewYork, 1977.

**PRETEST
ANSWERS**   1.   Cesarean section   2.   Apnea, associated with increasing cyanosis   3.   Pallor; empty cord vessels; shocklike condition; apnea   4.   Clear the nasopharynx   5.   Suction of nasopharynx; assisted ventilation with oxygen; administration of sodium bicarbonate

**POST-TEST
ANSWERS**   1. F   2. T   3. F   4. T   5. F   6. T

CHAPTER ELEVEN

EARLY POSTPARTUM HEMORRHAGE

OBJECTIVES   *Define postpartum hemorrhage.*

Identify a physical indication of uterine hemorrhage.

Identify four factors that predispose to postpartum hemorrhage.

Identify three factors that create a maternal high-risk situation.

Identify nursing intervention when the mother's postpartum period is complicated by hemorrhage.

Differentiate between early and late postpartum hemorrhage.

GLOSSARY   *Late postpartum hemorrhage:* Over 500 cubic centimeters of blood loss through the vagina during the puerperium, after the first 24 hours within the postpartum period

Polyhydramnios: An excessive amount of amniotic fluid

Early postpartum hemorrhage: Over 500 cubic centimeters of blood loss, due to parturition, between the third stage of labor and 24 hours after delivery

Secundines: The placenta and the amnion and chorion

Traumatic delivery: Any delivery that causes injury to the maternal tissues, i.e., the use of forceps, podalic version, or manual extraction of the placenta

Atony: Lack of normal muscle tone

PRETEST In the spaces provided, fill in the word or words that best complete(s) the statements. Then turn to page 363 and check your answers.

1. "Early postpartum hemorrhage" is _____

   _____

   _____

   _____

   _____.

2. It is essential that the delivery room staff palpate the mother's _____ for indications of bleeding.

3. If the mother is bleeding, often the uterus will be _____.

4. Postpartum hemorrhage is the _____ cause of postpartal morbidity and mortality.

5. Three factors that predispose to postpartum hemorrhage are _____

   _____, _____

   _____, and _____

   _____.

6. Situations that may lead to uterine atony are _____

   _____, _____, _____,

   _____, and _____.

7. If a mother is having increased uterine bleeding, the nurse will first

   _____ and then _____

   _____.

8. A chemical agent that may be used to help control bleeding is an

   _____.

9. Late postpartum hemorrhage occurs after _____ postpartum and during the period of the puerperium.

As labor progresses to its culmination and all interest becomes centered on the neonate, it is essential that the care of the mother not be neglected. The delivery room nurse must be aware that the fundus of the mother should be watched carefully during the first hour postpartum, called the fourth stage of labor. It is during this critical period that the mother is most prone to *postpartum hemorrhage*, usually due to uterine atony.

Postpartum hemorrhage is defined as maternal bleeding of more than 500 cubic centimeters after parturition. Sometimes this is difficult to estimate; a drop of 6 percent in the hematocrit from predelivery is significant.

Remember, immediately after delivery the uterus drops down to a position between the umbilicus and the _____   symphysis
_____ .   pubis

The fundus should be palpated as a _____ mass   firm;
that, by one hour postpartum, rises to about the level of the
_____ .   umbilicus

As long as the fundus remains contracted, there usually is no fear of uterine bleeding. Therefore, the nurse must be constantly vigilant concerning the condition of the fundus. It also must be remembered that blood can collect in the uterus and vaginal bleeding may not become evident for several hours. The only way that this type of insidious bleeding can be detected is by abdominal palpation of the fundus at frequent intervals.

Postpartum hemorrhage, the leading cause of maternal morbidity and mortality, can be effectively controlled by a vigilant staff. It is important that the course of labor and delivery be carefully recorded so that the delivery room staff and postpartum staff can be aware of those mothers that may be high-risk.

Postpartum hemorrhage may occur as a result of poor uterine tone; inability of the uterus to contract effectively, often due to retained secundines; lacerations of the cervix and/or vagina; or a perineal tear or episiotomy extension. In addition, the mother who has had a long or traumatic delivery, an overdistended uterus, or large amounts of anesthesia is more prone to this complication of the postpartum period than the mother who has not had these experiences.

The nurse in the delivery room is responsible for palpating the mother's fundus frequently during the first hour after the _____ .   delivery

If the fundus is firm this is an indication that the mother is not having undue _____ from the uterus.

bleeding

Should the uterus be relaxed and the mother bleed 500 cubic centimeters or more after the delivery, she is said to have _____.

postpartum hemorrhage

The leading cause of maternal morbidity and mortality during the maternity cycle is _____.

postpartum hemorrhage

A mother who has had a forceps delivery, a multiple pregnancy, polyhydramnios, or a long labor is considered to be _____.

high-risk

A vigilant staff can diminish the effects of hemorrhage. Recent studies show that most postpartum hemorrhage is of the insidious type rather than being due to an apparent massive amount of bleeding. It is necessary to intervene immediately, within five hours, to prevent maternal death. If other stressors, as well as hemorrhage, are operating the mother is more at risk.

The nurse must be aware of the signs of severe blood loss (shock); therefore frequent monitoring of the mother's vital signs is necessary.

If, while caring for a postpartal mother, you should become aware of a relaxed uterus, your first action would be to grasp the fundus and massage it firmly. This will cause the mother discomfort, and she should be given an explanation of the reason for your action. Most people are extremely fearful about bleeding and often exaggerate the amount of bleeding present because of their anxiety. It therefore is essential that the nurse remain calm and communicate to the mother complete control of the situation. When the uterus becomes firm, the massaging should be discontinued, for overmassage contributes to muscle fatigue and further uterine relaxation. The mother should be carefully watched, for bleeding may resume. Since the bleeding usually is a continuous trickle, it is important for the nurse to keep count of the number of perineal pads used and the amount of saturation. In order to control the bleeding, it sometimes is necessary for the nurse to administer the prescribed oxytocic after expelling clots from the uterus.

If the bleeding continues, an intravenous should be started and the mother should be typed and crossmatched with blood for transfusion in case a blood transfusion should become necessary. The physician should be notified of the bleeding at its onset and kept informed of the mother's condition.

If the nurse becomes aware of a relaxed uterus, the first action would be to _____.

massage it

Fundal massage should be discontinued when _____ | the uterus
_____. | becomes firm

Another way to assess the amount of bleeding is for the nurse to keep a _____. | peri-pad count

If the bleeding continues, the nurse may express clots from the uterus and administer a prescribed _____ to help the uterus to contract. | oxytocic

It is important for the mother to be informed, upon discharge, how she can reach her obstetrician or the hospital medical staff if she is a staff patient. Occasionally, a mother may not hemorrhage until after discharge. A *late postpartum hemorrhage* is one that occurs after the first 24 hours following delivery and within the puerperium. This type of hemorrhage usually is a sudden, massive blood loss from the vagina. It usually is due to retained placental fragments or subinvolution of the placental site. The mother usually is at home and alone when this occurs and needs immediate transportation to the hospital and someone to care for her infant. The mother must be examined, and a dilatation and curettage usually is performed to remove any retained placenta.

Late postpartum hemorrhage occurs _____ | 24 hours;
following delivery and within _____. | puerperium

Late postpartum hemorrhage usually is due to _____ | retained
_____ or _____. | placental fragments; subinvolution

If the mother develops late postpartum hemorrhage, treatment should be immediate _____. | hospitalization

Now, let us look at a situation in which you are caring for a woman who exhibits symptoms of this condition.

Olive Marks, a twenty-three-year-old, Gravida II, Para II, has just delivered a 7¾-pound boy ½ hour ago. The baby has been taken to the nursery for admission and care, while Jim, the father, has just left to notify the relatives. You are giving Olive postpartum care in the delivery room. Her vital signs are blood pressure 95/60, pulse 90, respirations 24. When you check her fundus, it is two fingerbreadths above the umbilicus and soft. When you massage the fundus, several big clots are expelled, and there is a large amount of bright red lochia.

You would do which of the following set of actions?

A.   Check Olive's lochia every five minutes when you check

the level and consistency of the fundus, explaining to her why it is necessary to do this.

Go to page 359.

B. Notify the physician, place Olive in Trendelenberg position, and have an intravenous setup ready to be started and oxytocics available. Monitor the blood pressure, and check the fundus and lochia.

Go to page 360.

C. Have Olive cross her legs, and then examine the maternal surface of the placenta to make sure that it is intact. Then check the vital signs and fundus again.

Go to page 361.

A is not the best choice, although you want to know Olive's current status. You have not assessed the situation adequately.

Return to page 355. Review the material and choose another response.

Your choice of *B* indicates a very good assessment of Olive's status. She is losing a large amount of blood with the clots and the lochia, and the body responses are attempting to adapt, as seen with the rapid pulse and lowering blood pressure. Your actions assist the body's attempt to increase the blood circulation through the brain and major organs. And you are getting medication ready for the physician in case he should order this to assist in keeping the fundus firm and to replace fluid volume.

Advance to page 362 and take the post-test.

Your choice of *C* is not good. The most important thing is to stay with Olive and initiate measures that are restorative, promotive, and preventive in nature.

Return to page 355. Review the material and choose another response.

POST-TEST   Indicate whether each statement is true or false by circling the appropriate letter. Then turn to page 363 and see how well you have done.

1. It is normal for a mother to lose between 450 and 550 cubic centimeters of blood during parturition.   T   F

2. As long as the mother's fundus is firm, there is no reason to be concerned about hemorrhage.   T   F

3. Postpartum hemorrhage really is no threat to the postpartal mother.   T   F

4. The most common cause of early postpartum hemorrhage is subinvolution of the placental site.   T   F

5. Multiple pregnancy, anesthesia, or extension of episiotomy may be causative factors in postpartum hemorrhage.   T   F

6. The first action of the nurse when the mother is having untoward bleeding is to massage the fundus.   T   F

7. An intravenous should be started, the mother's blood typed and crossmatched, and an oxytocic administered if the bleeding continues.   T   F

8. It is essential to keep the parents well informed about what is being done.   T   F

9. Postpartum hemorrhage is considered late when it occurs after the mother has left the delivery room.   T   F

10. Late postpartum hemorrhage often is due to retained placental fragments.   T   F

In the specific areas with which you had difficulty, return to the material and review.

BIBLIOGRAPHY   Pritchard, Jack and Paul MacDonald: *Williams Obstetrics*, 15th ed., Appleton-Century-Crofts, New York, 1976.

Romney, Seymour L., et al.: *Gynecology and Obstetrics: The Health Care of Women*, McGraw-Hill Book Co., New York, 1975.

PRETEST ANSWERS   1. Vaginal bleeding of over 500 cubic centimeters which occurs anytime following the delivery of the baby up to the first 24 hours postpartum   2. Fundus   3. Relaxed   4. Primary   5. Any of the following: uterine atony; retained placental fragments; lacerations of the cervix or vagina; extension of the episiotomy   6. Overdistended uterus; traumatic delivery; long labor; exhaustion; general anesthesia   7. Massage the uterus; notify the physician   8. Oxytoxic   9. 24 hours

POST-TEST ANSWERS   1. F   2. F   3. F   4. F   5. T   6. T   7. T   8. T   9. F   10. T

UNIT V
EXAMINATION
The following multiple-choice examination will test your comprehension of the material covered in the fifth unit of this program. Remember, you are not competing with anyone but yourself. Therefore, do not guess in order to answer the questions; if you are unsure, this means that you have not learned the content. Return to the areas that give you difficulty and review them before going on with the examination.

Circle the letter of the best response to each question. After completing the unit examination, check your answers on page 541 and review those areas of difficulty before proceeding to the next unit.

1. When the mother is in labor and the fetal heart is being monitored, a type I dip, or early deceleration, indicates that there is:
   a. Cord compression
   b. Placental insufficiency
   c. Head compression
   d. Tetanic contractions

2. If, while monitoring the fetal heart rate, during two consecutive contractions you noticed decelerations at the acme of each contraction, your first action would be to:
   a. Record it on the chart
   b. Reassure the mother that everything was fine
   c. Report to the doctor type II dips, late decelerations
   d. Report to the doctor type I dips, early decelerations

3. Upon identifying prolapse of the umbilical cord, the nurse's first action would be to:
   a. Notify the doctor
   b. Replace the cord in the vagina
   c. Cover the cord with saline-soaked sterile dressings
   d. Change the mother's position to knee-chest or Trendelenberg

4. The reason for changing the position of a mother when a prolapse of the cord is identified is to:
   a. Increase circulation to the mother's uterus
   b. Take pressure off the inferior vena cava
   c. Take pressure off the umbilical cord
   d. Increase the pressure on the fetal presenting part

5. You are caring for Mabel Holmes, who is in labor three weeks before her EDC. She is Gravida II, Para I, and the cervix is 4-centimeters dilated. As you plan her care, you will assess which of the following more frequently?
   a. Blood pressure
   b. Fetal heart rate
   c. Temperature
   d. Pulse and respirations

6. Premature rupture of membranes:
   a. Is most dangerous for the mother
   b. Is most dangerous for the fetus

    c. Is equally dangerous to the mother and fetus

    d. Causes no concern

7. An antibiotic given to the mother prophylactically following premature rupture of membranes:

    a. Can prevent fetal infection

    b. Can prevent amnionitis

    c. Can prevent maternal and fetal infection

    d. Is ineffectual for aiding in the prevention of either maternal or fetal infection

8. When you are in the labor room, you find that Mrs. S has been diagnosed as having dystocia. This means that:

    a. Labor is progressing very rapidly

    b. There is cessation of the progress

    c. The membranes have ruptured, but no contractions have begun

    d. The mother is overdue, but no labor has started

9. Hypertonic uterine inertia is characterized by:

    a. A long active phase

    b. Pain out of proportion to the type of contraction

    c. Treatment by the use of oxytocics

    d. The need to prepare the mother for cesarean section

10. A mother who has prolonged labor in the latent phase is treated by:

    a. Having her rest and giving her sedation

    b. Having her up walking around the unit

    c. Stimulating labor with Methergine

    d. Terminating the pregnancy by a cesarean section

11. If during labor the mother continually complains of severe back pain, the nurse might suspect which type of presentation?

    a. Posterior

    b. Transverse

    c. Anterior

    d. Oblique

12. Upon hearing the doctor say that she has complete breech presentation, the mother asks you what that means. Your best response would be:

    a. "It really is nothing to worry about, so don't be upset."

    b. "I understand how these strange words may be upsetting, but don't worry; everything is under control and you and the baby are fine."

    c. "Why do you seem so upset? Have you had an experience or heard anything fearful about breech deliveries?"

    d. "It means that the baby is in a squatting position rather than having the head down first."

13. The presence of meconium-stained amniotic fluid when there is a breech presentation usually is:

    a. Of no undue concern

       b.   Evidence of fetal distress
       c.   Evidence of fetal anoxia
       d.   Evidence of fetal and maternal intrauterine infection

14. When the mother is receiving a continuous epidural anesthesia, it is important that she should be:
       a.   In semi-Fowler's position
       b.   In Simm's position
       c.   Supine
       d.   Flat on her side

15. When the mother is receiving a saddle block, it means that the nurse must check more frequently:
       a.   Fetal heart rate
       b.   Blood pressure
       c.   Pulse rate
       d.   Contractions

16. When the mother receives general anesthesia during delivery, intubation is necessary since:
       a.   The mother needs assisted ventilation
       b.   The nitrous oxide is more effective
       c.   There is a danger of aspiration
       d.   The mother does not achieve complete relaxation without this

17. Induction of labor is done when the cervix is "ripe," with the use of:
       a.   An analgesic
       b.   An oxytocic
       c.   A hematinic
       d.   An antihistaminic

18. Forceps are applied to the fetal head only when the:
       a.   Presenting part is at station -2
       b.   Membranes are intact and the head at station 0
       c.   Cervix is 8 centimeters dilated and the presenting part at station $+1$
       d.   Membranes are ruptured and the cervix fully dilated

19. Low forceps are used when the baby's head is at the level of:
       a.   The spines
       b.   Station $+1$
       c.   Station -1
       d.   The perineum

20. Podalic version is when the baby is turned in utero to:
       a.   A vertex presentation
       b.   A breech presentation
       c.   An LOP position
       d.   An LOA position

21. When caring for a mother who has had a cesarean section delivery, you would expect her lochial discharge to be:
    a. Greater than after a vaginal delivery
    b. The same as after a vaginal delivery
    c. Less than after a vaginal delivery
    d. Completely absent

22. A second-degree laceration is one that:
    a. Involves the fourchet, the perineal skin, and the vaginal mucus membranes
    b. Extends through the skin, mucus membranes, rectal sphincter, and rectum
    c. Involves the skin, the mucus membranes, and the muscles of the perineal body
    d. Extends completely through the skin, mucus membranes, perineal body, and rectal sphincter

23. During labor, if the mother felt sudden severe cutting pain during a contraction and exhibited signs of shock, you would suspect that:
    a. She had placenta previa
    b. The uterus had ruptured
    c. She had a cardiac problem
    d. She has hypotonic inertia

24. A noncardiac mother who suddenly shows signs of dyspnea and cyanosis after amniotomy may have suffered:
    a. A ruptured uterus
    b. Uterine hemorrhage
    c. Precipitous delivery
    d. Pulmonary embolism

25. If a newborn shows signs of respiratory distress, the first action of the nurse in the delivery room would be to:
    a. Place the infant in a cool isolette with oxygen
    b. Administer oxygen under positive pressure
    c. Suction the nasopharynx
    d. Pass an endotracheal tube to make sure there were no mucus plugs

26. In order to control postpartum hemorrhage, the nurse would:
    a. Massage the fundus every 10 to 15 minutes for the first hour after delivery
    b. Massage the fundus when it felt soft
    c. Check the placenta for intactness before removing it from the delivery room
    d. Teach the mother how to palpate her own fundus and when to call the nurse

UNIT VI

INTERRUPTIONS IN HEALTH IN THE POSTPARTUM PERIOD

CHAPTER ONE

INTERRUPTIONS OF THE GENITOURINARY SYSTEMS

OBJECTIVES *Identify and define puerperal infections.*

Identify the dangers of puerperal infections.

Identify the factors that predispose to puerperal infections.

Identify the two major types of puerperal infections.

Identify nursing intervention to be instituted in the presence of a puerperal infection.

Define cystitis.

Identify signs and symptoms of cystitis.

Identify nursing intervention to be instituted in preventing and treating this condition.

Define subinvolution of the uterus.

Identify signs and symptoms of subinvolution.

Identify factors responsible for subinvolution.

Identify preventive and treatment measures for this condition.

Identify nursing intervention measures utilized in preventing and treating subinvolution.

Define mastitis.

Identify signs and symptoms of mastitis.

Identify nursing assessment and intervention measures for mastitis.

GLOSSARY   *Puerperal infection:* A postpartal inflammatory response of the genital tract accompanying invasion of pathogenic organisms, signaled by an elevation of temperature to 100.4°F during any two days of the postpartum period not including any elevation within the first 24 hours following delivery.

Local puerperal infection: Infectious process confined to a particular area: the endometrium, cervix, vagina, vulva, or perineum

Extended puerperal infection: Systemic spread of the original process occurring as the circulatory and lymphatic systems become involved

Endometritis: Inflammation of the lining of the uterus

Metritis: Inflammation of the musculature of the uterus

Pelvic cellulitis: Inflammatory process affecting the connective tissues of the uterus and/or the broad ligament, also termed ''parametritis''

Cystitis: Inflammation of the bladder

Residual urine: A volume of 60 cubic centimeters or more of urine remaining in the bladder following spontaneous voiding

Retention of urine: Inability to void or expel urine from the bladder

Mastitis: Inflammation of the mammary glands and their surrounding tissues.

Parenchymous mastitis: Inflammatory response of one or more lobes of the mammary glands

Periglandular mastitis: Inflammatory process taking place in the fat and loose tissues found between the mammary lobes

Subinvolution of the uterus: The failure of the uterus to return to a nonpregnant state in size and firmness and to descend progressively into the pelvic cavity

Submammary abscess: Inflammatory and suppurative process taking place within the connective tissues underneath the mammary glands

PRETEST In the spaces provided, fill in the word or words that best complete(s) the statements. Then turn to page 395 and check your answers.

1. The symptom generally accepted as signaling the onset of a puerperal infection is _____

_____

_____

_____ .

2. Factors that predispose to puerperal infections are _____ ,

_____ , _____ , and

_____ .

3. Puerperal infections are categorized as _____ and as

_____ of the original process.

4. The pathogenic organism most commonly responsible for the development of a puerperal infection is _____ .

5. Endometritis is _____

_____ .

6. Signs of parametritis include _____ , _____

_____ , and _____

_____ .

7. The danger that is present when thrombophlebitis occurs is _____

_____

_____ .

8. Peritonitis occurs as a result of _____

_____

_____

_____ .

9. When the mother develops puerperal infection, the baby is _____

_____ .

10. Treatment of the infectious process includes _____ ,

_____ , _____ , and

_____ .

11. During the postpartum period, a common alteration of the urinary tract is

_____ .

12. Conditions that predispose to the development of cystitis are _____ _____ and _____ .

13. Symptoms associated with cystitis are _____ _____ and _____ .

14. The best preventive measures for this condition are associated with close observation of the mother. Some of these preventive measures are
   a. _____ _____ _____ ; b. _____ _____ ; and c. _____ _____ _____ .

15. Therapeutic approaches consist of _____ , _____ , and _____ _____ .

16. Subinvolution of the uterus is a complication of the postpartum period defined as _____ _____ _____ _____ .

17. Causative elements of subinvolution are a. _____ _____ ; b. _____ ; c. _____ _____ ; d. _____ .

18. Symptoms of subinvolution are a. _____ ; b. _____ ; c. _____ .

19. When subinvolution occurs as a result of lack of muscle tone, _____ may be prescribed.

20. Mastitis is an _____ _____ .

21. Three types of mastitis are _____ , _____, and _____ _____.

22. Onset of mastitis usually takes place between the _____ and _____ weeks of the puerperium.

23. The organism most commonly responsible for this interruption is _____.

PUERPERAL INFECTIONS

The first volume of this series identified the fact that the period following the delivery of the baby and the placenta is characterized by rapid physiological and anatomical changes in the mother. Because of their sudden nature, these changes represent stressful situations for the woman as she mobilizes all her available resources in adapting and effecting restoration of a positive homeodynamic balance.

This period, usually referred to as the "postpartum period," also is known as the period of the _____ and generally lasts for _____ to _____ weeks.

> puerperium;
> five; six

Under normal circumstances, the postpartum period is a critical time for the mother since anatomical and physiological systems either rapidly alter to nonpregnant states, as in the case of uterine involution, or progress in a slower manner, as exemplified by the breast changes taking place in the lactating mother. Preexisting health interruptions or nonhealth states brought about by the pregnancy itself often can, and do, produce high-risk situations for the mother which require immediate assessment measures and call for specific intervention techniques to effect restoration to a positive homeodynamic balance. One of the most commonly found and most serious interruptions in maternal health during the puerperium is puerperal infection.

High-risk situations for the mother during the puerperium may be brought about by preexisting _____ _____ or by nonhealth states brought about by _____ _____.

> nonhealth
> states; the
> pregnancy

One of the most common interruptions in maternal health during this period is _____.

> puerperal infection

A *puerperal infection*, also known as "postpartum fever," "childbirth fever," or "puerperal sepsis," is the postpartal infectious process that develops when pathogenic organisms invade the genital tract. A puerperal infection is signaled by an elevation of body temperature to 38°C (100.4°F) during any two days of the postpartum period not including any elevation that may appear within the first 24 hours following the delivery of the baby and the placenta. The incidence of puerperal infection is statistically referred to as "puerperal morbidity."

When an inflammatory process develops in the genital tract as a result of _____ by _____ organisms, it is known as a _____.

invasion; pathogenic; puerperal infection

Historically, puerperal infections were the most common causes of maternal deaths. After the discovery of the fact that microorganisms introduced into the maternal genitalia were responsible for the presence of puerperal infections, the use of aseptic techniques and antibiotics led to the decreased incidence of maternal deaths. Nonetheless, puerperal infection is still a leading cause of death in childbearing.

Interruptions in health that occur during labor, such as prolonged traumatic labor, prematurely ruptured membranes, hemorrhage, anemia, and retention of placental tissues, are factors that predispose to the development of a puerperal infection.

Puerperal infection is one of the leading causes of _____.

maternal deaths

Three factors have been responsible for the decrease of mortality rates as a result of postpartum infections: (1) recognition that _____ entering the _____ _____ _____ _____ set up infectious processes, (2) application of _____ techniques, and (3) the discovery of _____.

microorganisms; tissues of the generative tract; aseptic; antibiotics

Factors that predispose to the development of a puerperal infection may be _____ _____, _____, _____ , _____ _____ , and _____ of _____tissue.

a prolonged traumatic labor; anemia; hemorrhage; prematurely ruptured membranes; retention placental

Puerperal infections generally are categorized under two major types: A *local* puerperal infection is one in which the infectious process may remain confined to a particular site or area; this usually is the case in situations in which the cervix, vulva, vagina, or perineum has been lacerated or traumatized. An *extended puerperal infection* is one in which a systemic spread of the infection occurs as the circulatory and lymphatic systems become involved.

Puerperal infection may be a _____ infection or

local;

an extension in which the _____ process spreads
through the _____ and _____ systems.

After the completion of the third stage of labor, the site of previous
placental attachment is a bleeding area and thus becomes an ideal portal
of entry for invading microorganisms. Susceptibility of this area is
increased by the fact that at this time the decidua is infiltrated with
blood and becomes an excellent medium for the growth and reproduc-
tion of invading bacteria.

Other anatomical structures may be subjected to an infectious
process if their integrity has been damaged during the processes of
labor and delivery. The perineal body is particularly susceptible to the
invasion of pathogenic organisms if it has sustained lacerations during
the delivery of the baby or if an episiotomy has been performed.

Injuries and contusions of the vulva produced by the utilization
of forceps during delivery and vaginal and cervical lacerations that may
have taken place as a result of a traumatic delivery also are susceptible
to infections.

There are several anatomical structures that are particularly
susceptible to the action of microorganisms and thus to the development of an infectious process. One structure is the site of
_____ attachment; this area is _____
and _____. It provides for an ideal portal of entry for
_____.

placental; open;

bleeding;

microorganisms

Since the lining of the uterus at this time is infiltrated with
_____, it provides an excellent medium for the
_____ of invading bacteria.

blood;

growth

Another structure that may be subjected to the development of
an infectious process is the _____ body if trauma such
as _____ has occurred during delivery or if an
_____ has been performed.

perineal;

lacerations;

episiotomy

Injuries and _____ of the _____
may be produced by operative obstetrical methods.

contusions; vulva

The bacteria that are known to produce an infectious process
during the puerperium can be *endogenous*, such as the anaerobic streptococcus organism frequently found in the vagina of pregnant women,
or *exogenous*, any number of pathogenic organisms that are introduced

into the birth canal by external sources. In the former case, the bacteria normally present in the external reproductive organs, although nonpathogenic as a rule, are activated by the presence of trauma or devitalized tissue. This type of infection accounts for over half of the cases of puerperal sepsis found. The latter type of infection usually is transferred by infected instruments, a break in surgically aseptic technique during vaginal examinations, organisms present in the nasopharynxes of those in attendance during labor, or contamination of the genital canal by fecal material during the second stage of labor.

Puerperal infections can be caused by two types of bacteria: _____ and _____.

    endogenous; exogenous

Endogenous bacteria usually are present in the _____;

    vagina;

these bacteria are not capable of producing infection under normal circumstances and therefore are usually _____.

    nonpathogenic;

However they can create an infectious process in the presence of _____. This type of bacterial invasion is responsible

    trauma;

for about _____ of the reported incidences of puerperal

    half

infections.

Bacterial contamination also can take place through invasion of _____ organisms not found within the female re-

    pathogenic;

productive organs. Contamination with external pathogens usually comes about by the utilization of _____,

    infected instruments;

through a break in _____ during

    surgical asepsis;

_____ of the mother while

    vaginal examinations;

she is in labor, from organisms present in the _____ of

    nasopharynxes;

the staff during labor, or by contamination of the genital canal by _____ material during the _____ stage

    fecal; second

of labor.

The symptoms of local inflammatory and infectious processes of the perineum, vulva, vagina, or cervix are pain, burning on urination, sensation of heat, discoloration of tissues, edema, and presence of purulent discharge. These reactions usually are accompanied by a temperature elevation ranging from 100.4 to 101°F (38.4°C).

Local inflammatory responses signaling the presence of a puerperal infection are _____, sensation of _____,

    pain; heat;

_____ on urination, _____ ,   burning; edema;

and the presence of _____ .   discharge

A fever of _____ to _____ may be   100.4; 101°F (38.4°C)

present.

If microorganisms have invaded the uterus and have set up an
infectious process at the site of placental attachment, *endometritis*, or
inflammation of the lining of the uterus, takes place. A rapid spread
of the infection to the musculature of the uterus is known as *metritis*.
If the infection has spread through the circulatory and lymphatic systems to the connective tissues surrounding the uterus and/or the broad
ligaments, it is called *parametritis* or *pelvic cellulitis*.

Endometritis is the _____ of the _____   inflammation; lining;

of the _____ .   uterus

Metritis occurs when there is a _____ spread of   rapid;

infection to the _____ of the _____ .   musculature; uterus

Pelvic cellulitis, also known as _____ , develops   parametritis;

when the infectious process spreads to the _____   connective;

tissues surrounding the uterus and/or to the _____   broad

_____ .   ligaments

The symptoms commonly found in mild cases of endometritis
include elevation of body temperature on or about the forty-eighth
postpartum hour, ranging from 101 to 103°F; increased pulse rate; chills;
general malaise; anorexia; and headache. More severe infectious processes of endometritis are characterized by sudden body temperature
elevations of from 104 to 105°F, and a marked increase of pulse rate.
The afterpains are prolonged and severe, and the uterus, when palpated,
is tender and usually enlarged. Changes in lochial discharge are noted,
although the appearance and the amount of the lochia are dependent
upon the type of microorganism producing the infectious process. Generally, however, the lochia is profuse, dark brown in color, and foul-
smelling.

A mild case of endometritis produces an elevation in body   101; 103°F;

temperature to _____ to _____ on or

about the _____ postpartum hour.   forty-eighth

Other symptoms may be _____ pulse rate, | increased;

_____, _____, | chills; general malaise;

_____, and _____. | anorexia; headaches

More severe endometritis is characterized by a _____ | sudden;
rise in body temperatures to _____ to _____. | 104; 105°F
The increase in body temperature is accompanied by
a marked increase in _____ rate, prolonged and severe | pulse;
_____, and a _____ and _____ | afterpains; tender; enlarged
uterus when palpated.

The lochia usually is _____, its color _____ | profuse; dark
_____, and its odor _____. | brown; foul

The placental site forms thrombuses or clots following delivery, and the placental site is a prime area for microorganisms, usually anaerobic streptococci, to invade. Should this happen, *thrombophlebitis* occurs along the venous system of the uterus and ovaries. This inflammatory process attempts to wall off the infection and prevent its spread. At times this adaptive mechanism is successful and the infection process resolves. At other times the venous system is the route by which the puerperal infection spreads to other parts of the body and other organs. *Pelvic thrombophlebitis* occurs when the ovarian, uterine, or hypogastric vein becomes inflamed. The mother will experience extremes in temperature ranging from normal to 105°F, and chills. These symptoms usually develop about two weeks following delivery. Problems occur when part of the thrombus breaks off and travels to the lungs; should this happen, the mortality rate is increased. The thrombus may travel to the legs also; this is *femoral thrombophlebitis* and is discussed in Unit VI, Chapter Two, page 401.

When the microorganisms invade the venous system, this infection
is called _____. | thrombophlebitis
The venous system may be _____ | the route by
_____ | which the puerperal infection
_____. | spreads

Pelvic thrombophlebitis occurs when the inflammatory response
spreads to the _____ | ovarian, uterine, or
_____. | hypogastric vein
The mother will experience _____ | chills and
_____ in pelvic thrombophlebitis. | fever

Complications arise when _____ | part of the thrombus
_____ | breaks off and travels to the
_____. | lungs

Pelvic cellulitis or parametritis develops following a cervical laceration or thrombophlebitis. The organism travels and usually locates
in the broad ligament. The mother develops a fever that persists and
is around 102°F when the infection is mild. She experiences abdominal
pain that may be localized on one side or may be found on both sides.
Often the exudate forms a mass that can be felt in the broad ligament
as the process continues. In the majority of cases, when the infectious
process has been limited by the body's adaptive response, the exudate
is gradually absorbed into the system and is eliminated. Sometimes an
abcess is formed, and then incision and drainage are necessary.

Pelvic cellulitis or parametritis develops after there are _____ | cervical
_____ or _____. | lacerations; thrombophlebitis
The temperature of the mother usually is about _____. | 102°F
The mother experiences pain _____. | in the abdomen
In the majority of instances, the infectious process _____ | resolves
_____ | through the body's adaptive
_____. | response

Metritis, the extension of the local puerperal infection to the my-
ometrium, is not a common occurrence. It can follow thrombophlebitis
or lymphatic involvement. Often adhesions occur following this
inflammation.

The development of metritis follows _____ or | thrombophlebitis;
_____. | lymphatic involvement

Peritonitis occurs when the infectious process extends to the peritoneum by way of the lymphatics or when thrombophlebitis or parametritis extends. It is one of the most serious complications, and the
mortality rate is high. Usually during the first 72 hours postpartum, the
mother will exhibit signs of the infectious process, these signs being
a temperature between 103 and 105°F, chills, and a rapid pulse of 140
or more per minute. The pain is severe, and paralytic ileus or diarrhea
may occur. The infection speads throughout the bloodstream, and the
lungs become involved. The mother often is delirious or unconscious
before death.

Symptoms of peritonitis usually appear within _____

_____ .   the first

                                                                           72 hours

The mother experiences _____ , _____ ,   fever; chills;

_____ , and _____ .   rapid pulse; pain

The infection travels through the _____ .   bloodstream

Before death the mother is _____ or   delirious;

_____ .   unconscious

Preventive and promotive measures are extremely important. Good prenatal care ensures that the mother's health status is optimum before labor begins and that there is no anemia. The obstetrical staff must be healthy. Frequent nose and/or throat cultures will determine whether anyone is a carrier of pathogenic organisms. Aseptic technique in all aspects of care of the mother during labor and delivery will reduce the incidence of infection. Should the mother's temperature rise after the rupture of membranes during labor, prophylactic antibiotics are administered.

The mother who undergoes a long and traumatic delivery needs rest, replacement of fluid and blood loss, and adequate nutritional intake to restore her homeodynamic balance. These measures may help prevent the development of puerperal infection.

If the mother develops a puerperal infection, she usually is isolated from the other mothers; at times she is transferred to another unit. This means that she does not have the baby to care for or even see. As well as dealing with the stressor of the inflammatory process, the mother must cope with her feelings of inability to control the situation and to begin her mothering role. The nurse can be very effective by informing the mother of the baby's well-being and daily activities such as sleeping and eating.

If the mother develops a puerperal infection, she is

_____ .   isolated from others

The nurse can provide support by _____   informing

_____   the mother about the baby's

_____ .   activities

Restorative measures in puerperal infections may involve treatment with antibiotics that when used singly or in combination are effective in destroying the organism involved once its type has been identified by means of culture and sensitivity laboratory examinations. The staff should try to increase the mother's resistance to infection by keeping her on a fluid intake of 3,000 to 4,000 milliliters within a 24-hour period, providing her with a diet high in calories and vitamins, and ensuring rest and sleep.

The mother should be placed in a semi-Fowler's position which will ensure lochial drainage and prevent upward extension of the infectious process. The uterus should be checked for firmness and state of contraction through firm palpation and massage; thus extension of microorganisms through the muscles of the uterus will be prevented and blood clots or any remaining placental pieces will be expelled.

If the mother develops thrombophlebitis, then often anticoagulants are given to prevent the further formation of thrombi and hopefully to reduce the chances of the formation of any emboli. Because of the presence of the healing placental site, the mother must be carefully observed for signs of bleeding while she is receiving the anticoagulant medication.

Chemotherapeutic agents such as _____ are given | antibiotics;

to the mother to treat the infection. Fluid intake of _____ | 3,000;

to _____ per _____ hours | 4,000 milliliters; 24

should be provided to further support her resistance.

Diet should be rich in _____ and _____, | calories; vitamins

and rest and sleep should be encouraged.

To prevent upward _____ of the infectious process | extension;

and to ensure and promote free drainage of _____, the | lochia;

nurse should place the mother in a _____ | semi-Fowler's

position.

The nurse should massage the uterus to maintain its _____, | firmness;

prevent extension of microorganisms through the _____, | muscles;

of the _____, and promote expulsion of _____ | uterus; blood

_____ or _____. | clots; placental pieces

If thrombophlebitis develops, then, so that further thrombus

formation can be prevented, _____ are given. | anticoagulants

CYSTITIS

Cystitis is the inflammation of the bladder. When cystitis develops during the postpartum period, it usually is due to stagnation of urine in the bladder. The stagnant urine acts as a good medium for the growth of bacteria. There are two major reasons that urine may stay in the bladder for a period of time: retention of urine and residual urine.

Retention of urine is the inability to void; it often results after trauma to the bladder during delivery has caused obstruction of the urethra. Another cause of retention of urine is that the analgesia and anesthesia of labor and delivery decrease bladder sensitivity. This condition may continue for about five to six days or even longer. *Residual urine* is a volume of urine greater than 60 cubic centimeters which remains in the bladder each time the mother voids; when the bladder has poor tone, each time the mother voids a small amount spills over and the rest of the urine remains in the bladder.

Symptoms associated with cystitis are a painful or burning sensation upon urination, a temperature rise between 100 and 101°F, and a tenderness over the bladder.

Trauma to the bladder during delivery or surgical intervention may produce obstruction of the _____.

         urethra

When this occurs, there is urinary _____.

         retention

If stagnation of urine occurs and if bacteria have found a portal of entry into the bladder, _____ may develop.

         cystitis

Symptoms associated with this interruption are _____ or _____ upon urination, temperature rises to from _____ to _____ F, and maternal complaints of tenderness over the bladder.

         pain;
         burning;
         100; 101°

Preventive measures against cystitis include close observation of the mother's urinary output and of signs and symptoms of bladder distension. Distension can be ascertained by palpation of the abdomen above the symphysis pubis; a full bladder tends to displace the fundus of the uterus to the side and thus prevent the processes of involution. If the mother is encouraged to void frequently during labor and the immediate postpartum period, there is less chance of trauma and distension leading to retention.

When voiding has not occurred within eight hours after delivery, a catheterization may be ordered. This procedure, however, generally is avoided unless absolutely necessary because there is the danger of introducing bacteria into an otherwise sterile system.

Accurate measurement of the mother's voiding each time gives an indication of the bladder function. If the mother voids frequently in small amounts, residual urine should be suspected, and this can be confirmed by catheterization immediately after the mother has voided. At times it is necessary to place an indwelling catheter until bladder function returns.

Treatment of cystitis includes the administering of chemotherapeutic agents to combat the microorganism, ensuring that the bladder remains empty, and forcing fluids.

⬇

Cystitis may be prevented by maintaining close observation of the mother's urinary _____; checking for presence of bladder _____; and paying heed to maternal complaints of _____, constant _____ to urinate, or frequent voiding in _____ amounts.

output;

distention;

discomfort; desire;

small

Postpartally, voiding should occur within the first _____ hours. If the mother is unable to void within eight hours, a _____ may need to be done. Maintaining strict, surgically aseptic techniques during this procedure is of the essence because _____ may be introduced.

eight;

catheterization

microorganisms

If cystitis is present, therapy consists of administering _____, ensuring that the _____ remains _____, and _____ fluids.

chemotherapeutics; bladder;

empty; forcing

SUBINVOLUTION OF THE UTERUS

If you recall, under normal circumstances the uterine muscle starts to adjust to a nonpregnant state immediately postpartally. This process is referred to as _____.

involution

When this fails to occur, that is to say, when the uterine muscle does not return to a nonpregnant state in size and firmness and fails to descend progressively into the pelvic cavity within the usual period of one week, this condition is termed *subinvolution*. There may be many causes for subinvolution. Placental tissue and membranes may have been retained, atony of uterine muscle may be present, an endometritis process may be occurring, or uterine fibroids may be present.

Generally, symptoms of this condition are a large, soft, flabby uterus; a lochial discharge that is profuse, redder than usual, prolonged beyond the usual period of time, and sometimes resembles profuse bleeding; and pelvic discomfort. Other symptoms indicating that an interruption in health may be present are fever or signs of severe hemorrhage.

When the uterine muscle fails to return to a nonpregnant state, this condition is termed _____.

subinvolution

Factors that may be responsible for such a condition are
_____ of _____ and
membranes, _____ of uterine muscle, postpartum infection
such as _____, or presence of uterine _____.

retention; placental tissues;

atony;

endometritis; fibroids

Symptoms exhibited when subinvolution is present are
_____, _____, _____ uterus;
prolonged _____ discharge which may be more
_____ and brighter red in color than usual; and _____
discomfort.

large; soft; flabby;

lochial;

profuse; pelvic

Medical management of this condition is directly related to the
causative element. For example, if subinvolution is caused by atony
of the uterine muscle, then oxytocic preparations, which promote uterine tone and thus ensure firm contraction, are administered so that the
accumulation of blood clots and hemorrhage are prevented. If the
condition has come about as the result of tissue retention, surgical
intervention in the form of dilatation and curettage is necessary to
remove this tissue. Antibiotic therapy to prevent the emergence of a
postpartum infection may be prescribed.

Treatment of subinvolution caused by atony is administration of
_____ that will aid in promoting the restoration of
uterine muscle tone.

oxytocics

When subinvolution is due to retention of part of the secundines,
surgical intervention by _____ and _____
is needed in order to remove the retained tissue.

dilatation; curettage

Concomitantly, chemotherapeutic agents such as _____
may be administered so that _____
can be prevented.

antibiotics;
postpartum infections

Nursing observations during the postpartum period are geared to
assessing the size, descent, and consistency of the uterus in order to
prevent serious interruptions such as hemorrhage and shock. There
are two important nursing assessment measures that will yield
information as to the progress of involution. These are_____
the fundus and observing the _____ and _____
of lochia.

palpating;
type; amount

If the nurse feels a soft, boggy uterus, her first action should be firmly _____ the fundus. If this fails to restore the | massaging

organ to a firm state and if the lochia is profuse and redder than usual

beyond the period of the lochia rubra, the physician should be notified

immediately.

It is believed that ambulation during the early postpartum period
does much to prevent interruptions in the involution process. Therefore,
mothers should be encouraged to get out of bed as soon as possible.

Nursing measures include _____ the uterus, | palpating;

observing the _____, and massaging the _____. | lochia; fundus

The mother should be encouraged to _____ | get out of

_____ as soon as possible because early _____ | bed; ambulation

has been found to decrease the incidence of subinvolutional complica-

tions.

INTERRUPTIONS AFFECTING THE BREAST

Mastitis   A serious puerperal complication affecting the breast is mastitis. *Mastitis* is an inflammation of the mammary glands or their tissues
which may occur any time while the mother is lactating but is found most
commonly between the first and fourth postpartum weeks. Mastitis
develops as a result of an invasion by pathogenic organisms, usually
Staphylococcus aureus, which sets up an infectious process that gives
rise to the inflammatory response. Common predisposing factors may
be improper hygiene; erosions or fissures of nipples, which become an
entry point into the subcutaneous tissue or lymphatic system; or conditions favorable to bacteria already present in the mammary ducts.
Bruising or injuries to the breast may predispose to the invasion of
deeper mammary tissues by such bacteria.
    Although engorgement of the breast is not in itself a cause of
mastitis, the overdistension and edema produced by stasis of the lymphatics and venous supplies may produce injury to the tissues, which in
turn become more susceptible to the invasion of microorganisms and
thus to the appearance of infection.

Mastitis is an _____ of the _____ | inflammation; mammary

_____ or their _____. | glands; tissues

Usually the onset of this interruption occurs between the

_____ and _____ postpartum weeks. | first; fourth

The organism most commonly responsible for this inflammatory response is _____, although other endemic bacteria may set up an infectious process if the breast has been _____ or _____.

⬇

Staphylococcus aureus;

injured; bruised

It is important that breast engorgement be relieved as soon as its signs are detected so that the injuries that may render breast tissue susceptible to bacterial invasion may be prevented.

An infectious process of the mammary glands either may be a local inflammatory response or may be of the suppurative kind, which in turn may lead to abscess formation in the glandular tissues. Several types of mastitis have been identified. Inflammatory processes may arise around the areola, and small abscesses of the tubercles of Montgomery may develop. A *parenchymous* or *glandular mastitis* may develop as the inflammatory process affects one or more lobes of the mammary gland. A *periglandular cellulitis* may appear if the inflammation takes place in the fat and loose tissues found between the lobes. When the infectious process progresses into the connective tissues underneath the gland, a *submammary abscess* develops, with the subsequent presence of purulent material. Of these, the parenchymous type is the most common and has been found to be most amenable to treatment, whereas submammary abscesses, although rarer, are most serious to the welfare of the mother.

Mastitis may vary from local inflammatory and infectious processes to the _____ kind. This latter type may lead to _____ formation in the _____ tissues.

suppurative;

abscess; glandular

Several varieties of mastitis have been identified. Inflammation may be present around the _____, and small abscesses of the _____ may develop.

areola;

tubercles of Montgomery

A second type is the _____ form or _____ mastitis. This involves the _____ of the mammary glands, is the most _____ type of mastitis, and is found most amenable to _____.

parenchymous;

glandular; lobes;

common;

treatment

A third type of mastitis is _____. This inflammatory response develops in the _____ and _____ tissues found between the glandular lobes.

periglandular;

fat; loose

A fourth and most serious type of mastitis gives rise to a _____ abscess, affecting the connective tissues underneath the gland.

⬇
submammary

Mastitis generally appears between the first and fourth weeks of the postpartum period. Its symptoms are marked engorgement, severe and acute tenderness and pain in the breast, chills, general malaise, and a sudden elevation of body temperature to between 103 and 104°F. There is an increase of pulse rate, and upon palpation, the breasts are felt to be quite hard and appear red.

Typical symptoms of mastitis are _____ _____, severe _____, and a sudden rise of _____ ranging from _____ to _____ F. The pulse rate is _____, and upon visual and tactile inspection the breasts appear _____ and _____.

marked
engorgement; pain;
body temperature; 103;
104°; increased;

hard; red

The most important measures instituted against mastitis are those classified as prevention. Beginning during the later months of her pregnancy as part of her antepartum care, the mother should be taught breast hygiene. The development of lesions or fissures can be prevented through avoidance of excessive manipulation; early detection of small cracks in the nipples; and attention to maternal complaints of raw, tender nipples, the soreness of which, if undetected, eventually may lead to fissures, thus providing an ideal portal of entry for any bacteria present.

Once mastitis is present, it may be brought under control through the administration of antibiotics if these chemotherapeutic agents are started early. Pain and swelling may be relieved through the application of breast binders or support provided by a tight-fitting brassiere. Applications of ice may be indicated; however, once suppuration is present, heat applications to localize the infectious process are ordered. For the breast-feeding mother, mastitis becomes a problem because this method of feeding must be discontinued once the diagnosis has been established.

Should the infectious process not respond to these conservative medical and nursing interventions, that is to say, if the inflammatory response develops into a purulent abscess formation, surgical intervention in the form of incision and drainage of the abscess may be necessary.

Mastitis can be avoided through the institution of measures that are _____ in nature. These include _____ hygiene, which should be taught during _____ _____.

> preventive; breast; antepartum care

Fissures, lesions, and cracks can be prevented through avoidance of _____ manipulation. Early detection of lesions and attention to maternal complaints of _____, _____, and tender _____ may lead to the prevention of injuries to the breast which may become _____ of entry for invading microorganisms.

> excessive; sore; raw; nipples; portals

Therapy for mastitis includes the administration of _____ early. Relief for the _____ and the _____ accompanying this condition may be provided by the application of a _____ or a tight-fitting _____. Applications of _____ may be indicated if no suppuration is present. However, if purulent material is apparent, applications of _____ are ordered so that the abscess can be _____. If the mother is breast-feeding, she may be asked to _____ this activity immediately.

> antibiotics; pain; swelling; breast binder; brassiere; cold; heat; localized; discontinue

In many circumstances, the newborn infant is a carrier of the organism responsible for the onset of mastitis. Therefore, it is essential that strict nursery and obstetric techniques be enforced so that the development of epidemic infections such as those seen in nurseries and maternity wards can be prevented. Extreme care should be observed, particularly when outside visitors are admitted into the maternity units. It is known that staphylococcus organisms are becoming increasingly resistant to many of the antibiotics in present use, thus making it increasingly difficult to treat infectious processes produced by these microorganisms. Health teaching, therefore, should not only include the mother and the infant but should also include other family members so that the occurrence of infections can be prevented.

Any interruption affecting the normal course of the postpartum period will have the effect of significantly altering the relationships between the infant and the mother. Since the infant's immunological systems at birth are immature and therefore unable to deal with the stresses imposed by exposure to infectious organisms, the mother who is affected by a postpartum infection will not be able to see the baby for as long as the infectious process has not been brought under control. As previously seen, this period of time may vary; however limited in duration, the separation from the baby forcibly imposed upon her may add new stressors to a mother in a physiological crisis. The normal events of the taking in and taking-hold phases* are interrupted or delayed. If she has planned to breast-feed, for example, she may perceive her condition as a failure in her ability to nurture and care for the infant.

The rigid treatment measures that a postpartum interruption imposes upon the mother may add to her depression and discouragement. It is up to the nurse, therefore, to anticipate the needs of mothers at this time, particularly the need for verbalization of feelings, and at the same time keep the mother informed regarding her infant's progress and appearance. Information such as any weight gain or loss of the baby, the amount of formula being ingested, the general appearance, and the care the baby is receiving will do much to alleviate the mother's anxiety and apprehension. Whenever possible, she should be allowed to view the baby from a distance so as to maintain the ties that were so suddenly interrupted by the complication.

*These phases are discussed in the first volume in this series, on pp. 393–396.

POST-TEST Indicate whether each statement is true or false by circling the appropriate letter. Then turn to page 395 and see how well you have done.

1. Hemorrhage is a predisposing factor of infection. T F

2. Infection of the perineum is considered to be an extension of the local puerperal infection. T F

3. Extensions of the local puerperal infection always are through the lymphatics. T F

4. The placental site is an area very vulnerable to invading microorganisms. T F

5. The organism most often responsible for the infectious process in puerperal infections is *Staphylococcus aureus*. T F

6. Signs and symptoms of endometritis include burning on urination. T F

7. If the mother develops endometritis, the lochia often changes to a dark brown color. T F

8. Thrombophlebitis usually begins at the placental site. T F

9. There is a danger of pulmonary embolism occurring if thrombophlebitis develops. T F

10. Parametritis is the same as peritonitis. T F

11. Antibiotics are effective when used in instances of puerperal infection. T F

12. If a mother develops puerperal infection, she is isolated from the other mothers. T F

13. Urine remaining in the bladder is of no significance. T F

14. Retention may result from decreased sensitivity due to anesthesia. T F

15. To determine if there is residual urine, one needs to catheterize the mother. T F

16. Poor tone of the bladder predisposes to residual urine. T F

17. There is no discomfort perceived by the mother when she develops cystitis. T F

18. Part of the treatment for cystitis is forcing the fluid intake. T F

19. If the uterus is soft, this is an indication that involution is progressing well. T F

20. If the mother has a heavy flow of lochia and it is bright red, this may be a sign of subinvolution. T F

21. A uterine fibroid may interfere with involution processes. T F

22. The mother should be encouraged to ambulate early to help prevent subinvolution.   T   F

23. Postpartum hemorrhage may occur if there is uterine atony.   T   F

24. The usual organism causing mastitis is streptococcus.   T   F

25. Poor hygiene may predispose to the development of mastitis.   T   F

26. Periglandular cellulitis is an infection of fat and loose tissues.   T   F

27. The baby may be the carrier of the pathogenic organism causing mastitis.   T   F

28. Signs of mastitis include redness of the breast and fever.   T   F

In the specific areas with which you had difficulty, return to the material and review.

BIBLIOGRAPHY

Clausen, Joy, Margaret Flook, and Bonnie Ford: *Maternity Nursing Today*, 2d ed., McGraw-Hill Book Co., New York, 1977.

Dickason, Elizabeth J. and Martha Schult (eds.): *Maternal and Infant Care*, McGraw-Hill Book Co., New York, 1975.

Friedman, Emmanuel A. and J. P. Greenhill: *Biological Principles and Modern Practice of Obstetrics*, W. B. Saunders Co., Philadelphia, 1974.

Pritchard, Jack and Paul MacDonald: *Williams Obstetrics*, 15th ed., Appleton-Century-Crofts, New York, 1976.

Reeder, Sharon R., et al.: *Maternity Nursing*, J. B. Lippincott Co., Philadelphia, 1976.

PRETEST ANSWERS

1. An elevation of temperature to 100.4°F for a period of 48 hours after the first 24 hours following the delivery   2. Hemorrhage; anemia; traumatic delivery; retention of placental fragments   3. Local; extensions   4. Anaerobic streptococcus   5. An inflammatory response of the endometrium   6. Fever; pain in the abdomen; a mass that may be felt   7. The development of a pulmonary embolism   8. Extension of the infectious process from the parametrium through the lymphatics or by thrombophlebitis   9. Kept isolated from her   10. Antibiotics; rest; fluids and nutrients; sometimes anticoagulants   11. Cystitis   12. Retention of urine; residual urine   13. Pain or burning on urination; fever   14. a. Observe for bladder distention during labor and during the postpartum period; b. keep an accurate measurement of the urinary output; c. make sure that the mother voids within the first eight hours after delivery   15. Chemotherapy; forced fluids; keeping the bladder empty   16. Failure of the uterus to return to a nonpregnant state in size and to descend progressively into the pelvic cavity   17. a. Atony of the muscle; b. endometritis; c. retained membranes and placental tissue; d. uterine fibroids   18. a. Soft, flabby uterus; b. profuse lochia, redder than usual; c. pain   19. Oxytocics   20. Inflammation of the mammary glands   21. Glandular mastitis; periglandular cellulitis; submammary abscess   22. First; fourth   23. *Staphylococcus aureus*

POST-TEST ANSWERS

1. T	2. F	3. F	4. T	5. F	6. F	7. T	8. T	9. T
10. F	11. T	12. T	13. F	14. T	15. T	16. T	17. F
18. T	19. F	20. T	21. T	22. T	23. T	24. F	25. T
26. T	27. T	28. T						

CHAPTER TWO

INTERRUPTIONS OF THE CARDIOVASCULAR SYSTEM

OBJECTIVES   *Define late postpartum hemorrhage.*

Identify its danger in relation to its typical period of onset.

Identify nursing intervention measures with late postpartum hemorrhage.

Define thrombophlebitis.

Identify its dangers to the mother.

Identify nursing intervention measures to be instituted in the presence of throm-bophlebitis.

GLOSSARY   *Late postpartum hemorrhage:* A loss of blood exceeding 500 cubic centimeters which occurs after the first 24 hours postpartum and may be as late as the end of the first postpartum week or later on during the postpartum period

Phlegmasia alba dolens: Painful white inflammation; another name given to femoral thrombophlebitis. It also is referred to as "milk-leg"

Thrombophlebitis: Inflammation response of the lining of the veins followed by the formation of a thrombus

PRETEST In the spaces provided, fill in the word or words that best complete(s) the statements. Then turn to page 404 and check your answers.

1. A late postpartum hemorrhage occurs from after _____ _____ up to _____ of the puerperium.

2. This loss of blood is usually about or over _____ cubic centimeters.

3. Causative elements for a delayed postpartum hemorrhage are _____ _____ and _____ _____.

4. Signs and symptoms of a hemorrhage are a. _____ _____; b. _____ _____; and c. _____ _____.

5. ''Thrombophlebitis'' is defined as _____ _____.

6. Two types of thrombophlebitis are _____ and _____ .

7. A lay term for ''phlegmasia alba dolens'' is _____.

8. Symptoms of thrombophlebitis are _____, _____, and _____.

9. Medical management of this condition includes prescribing _____ and _____ .

LATE POSTPARTUM HEMORRHAGE

Late postpartum hemorrhage occurs after the first 24 hours postpartum and may be seen either at the end of the first week following delivery or later on during the postpartum period. Usually, a late postpartum hemorrhage tends to occur between the sixth and tenth days of the puerperium.

If you recall, we defined a hemorrhage as being a blood loss of _____ cubic centimeters or more. As a rule, the   500
greatest danger of this complication arising generally is past if there has been no significant blood loss during the first hour following delivery. Nevertheless, the risk of this occurrence continues thereafter and should be anticipated, since other circumstances and interruptions such as uterine atony and retention of placental tissue can be causative elements.

The incidence of a late postpartum hemorrhage is greatest between the _____ and _____ days of   sixth; tenth;
the _____.   puerperium

Generally, the causative factors leading to a delayed postpartum hemorrhage have been identified, as briefly mentioned before, as being (1) abnormal involution of the placental site, that is, retardation of the process of reduction of the placental site and the process of exfoliation due to the growth of endometrial tissue over the placental site, and (2) retention of placental tissues which has gone undetected up to this time. At times, when a section of placental tissue has been retained, it may begin to undergo changes leading to the formation of a placental polyp, which, since it becomes an obstruction to the processes of uterine involution, may culminate in a late hemorrhage.

Two factors have been identified as being the causative elements of late postpartum hemorrhage: (1) _____   abnormal
_____   involution of the placental site;
and (2) _____.   retention of placental tissue
Retention of _____ tissue eventually may lead to   placental;
the formation of a _____ and thus may interrupt the   polyp
process of involution; it is a causative element of a late postpartum hemorrhage.

If either of these factors exists, the health of the mother is impaired and there is a danger that late postpartum hemorrhage may occur after she has been discharged from the hospital, particularly if other health interruptions have been present during the pregnancy and postpregnancy cycles. In such cases, before discharge the mother and other family members should be given instructions concerning the symptoms of possible complications. These include the following items: (1) a soft, boggy uterus that fails to contract when massaged or expels large amounts of clots after massage is instituted and (2) an unusually large amount of lochia, bright red in color.

This last observation may be an indication of a complication, because at this time the lochia should be _____ _____ in color and quite moderate in amount.

whitish
yellow

When late postpartum hemorrhage occurs, the treatment is blood replacement and then curettage of the uterus to remove the causative agent, either a polyp or a placental fragment. Doing this may require that the mother be hospitalized for a period of time, thus introducing a stressor that will disrupt the beginning interactions with the newborn baby. Whenever possible, rooming-in arrangements should be made so that the infant can remain with the mother during the short-stay hospitalization required. Should this not be possible, the nurse must keep in mind that the mother's recovery may be complicated by anxieties generated by separation from the baby. She will wish to return home as soon as possible and will overlook the importance of getting appropriate rest and relaxation. Enlisting family members to help in the care of the infant during this time will ensure that these measures are carried out.

THROMBOPHLEBITIS

Thrombophlebitis is a condition generally categorized as a puerperal infection which develops when an inflammatory response begins to take place within a vein and a thrombus or a vascular clot then is formed. Thrombophlebitis may come about as a result of blood stagnation due to overstretching of the vessels or due to the development of thrombi at the placental site, which becomes infected. When organisms invade the placental site, an inflammatory response is set up in the pelvic veins. As previously stated, extension into other organs and parts of the body is a characteristic of puerperal infections; therefore thrombophlebitis may extend into the femoral veins, causing a condition usually referred to as "phlegmasia alba dolens" or "milk-leg," or may extend into other venous structures such as the venous systems of the ovary and uterus, causing a pelvic thrombophlebitis.

Since thrombophlebitis directly affects the cardiovascular system, this complication of the puerperal period requires special medical management to prevent the greatest danger to the mother, that is, the development of a pulmonary embolism. In a pulmonary embolism, a small part of the thrombus formation present in the uterine or pelvic veins or the femoral vessel may become dislodged, be carried away by the bloodstream, and occlude the pulmonary artery. Occlusion of the pulmonary artery usually proves to be fatal to the patient because circulatory processes to the lungs are obstructed. It is essential, therefore, that any mother who has had a diagnosis of thrombophlebitis or who has suffered a postpartum hemorrhage be closely observed for signs or symptoms of pulmonary occlusion such as severe cardiac pains, dyspnea, irregular or difficult-to-obtain pulse, pallor or cyanosis, and increased feelings of apprehension.

Circulatory alterations in which clot formation and inflammatory responses of the veins occur are referred to as _____.

| thrombophlebitis

Should this condition develop during the postpartum course, it generally is categorized as a _____.

| puerperal infection

Thrombophlebitis may come about as a result of _____ of blood due to _____ of blood vessels or due to _____ at the placental site.

| stagnation;
| stretching;
| infected thrombi

This inflammatory response may extend into venous systems surrounding pelvic organs such as the _____ and the _____, thus causing a _____ thrombophlebitis, or may extend into the femoral veins, setting up an inflammatory response often referred to as _____ _____ or _____ leg.

| ovaries;
| uterus; pelvic;
|
| phlegmasia
| alba dolens; milk-

The greatest danger to the mother who is affected by thrombophlebitis is the development of a _____.

| pulmonary embolism

Signs of a pulmonary embolism include _____ _____, _____, _____, _____, and _____.

| severe
| cardiac pain; dyspnea;
| irregular pulse; pallor or
| cyanosis; apprehension

The development of thrombophlebitis usually follows complications of the intrapartum period such as placenta previa, complications of the third stage of labor, or surgical interventions such as cesarean section.

Femoral thrombophlebitis is characterized by signs and symptoms such as pain, heat, swelling tenderness, and redness along the vein that is being affected. This indicates that a clot has been formed in the femoral vein and that return circulation is being interfered with. The arterial circulation in the leg constricts, causing the limb to appear white. These signs and symptoms tend to appear around the tenth postpartum day. However, their onset may be delayed up to the twentieth postpartum day. At times, severe pain in the groin, which often interferes with the woman's ability to sleep, may last several weeks, gradually subsiding over a period of four to six weeks. However, the condition may cause her discomfort in years to come.

Characteristic symptoms of femoral thrombophlebitis are
_____, _____, _____
_____, and _____ along the _____
vein.

pain; heat; swelling

tenderness; redness; femoral

Symptoms of this condition tend to appear between the
_____ and the _____ days of the puerperium, and the symptom of pain may last for _____ weeks but gradually subside.

tenth; twentiuth

several

The chances of recurrence of this condition are increased with each subsequent pregnancy, and thus a history of thrombophlebitis becomes significant during succeeding antepartal visits.

Pelvic thrombophlebitis becomes quite a serious complication of the puerperium (see page 381).

Femoral thrombophlebitis may affect the mother for a period of time generally ranging from _____ to _____ weeks, and chances of recurrence of this condition with subsequent pregnancies are _____.

four; six;

increased

Occasionally, anticoagulants may be prescribed as a prophylactic measure against thrombi formation. Medical management of mothers affected by thrombophlebitis includes the administration of anticoagulants to prevent further clot formation and antibiotics to combat the microorganism responsible for the infectious process.

Nursing intervention measures are geared to maintaining bed rest until several days or weeks after the temperature elevation has subsided, elevating the affected part, applying moist heat along the affected vessel, and maintaining the affected part immobilized while preventing pressure created by bed covers. Under no circumstances should massage of the affected part be instituted since the dangers of emboli are ever present in this condition.

Once the mother is allowed out of bed, she may wear elastic stockings to prevent swelling of the legs.

Treatment for thrombophlebitis includes the administration of _____ and _____, while the nursing care given to the mother at this time should take into consideration maintenance of absolute _____, _____, _____ of the affected part, and application of _____ along the affected vessel.

anticoagulants; antibiotics;

bed rest; elevation;

immobilization;

moist heat

POST-TEST Indicate whether each statement is true or false by circling the appropriate letter. Then turn to page 404 and see how well you have done.

1. Late postpartum hemorrhage occurs 24 hours following delivery. T F

2. Part of the placental site can alter and form a polyp. T F

3. The uterus remains contracted at all times before a postpartum hemorrhage occurs. T F

4. Treatment of the postpartum hemorrhage includes curettage of the uterus. T F

5. Phlegmasia alba dolens is the same as pelvic thrombophlebitis. T F

6. The danger of thrombophlebitis is the possible formation of emboli. T F

7. Femoral thrombophlebitis is treated with moist heat. T F

8. The mother does not have her activity restricted if she develops femoral thrombophlebitis. T F

In the specific areas with which you had difficulty, return to the material and review.

BIBLIOGRAPHY   Clausen, Joy, Margaret Flook, and Bonnie Ford: *Maternity Nursing Today*, 2d ed., McGraw-Hill Book Co., New York, 1977.

Dickason, Elizabeth J., "Problems Causing Bleeding in Pregnancy," in Elizabeth J. Dickason and Martha Schult (eds.): *Maternal and Infant Care*, McGraw-Hill Book Co., New York, 1975.

————, "Cardiovascular Problems in Pregnancy," op. cit.

Hammond, H., "Death from Obstetrical Hemorrhage," *California Medicine*, pp. 16–20, 1972.

Malvern, J., et al., "Ultrasonic Scanning of the Puerperal Uterus Following Secondary Postpartum Hemorrhage," *Journal OB-GYN British Commonwealth*, pp. 320–324, April 1973.

Pritchard, Jack and Paul MacDonald: *Williams Obstetrics*, 15th ed., Appleton-Century-Crofts, New York, 1976.

Reeder, Sharon R., et al: *Maternity Nursing*, J. B. Lippincott Co., Philadelphia, 1976.

**PRETEST
ANSWERS**
1. The first 24 hours; the end 2. 500 3. Retained placental fragments; abnormal involution of the placental site 4. a. A soft, boggy uterus; b. large amounts of clots or tissue; c. an unusual amount of lochia that is bright red 5. An inflammation of the vein 6. Pelvic; femoral 7. Milk-leg 8. Pain; fever; swelling of affected limb 9. Antibiotics; anticoagulants

**POST-TEST
ANSWERS**
1. T 2. T 3. F 4. T 5. F 6. T 7. T 8. F

CHAPTER THREE

PSYCHOLOGICAL INTERRUPTIONS

OBJECTIVES   *Identify factors that may lead to the development of psychological interruptions during the postpartum period.*

Identify signs, symptoms, and behavioral changes that occur as a result of psychosis during the postpartum period.

Identify nursing intervention measures to be instituted during this time.

GLOSSARY   *Defense mechanisms:* Unconscious psychological attempts to deal with anxiety and conflicts so as to preserve the integrity of the personality
Psychosis: A severe disturbance in thinking, feeling, and behavior manifested by distortion and/or detachment from reality. Psychosis may be organic or emotional in origin

PRETEST   In the spaces provided, fill in the word or words that best complete(s) the statements. Then turn to page 415 and check your answers.

1. Factors that may predispose during a time of stress to psychological difficulty are _____ and _____.

2. Mothers who develop psychoses during the postpartum period are unable to deal with _____ _____.

3. During the postpartum period, if the nurse observes signs in the mother's behavior which indicate a psychosis, these might include _____ , _____ , _____ , _____ , _____ , and _____ .

4. When the mother becomes psychotic, the nursing intervention is geared toward _____ , _____ , _____ , and _____ _____ .

5. Nursing care of the family provides _____ _____ , _____ , and _____ .

Throughout this book and in our previous volume, we identified the many psychological and social adaptations required of mothers during the pregnancy cycle. As a rule, the processes of role identification, the psychological adaptations, and all of the emotional discomforts associated with a pregnancy have been dealt with shortly after the arrival of the new baby. However, conflicts arising out of deeply ingrained neurotic methods of coping may be exacerbated by the pregnancy and by the delivery itself; the up-to-now efficient defense mechanisms employed by the mother as she dealt with daily psychological difficulties may become insufficient or may fail to function for the maintenance of the integrity of the personality, and psychological interruptions may ensue.

Much research has been done regarding the nature and contributing factors of a psychotic episode either during the pregnancy itself or postpartally. Although there is some evidence that hormonal imbalances have influences upon the psychological state of the individual, this research is as yet inconclusive.[1] A psychosis occurring during the postpartum period sometimes has distinct toxic and organic features.

It is thought, however, that existing personality traits, unconscious conflicts, and unresolved and unmet maturational needs may give rise to the onset of psychological difficulties at a time of stress. During the postpartum period or in the following year, the new adaptation requirements of this period may precipitate a psychological crisis. Rather than being the causative agent, the birth of the baby seems to act as a catalyst triggering the emergence of a psychotic episode.

Causative elements of a postpartum psychosis are _____. However, it is thought that factors such as _____, unconscious _____, unmet _____ needs, and _____ may be elements triggering psychotic episodes during the postpartum period.

unknown;

anxiety;

conflicts; maturational;

personality traits

Some research indicates that _____ imbalances exert some influence in generating a psychotic _____; however, this evidence is inconclusive. It is known, however, that the birth of the baby may act as a _____ to the emergence of a psychosis during the postpartum period.

hormonal;

episode;

catalyst

Some emotional problems, such as the common "postpartum blues," are seen frequently, especially in the immediate postpartum period. Frank psychotic episodes, however, are rare. A psychosis appearing postpartally is seen by most experts as not being different from

a psychotic episode at any other time in life except for the fact that the
precipitating event is pregnancy and/or delivery.

⬇

"Postpartum blues" occurs _____ during the
puerperium; psychotic reactions during the same period are _____.

commonly;

rare

It is very difficult to predict which mothers may develop severe
psychological disturbances resulting in the crisis state of psychosis.
The nurse must keep in mind the importance of the mother's homeodynamic balance, which may be influenced by such stressors as physical
disturbances or psychosocial, economic, or family pressures. A mother
who has had a stressful, tumultuous pregnancy and a difficult labor
may go through the puerperium quite comfortably, while one who has
enjoyed a relatively smooth pregnancy and labor may become overwhelmed by her new responsibilities and feelings and become psychotic
because her adaptive mechanisms are ineffective during the postpartum
period. The timing, number, and intensity of the stressors affecting the
mother's homeodynamic balance may so deplete her resources or immobilize her emotional responses as to result in a psychotic crisis.

The nurse can be instrumental in differentiating between the normal postpartum blues and a psychotic reaction. Usually, the first signs
and symptoms of both occur within two to three days after delivery.
Whereas many mothers may experience the usual crying spells and
blues without clearcut cause, they usually respond to extra rest, reassurance that this is normal and will pass, and attention from the
family. A mother experiencing a prepsychotic or psychotic episode,
however, will become increasingly unable to find comfort within her
realistic situation.

The conflict and psychological stresses affecting the mother find
expression in her behavior; she becomes increasingly irritable, is unable
to sleep, may suffer from anorexia, may be given to extreme feelings
of depression, may become suspicious, and generally exhibits symptoms of agitation and tenseness. Other behavioral signs commonly
found are her total rejection of and hostile feelings toward the baby
and/or her husband. She may become delusional and may deny the
existence of the baby. She may avoid any contact or any interpersonal
exchange with the infant.

Generally, symptoms indicating psychological imbalances may
be found in behaviors such as _____, inability to
_____, increased _____, extreme feelings
of _____ and _____, _____,

anorexia;

sleep; irritability;

depression; suspicion; agitation;

and tenseness. All other behaviors associated with extreme anxiety are quite common.

In addition, the mother may _____ and become quite _____ toward the _____ and/or the _____. She may become _____ and deny the _____ of the baby, typically avoiding any _____ with the infant.

reject;

hostile; father;

baby; delusional

existence;

contact

Nursing intervention with the mother undergoing a psychotic episode is geared first toward prompt identification of the crisis state. Nurses, in their close contact with patients while providing 24-hour care, are the ones who first will observe and identify the occurrence of this disruption in health. Nursing care should be primarily supportive, with emphasis on accepting the mother's feelings yet reinforcing reality in a nonjudgmental way. Maintaining a safe environment also is important, since a mother who is delusional often may be destructive toward herself or others.

If a mother has become psychotic on a postpartum unit, one of the initial responsibilities of the nurse is to promptly _____ and _____ the occurrence of the disruption to other members of the health team. Maintenance of a _____ environment and _____, _____ nursing care are important.

identify

communicate

safe

supportive; nonjudgmental

It is important that a psychiatric consultation be arranged as soon as possible, since tranquilizers, intensive psychotherapy, and/or electroconvulsive therapy frequently are utilized in treatment of this condition as they are in any other severe psychosis.

A mother who has become psychotic during her postpartum hospitalization may be transferred directly to a psychiatric in-patient service. Sometimes, however, a psychotic reaction may not become distinct for several weeks or even months after delivery, especially when such postponing measures are taken as another family member or baby nurse assuming most of the direct infant care. In this type of situation, it may be the nurse in a postpartum clinic or doctor's office who, after talking with the mother and/or family, suggests a psychiatric consultation.

The impact that such an interruption in the mother's health will have on the family is great. For the most part, it can be surmised that an uneventful postpartum course and the resumption of family living was expected by the members of the family unit. To them, therefore, the unexpected reactions exhibited by the mother become frightening and threatening to the stability of the family system.

The nurse must make appropriate nursing intervention at this time to support the strengths of the family unit. Primarily, the nurse's efforts should be directed toward listening to the family's expression of feelings, attempting to explain what is going on, and assisting them to adjust to this crisis without rejecting the woman on the basis that she is a "bad mother."

If the crisis continues and is unresolved, appropriate referrals to family therapy centers that will assist family members to deal with and adapt to the problems presented by this stressful situation may be required.

Now, let us see how you would respond to a new mother who seems to be psychologically disturbed.

Sally Glynn, a twenty-two-year-old primipara, delivered a 7-pound girl. This is the third postpartum day, and you meet Sally in the morning. She appears tired and irritable, and she complains that she does not feel hungry. She says that she has been unable to sleep for two nights. As you make her bed, you note that she seems very disorganized. She asks the same questions repeatedly; seems anxious; and cannot decide whether to comb her hair, brush her teeth, or shower first. Although Sally has seen her normal baby at each feeding time, she keeps asking you if "it" is all right and has all four limbs. Which of the following is the best response to Sally's behavior?

A. You reassure Sally that the baby is fine and that if she takes her sleeping pill and gets some good rest, tomorrow everything will be all right.

Go to page 411.

B. You take Sally to the nursery and show her the baby so that she is not confused about the baby's status and so that she will be relieved.

Go to page 412.

C. You recognize that Sally's behavior indicates an unusual amount of psychological difficulty. After helping her specifically organize her morning care, you notify the physician of her unusual behavior.

Go to page 413.

If you chose A, you did not correctly assess the type of behavior that Sally was exhibiting, since your response was based on the assumption that her inability to sleep was the only difficulty inherent in this situation.

Return to page 407. Review the material and choose another response from page 410.

Your choice of *B* indicates that you have not clearly evaluated Sally's status. You did not realize that Sally had seen her child numerous times before, so that this is not the problem.

Return to page 407. Review the material and choose another response from page 410.

Excellent assessment is indicated by your choice of *C*. You have recognized that Sally's behavior is indicative of her inability to deal with this stress situation, and you have supported her by structuring her activities. You have communicated her status to the physician so that further intervention measures will be instituted.

Advance to page 414 and take the post-test.

POST-TEST Indicate whether each statement is true or false by circling the appropriate letter. Then turn to page 415 and see how well you have done.

1. Postpartum blues is an indication of psychotic behavior. T F

2. Unmet maturational needs may contribute to the production of a crisis state. T F

3. Psychoses occurring in the postpartum period always become resolved without psychiatric intervention. T F

4. Stressors acting in combination can produce a crisis situation. T F

5. It always is possible to predict that a mother will develop a psychosis during the postpartum period. T F

6. If the mother becomes psychotic, she may become suspicious. T F

7. It is important to make the environment safe for the psychotic mother. T F

8. If a mother has another person who takes complete care of the baby, a psychotic reaction may be postponed. T F

9. When the mother has a psychotic reaction, the nursing intervention with the family is to support the family strengths. T F

In the specific areas with which you had difficulty, return to the material and review.

REFERENCES   1.   Elise Fitzpatrick, J. Eastman Nicholson, and Sharon R. Reeder: *Maternity Nursing*, 11th ed., J. B. Lippincott Co., Philadelphia, 1966, p. 200.

BIBLIOGRAPHY   Arieti, Silvano: *American Handbook of Psychiatry*, Vol. III, Basic Books, New York, 1966.

Caplan, Gerald: *Concepts of Mental Health and Consultation*, U.S. Department of Health, Education and Welfare, 1959.

Freedman, Alfred M. and Harold I. Kaplan (eds.): *Comprehensive Textbook of Psychiatry*, Williams and Wilkins Co., Baltimore, 1967.

Noyes, Arthur P. and Lawrence C. Kolb: *Modern Clinical Psychiatry*, 6th ed., W. B. Saunders Co., Philadelphia, 1963.

Redlich, Frederick C. and Daniel X. Freedman: *The Theory and Practice of Psychiatry*, Basic Books, New York, 1966.

PRETEST ANSWERS   1.   Assumption of a new role; assumption of new responsibilities   2.   The number and the combination of stressors   3.   Irritability; anorexia; depression; suspicion; agitation; sleeplessness   4.   Support; acceptance of feelings; reinforcement of reality; provision of a safe environment   5.   Opportunity for expression of feelings; information; support of strengths

POST-TEST ANSWERS   1.   F   2.   T   3.   F   4.   T   5.   F   6.   T   7.   T   8.   T   9.   T

Student _____

INTERRUPTIONS IN HEALTH IN THE POSTPARTUM PERIOD

When caring for postpartal mothers in a secondary-care facility, in the home, or during a simulated experience, the student will:

			Satisfactory					Unsatisfactory				
*	1.	Identify three mothers who may be classified as high-risk because of any of the following: a. Antepartal course										
		b. Intrapartal course										
		c. Pelvimetry										
		d. Previous obstetrical history										
		e. Previous medical history										
		f. Postpartal status										
		g. Age										
*	2.	Select a mother whom you consider to be high-risk, and determine priorities of care by synthesizing all available data										
*	3.	Discuss nursing intervention or directly intervene when aberrations in the normal postpartal status are detected										
A	4.	Present a case study involving a high-risk postpartal mother, nursing data, nursing diagnosis, and intervention in a pre or post conference to a group of peers and/or staff										
*	5.	Identify special nursing measures related to a specific high-risk situation										
B	6.	Determine the meaning (to a specific mother/family) of a high-risk situation										
A	7.	Include appropriate members of the health team in meeting identified maternal/family needs in a postpartal high-risk situation										
*	8.	Accept a report concerning the status of the neonate, and/or audit the chart of the neonate										
*	9.	Assist the mother/family in preparing for discharge or in making special home preparations										

Instructor Comments:

Student _____

			Satisfactory					Unsatisfactory				
*	10.	Discuss drugs and/or other therapy being utilized in the care of a specific high-risk mother										
*	11.	Administer drugs and/or other therapeutic measures safely										
B	12.	Explain medications and/or other therapeutic measures to a high-risk mother/family										
B	13.	Keep a mother who is separated from her baby because of a high-risk situation informed of the progress of the baby										

Instructor Comments:

The following multiple-choice examination will test your comprehension of the material covered in the sixth unit of this program. Remember, you are not competing with anyone but yourself. Therefore, do not guess in order to answer the questions; if you are unsure, this means that you have not learned the content. Return to the areas that give you difficulty and review them before going on with the examination.

Circle the letter of the best response to each question. After completing the unit examination, check your answers on page 541 and review those areas of difficulty before proceeding to the next unit.

1. Puerperal infection occurs when there is an infectious process occurring in the:
   a. Genital tract
   b. Urinary tract
   c. Pulmonary system
   d. Breasts

2. Puerperal morbidity occurs when the mother after delivery:
   a. Develops a temperature of 100.4°F (38°C) or higher within the first 24 hours
   b. Develops a temperature of 100.4°F (38°C) or higher after the first 24 hours, and it persists for 48 hours
   c. Develops a temperature of 100°F or higher on the third day postpartum, and it lasts for 24 hours
   d. Develops a temperature of 100.8°F or higher for any two consecutive days during the postpartum period

3. A localized infection of the lining of the uterus is termed:
   a. Parametritis
   b. Pelvic cellulitis
   c. Endometritis
   d. Peritonitis

4. If the mother develops endometritis, the lochia often will be:
   a. Fleshy-smelling and pale
   b. Foul-smelling and dark
   c. Odorless and pink
   d. Fleshy-smelling and pink

5. Factors that predispose the development of puerperal infection include:
   a. Age
   b. Multiparity
   c. Blood type
   d. Trauma during delivery

6. The organism most often responsible for the development of puerperal infection is:
   a. Anaerobic streptococcus
   b. *Staphylococcus aureus*

    c. *E. coli*

    d. Beta hemolytic streptococcus

7. If the mother develops pelvic cellulitis, she will experience:
   a. Pain and swelling in her leg
   b. Inflammation of the perineum
   c. Fever and pain in the abdomen
   d. Pain in the chest radiating down the arm

8. Pelvic thrombophlebitis is treated with:
   a. Warm, moist heat
   b. Sedation and an antipyretic
   c. Antibiotics and anticoagulants
   d. Dilatation and curettage

9. If, during the postpartum period, the mother is walking about, complains of pain in her leg, and has a fever, you would suspect that she may have:
   a. Dehydration and stiffness from being in bed so long
   b. Femoral thrombophlebitis
   c. Pelvic cellulitis
   d. A leg cramp and slight elevation of temperature due to excitement

10. If during the postpartum stay the mother develops puerperal infection, she needs much support because:
    a. You must teach good asepsis when she is handling the baby
    b. You must teach her how to give care to the baby so that she does not become tired
    c. You must keep her informed about the baby since she is isolated from the baby
    d. She must have rest as much as possible, and therefore when the baby comes out, you will give the care to the baby

11. If there are retained placental fragments inside the uterus, these often are a factor in producing:
    a. Postpartum hemorrhage
    b. Discomfort during intercourse
    c. Difficulty in becoming pregnant the next time
    d. Poor bladder function

12. The mother in the postpartum period who voids frequently in amounts of 60 to 100 cubic centimeters should be observed for:
    a. Retention of urine
    b. A kidney stone
    c. Diarrhea
    d. Residual urine

13. If the mother develops cystitis, she will experience:
    a. Blurring of vision
    b. Burning on urination and fever

    c. Pain in the abdomen

    d. Tenderness of the femoral vein

14. Subinvolution of the uterus occurs when the mother's uterus:
    a. Contracts readily during the first ten days so that it no longer is palpable
    b. Contracts especially at feeding times during the first several days of the postpartum period
    c. Does not contract as the uterus normally does at this time, and there is a slowing of the process
    d. Contracts when the mother is up and walking around during the first three days postpartum

15. Mastitis can develop in the postpartum period, and if the mother is breast-feeding, she will be more prone to develop this if:
    a. The baby comes out every feeding
    b. She alternates the breast with which she begins the feedings
    c. She has fissured or cracked nipples
    d. She has the baby in with rooming-in

16. A mother who becomes psychotic in the postpartum period may show:
    a. A desire for complete independence
    b. Total comfort in handling the baby and a desire to have more children as soon as possible
    c. Disorganization and disorientation
    d. Brief crying spells, comforted easily by the father

17. Nursing intervention with the mother who has become psychotic during the postpartum period is primarily geared to:
    a. Maintaining the mother in an isolated environment with no contact with others
    b. Moving the baby into the mother's room for rooming-in so that she can assume complete care of the baby
    c. Immediately discharging her from the hospital as this is primarily a reaction to hospitalization
    d. Establishing a safe environment and providing support and structure

UNIT VII

INTERRUPTIONS IN HEALTH IN THE NEONATAL PERIOD

Chapter 8
Down's Syndrome

Chapter 9
Preparation for Returning to the Family

CHAPTER ONE

PARENTAL REACTIONS TO THE NEONATE WITH HEALTH PROBLEMS

OBJECTIVES   *Identify the primary need of the family in which the mother has given birth to a child with health problems.*

Identify three stages of parental positive adaptation.

Identify the need for the parents to begin to assume parental tasks.

Identify some of the feelings parents may have when faced with a child with health problems.

Describe parental behaviors after the birth of a defective infant.

Identify the feelings of nurses and doctors when involved in the birth of a child with health problems.

Identify nursing intervention when involved with the parents of a child with health problems.

PRETEST In the spaces provided, fill in the word or words that best complete(s) the statements. Then turn to page 438 and check your answers.

1. The parents should be told that their baby has a problem _____

    _____.

2. The birth of a baby with health problems creates for the family _____

    _____.

3. The parental tasks and roles should be established _____

    _____.

4. If the infant is in specialized equipment such as an incubator, it is important

    to _____

    _____.

5. Expected reactions of the parents following the birth of a child with

    interruptions in health include _____, _____,

    _____, and _____.

6. Genetic counseling will provide _____

    _____.

We already have discussed many types of stressors: those that occur because of loss of family equilibrium following some kind of emergency situation during the pregnancy cycle, those that occur when fears for the unborn child are intensified, and those created by the termination of a wanted or an unwanted pregnancy. We now will discuss some of the events that create a crisis state when a baby is born with interruptions in health.

Unless the parents already have had a handicapped child born to them, they rarely expect this type of crisis to occur in their lives. They are prepared to accept a beautiful, normal baby and are totally unprepared to handle the effects created by anything less. How to tell the parents that their baby is not normal is a problem that has long plagued doctors and nurses. They, too, often lose their equilibrium when present at the birth of children with health problems. In the past doctors often have signaled their anesthesiologists to quickly put the mother under deep anesthesia, because they thought it would be too traumatic to disclose the information at the time of delivery. However, it is a rare occurrence that the mother does not sense that something is wrong.

In the past nurses also have felt that they had no responsibility to give the mother any information about the condition of her child. "It is her doctor's job." "The doctor would get furious if I said anything." This occurred because nurses were unable to handle the stress situation created by their feelings.

Many studies have been done, many mothers interviewed . . . and the results are the same. The mothers know something is wrong; they want and need clarification about the extent of the problem. The unknown is traumatic to the mother and the family when they suspect that something is wrong. They are subjected to prolonged fears and anxieties that often prove more overwhelming than the reality. Parents cannot begin to look at or deal with the stressor unless they know what it is. They must be told exactly what is wrong with their child and what, if anything, can be done to alter or improve the condition.

It is essential that the nurse recognize that the parents will go through a stage of shock, follow that stage with a search for some magical cure or treatment, and eventually end with positive adaptation. The resolution of the crisis, however, may not occur until after the death of the child. During the lifetime of the child the parents are said to suffer "chronic sorrow."

Parents should be permitted, and even encouraged, to see the child as soon as possible. When possible, both parents should be told together about the prognosis for their child. The optimum time and place for them to be told is after the birth in the delivery room because experience has shown that acceptance is easier for the parents at this time. It often is the nurse who explains simply to the parents the apparent disorder their child has and the immediate treatment that will be done. It is important to recognize that the nurse and other health team members have feelings, and expression of sadness and empathy can be a sharing that is supportive to the family as long as the health team member is not overwhelmed and unable to function.

The babies often are separated from the parents by physical distance, either by separation within the institution or by transfer to another institution. This separation wreaks havoc with the need for the parents to begin their parental tasks. As a result, often they start grieving before the loss of their child is a reality. It is almost as though they are afraid to accept the possibility of its life continuing. This mother and father should be brought to the area where the child is as soon as possible. They should be carefully told what the baby will look like, what type of crib or isolette it will be in, and what the purpose is of any equipment that might be surrounding the child (explain this in very simple language). The parents should be allowed to touch their child as soon as possible, thus making it a reality, a living child.

Prior to the initial contact, the mother may fantasize the extent of the handicap. Even when the medical team has attempted to carefully explain the extent of the problem and what medical help is available, the mother may not have heard. It has been found that parents often do not hear anything after the diagnosis statement. They seem to go into shock. It takes time to adjust to the loss of a perfect child and to attempt to accept and cope with one that is imperfect. The family's equilibrium is completely disrupted.

After the initial contact with their child, the parents then begin to seek more information about the status of the baby. The nurse at this time can clarify the information about the baby's condition and the immediate treatments that are being instituted. The parents should be constantly informed of the baby's status so that they can deal with the reality. If the condition of the baby is one that will involve long-term problems, the parents have to accept the prognosis before they can explore the type of care necessary for their child. At this time, the nurse can be supportive by explaining the various aspects of the baby's condition and referring the family to appropriate agencies. Often if the child has something such as cerebral palsy, the official organization of parents of children who have this disability can be involved, and these parents can effectively relate to and provide support for the family.

The nurses must expect grief, guilt, anger, sadness, and tears. They should allow the parents to explore their feelings, communicating to them that they understand, that they accept their feelings, and that they will tell the parents where to get help if it is needed.

It is also unrealistic for the nurse to expect the father to be immediately "strong and supportive." He, too, has many feelings to work through.

However, it often is the father who seems to deal with the stressor first. The nurse can then encourage him to help the mother reach the same level of equilibrium by open communication and exploration of feelings. Then the parents can move together into small parental-task situations as the condition of the baby permits. It is essential that mothering and fathering actions be allowed to take place as soon as possible; should the child die, the parents will have had some contact with him. In this way the parents' fantasies and feeling that the baby is not real will be dispersed, so that the parents can begin to achieve a homeodynamic balance.

The nurse must understand the mechanisms that individuals use in response to severe stress. The verbal and nonverbal communication between father and mother and parents and nurse must be clearly identified. Accurate observations must be made, inferences on data developed, and nursing action planned. Parents are influenced by nursing actions, which begin the first time either parent is shown the child. Perceptual biases of both nurse and family must be carefully identified and dealt with.

After the parents have dealt with the reality of their child's condition, this question often arises: "If we have another child, will the same difficulty or condition result?" The answers may be determined by genetic counseling, which will interpret the chances of recurrence. The nurse can help in explaining the results of genetic counseling. If the condition is a result of an accident that happened during development, then the family can be reassured that recurrence would be extremely rare; whereas if it is a genetic disorder, it follows patterns of inheritance and the family should be helped to understand the implications before they make their decision about future children.

The nurse must be cognizant of the financial stress that has been placed on the family due to all the specialized care and long hospitalization; thus referral to agencies that will help the family to apply for the necessary funds, equipment, and help is very important.

Let us see how you would respond to a mother you might meet in the hospital.

When you report to duty on the postpartum unit, you are assigned to care for Maria Cruz. You are told that she delivered a 7-pound boy with a spinal defect two days ago. Since the baby had signs of respiratory distress, he was placed in an isolette and could not be brought to the mother's room. The staff reports that Maria has consistently found reasons why she could not visit the nursery to see her baby. In devising your nursing care plan, you decide to approach the Cruzes together and make which of the following suggestions?

A. That it is important for them to see their baby and that putting it off any longer will not help the situation.

Go to page 433.

B. That maybe they ought to wait to see the baby until the mother feels stronger, since sometimes it is a shock when you aren't used to these things.

Go to page 435.

C.   That it often is difficult to realize that something is wrong
     with a baby that they have already pictured as perfect,
     that it becomes even more difficult when they really have
     no experience to help to prepare them, but that you will
     stay with them and explain about the baby and what is
     being done.   Go to page 434.

If you chose A, you have not clearly identified the entire scope of the stress. True, you are aware of the importance of the parents' seeing the baby as soon as feasible, but you have not taken their needs into consideration nor helped them to begin to resolve the conflicts.

Return to pages 429–431. Review the material and choose another response from page 431.

Good! In your choice of C you have identified the parents' need for reassurance about their feelings. You have recognized and accepted their reluctance to accept the fact that their baby is not what they wanted and expected. You also have indicated to them that you are not shocked by their baby since you are able and willing to go with them, to discuss the problem, and to explain what is being done to help their child. You have created an atmosphere of reality and acceptance, thereby helping the parents begin to move toward a more harmonious homeo-dynamic family interaction.

Advance to page 436 and take the post-test.

If you chose *B*, you have chosen incorrectly. You have reinforced the stress factor dealing with the possibility of the baby's looking so bad that it will be hard to tolerate. You, yourself, seem to be having difficulty dealing with the stressor. We often use this type of ''cop-out'' to keep from dealing with our own feelings of inadequacy in the situation.

Return to page 429. Review the material, examine your own feelings, then choose another response from page 431.

POST-TEST Indicate whether each statement is true or false by circling the appropriate letter. Then turn to page 438 and see how well you have done.

1. The parents may have fears and fantasies that become overwhelming if they are not informed about the child's status.   T   F

2. The nurse must let the physician inform the parents of the child's status.   T   F

3. The parents are able to cope better with the crisis of a child born with anomalies if informed of them at the time of delivery.   T   F

4. The parents should begin their parental tasks when the baby is well.   T   F

5. The parents often have feelings of guilt that they were responsible for their child's having this problem.   T   F

6. The parents do not need ongoing information about the infant's health status.   T   F

7. Genetic counseling may be helpful in predicting the chances of recurrence.   T   F

In the specific areas with which you had difficulty, return to the material and review.

BIBLIOGRAPHY   Aquilera, Donna, Janice Messick, and Marlene Farrell: *Crisis Intervention: Theory and Methodology*, C. V. Mosby Co., St. Louis, Mo., 1970.

"Childhood Mortality in the Americas," *WHO Chronicle*, reported in *Nursing Digest*, pp. 52–54, March/April 1975.

Christensen, Ann, "Coping with the Crisis of a Premature Birth: One Couple's Story," *Maternal Child Nursing*, Vol. 2, pp. 33–37, Jan.–Feb. 1977.

Clausen, Joy, Margaret Flook, and Bonnie Ford: *Maternity Nursing Today*, 2d ed., McGraw-Hill Book Co., New York, 1976.

Codden, Patricia, "The Meaning of Death for Parents and the Child," *Maternal-Child Nursing Journal*, Vol. 6, No. 1, pp. 9–16, Spring 1977.

DuBois, Don, "Indications of an Unhealthy Relationship Between Parents and Premature Infant," *Nursing Digest*, Vol. 4, pp. 56–59, Fall 1976.

Farrell, Helen, "Crisis Intervention Following the Birth of a Handicapped Infant," *Journal of Psychiatric Nursing and Mental Health Services*, Vol. 15, pp. 32–36, March 1977.

Harvey, Karen, "Caring Perceptively for the Relinquishing Mother," *Maternal Child Nursing*, Vol. 2, pp. 24–28, Jan.–Feb. 1977.

Johnson, Joan Marie, "Stillbirth, a Personal Experience," *American Journal of Nursing*, Vol. 72, pp. 1595–1596, Sept. 1972.

Kaplan, David and Edward Mason, "Maternal Reactions to Premature Birth Viewed as an Acute Emotional Disorder," in Howard Parad (ed.): *Crisis Intervention*, Family Service Association of America, New York, 1965.

Klaus, Marshall and John Kennell, "Mothers Separated from Their Newborn Infants," *Pediatric Clinics of North America*, Vol. 17, No. 4, pp. 1031–1035, Nov. 1970.

Korones, Sheldon: *High-Risk Newborn Infants*, C. V. Mosby Co., St. Louis, Mo., 1976, pp. 236–241.

Kübler-Ross, Elisabeth: *Death, The Final Stage of Growth*, Prentice-Hall, Englewood Cliffs, N.J., 1975.

Owens, Charlotte, "Parents' Reaction to Defective Babies," *American Journal of Nursing*, Vol. 64, No. 11, pp. 83–86, Nov. 1964.

Scipien, Gladys, et al.: *Comprehensive Pediatric Nursing*, McGraw-Hill Book Co., New York, 1975, pp. 347–353.

Wade, Nicholas, "Crib Death," *Nursing Digest*, Vol. 3, pp. 23–24, March/April 1975.

Waechter, E., "Developmental Consequences of Congenital Abnormalities," *Nursing Forum*, Vol. 14, No. 2, pp. 108–129, 1975.

Yates, Susan A., "Stillbirth, What a Staff Can Do," *American Journal of Nursing*, Vol. 72, pp. 1592–1594, Sept. 1972.

Young, Ruth, "Chronic Sorrow: Parents' Response to the Birth of a Child with a Defect," *Maternal Child Nursing*, Vol. 2, pp. 38–42, Jan.–Feb. 1977.

PRETEST
ANSWERS   1. Following delivery   2. A crisis state   3. As soon as possible   4. Explain to the
parents all the equipment and how it works   5. Grief; guilt; sadness; anger   6. Information
about the chances of recurrence

POST-TEST
ANSWERS   1. T   2. F   3. T   4. F   5. T   6. F   7. T

CHAPTER TWO
PREMATURITY

OBJECTIVES   *Define prematurity.*

Identify four reasons for disequilibrium to occur in the parents during and immediately after a premature delivery.

Identify four tasks that the parents must accomplish for adaptation to occur after the birth of a premature infant.

Identify length and weight variations in the premature neonate.

Identify seven characteristics of the premature neonate.

Identify alterations from those of the normal neonate in the respiratory, circulatory, digestive, excretory, and neurological systems of the premature infant.

Identify specific hospital care of the premature neonate in response to systemic alterations.

Identify three feeding techniques and four variations in formula.

Define retrolental fibroplasia and identify its cause.

Identify emotional needs of the premature neonate.

Identify nursing intervention in the care of the premature infant and the parents.

PRETEST In the spaces provided, fill in the word or words that best complete(s) the statements. Then turn to page 460 and check your answers.

1. Prematurity is defined according to _____ and

    _____.

2. During a premature labor and delivery, the atmosphere becomes one of an

    _____ situation.

3. The parents of a premature infant often believe that the baby is or shortly

    will be _____.

4. The four tasks that a mother of a premature infant must accomplish in order

    to adapt to the disequilibrium caused by the stress situation are to

    a. _____;

    b. _____; c. _____

    _____

    _____

    _____

    _____; and d. _____

    _____

    _____.

5. The weight of a premature infant is _____ grams or less.

6. The length of a premature infant is usually under _____ inches.

7. The appearance of a premature infant in regards to activity, cry, and skin

    color is _____; _____

    _____; _____.

8. The respiratory system, as are other systems in the premature infant, is

    _____, which causes symptoms of _____

    _____.

9. The premature infant is prone to bleeding because of a. _____

    _____ and b. _____

    _____.

10. Feeding is a problem because the _____ and _____

    reflexes are weak or absent.

11. The reflexes of the neurological system which are present in both the normal

    full-term neonate and the premature infant are _____, _____

    _____, and _____.

12. The premature infant is fed according to its ability to handle the feeding. Food may be given by _____, _____ _____, or _____.

13. Formula may be made of a. _____ _____; b. _____; c. _____; or d. _____ _____.

14. Formula should be enriched with the two minerals _____, and _____. It should be higher in the nutrient _____ and lower in the nutrient _____ than the formula given to a full-term baby, and the baby should be given replacement _____.

15. The baby is placed in an incubator, which provides _____ _____, _____, _____, and _____.

16. Retrolental fibroplasia is caused by _____ _____ and causes permanent _____.

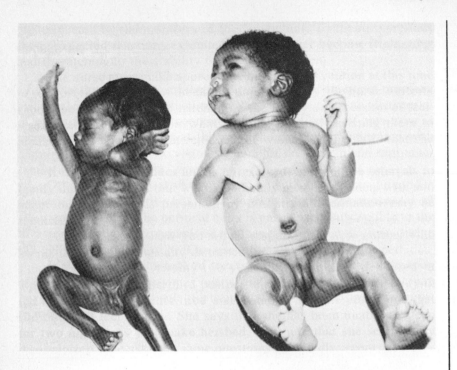

(Left) Premature infant, birth weight 1,300 grams (2 pounds, 14 ounces), 32 weeks gestation.
(Right) Full-term infant, birth weight 3,140 grams (6 pounds, 14 ounces), 40 weeks gestation.
(*From Comprehensive Pediatric Nursing by G. Scipien et al. Copyright © 1975 McGraw-Hill Book Company. Used with the permission of McGraw-Hill Book Company.*)

The premature infant is defined as an infant who is born before intra-uterine growth is completed so that all physiological systems are not fully developed. In the past an infant was classified as premature according to weight, the criterion being any neonate weighing less than 2,500 grams or $5\frac{1}{2}$ pounds. This criterion was insufficient since it made no distinction between the low-birth-weight, or dysmature, infant and the premature infant. A gestation period of between 26 and 37 weeks became the accepted criterion for prematurity. Determination of prematurity rests primarily on the neurological function of the reflexes (behaviors). Korones suggests that an infant born prior to the end of the thirty-seventh week of gestation is only small because of gestation.[1] These infants are of appropriate weight for their gestational age. Those infants who were born after the thirty-seventh week of gestation but who weigh under 2,500 grams are considered small for gestational age (SGA). It is possible for an infant to have retarded intrauterine growth (SGA) and also be born prior to the end of the thirty-seventh week of gestation. These infants are "small-for-dates, premature infants." Both prenatal and postnatal assessments of gestational age are possible.

The premature infant's physiological systems are _____ _____.

not

fully developed

Prematurity is defined as _____

birth between the

_____

_____.

    The infant's prematurity can be determined by _____

_____.

⇨

twenty-sixth and thirty-seventh

weeks of gestation

neurological

function

    A state of disequilibrium for the family is created by the birth of a premature infant. The family's adaptive mechanisms and resources must be mobilized to deal with this stress situation. Often due to the unexpectedness of the situation, a state of crisis arises, and the family needs intervention and support in order to deal adequately with this situation. The intervention and support begins as the family is admitted to the labor and delivery suite. The parents' normal concern about the labor process is heightened because of fear for the well-being of the baby. Many parents fear that the baby will die or is dead. Explaining to them what is currently happening and allowing them to hear the fetal heart rate reassures the parents and helps them to cope with this emergency situation.

    Admission to the labor and delivery suite, an anxiety-producing situation for women beginning labor under normal circumstances, becomes an emergency situation with premature labor. The staff, usually aware, calm, and communicative, is hurried, quiet, and uninformative, while the parents become frightened and feel that their baby, if not already dead, will soon be so. The mother is given little medication and thus is aware of what is taking place. The father, even when prepared, may be excluded from the delivery room; this fact heightens the suspense, fear, and atmosphere of emergency. If the parents do see the child briefly before he or she is removed to a special nursery or possibly another institution, both parents may be left with the memory of a very small, bluish, limp, unattractive-looking infant, a completely different experience from that which was expected.

    After the delivery the mother may be placed in a part of the hospital reserved for mothers who, for some reason, are without their newborn. The mother may be given very little information concerning the condition of her child. Staff does not wish to raise or diminish parents' hopes concerning the baby, and parent interaction may be missing entirely. It is, therefore, completely predictable that many parents will start the grieving process and separate emotionally from the child whom they feel will not live.

    When the mother is admitted to a postpartal unit, she has additional stressors with which to cope. She is involved with other mothers who are interacting with their newborn infants, causing her to be more concerned about her own child. Often she worries that the other mothers may feel inhibited in their mother-child interactions because of her plight. The astute nurse will observe the mother's behaviors for cues that would indicate decreased ability in utilizing her adaptive coping mechanisms, in order to plan nursing actions that will assist the mother to move to a state of equilibrium.

The atmosphere in a premature labor is one of an _____ situation.   emergency

The parents are given little _____.   information

Fathers usually are not allowed into the _____   delivery
room.

Medication for the mother is kept to a _____.   minimum

The baby, instead of looking like a normal, healthy newborn, appears frightening and _____ to the parents.   unattractive

The parents feel that the baby will probably _____   die
or be physically or mentally defective.

Mothers are _____ from the premature newborn,   separated
and thus the exploration of the baby so necessary to the start of the maternal role is prevented.

If staff members are not aware of the outward signs of crisis and their role in helping the family to utilize adaptive mechanisms, the adaptation may not take place for weeks, months, or ever.

It is felt that the mother must accomplish four tasks in order to regain a state of equilibrium: (1) She must accept the fact that she may indeed lose the baby before the anticipatory grief and withdrawal can begin. (2) She must recognize, examine, and accept the feelings of failure. She has failed to give birth to a normal, healthy baby. (3) After having to leave the hospital without the baby, she again must look at and begin to resume her maternal role in preparation for the homecoming of the baby after a prolonged hospital stay. (4) She must be realistic in her preparations for the care the baby will need and must have a realistic understanding of the special needs and some of the alterations in growth patterns.[2] The father not only can be supportive of the mother, but also must accomplish these same tasks in a similar way.

The first task that must be accomplished by the mother is the realization that she may indeed lose the child; she begins her anticipatory _____ and _____.   grief; separation

The second task involves the acceptance of her feelings of _____ failure.

The third task is concerned with her _____ for the homecoming of the child and her ability to start again to _____ to the infant.

The fourth and final task is one that is involved with her ability to be realistic in her preparations for the _____ of this baby and her ability to accept the differences in _____ and _____ patterns.

⬇

maternal preparation;

relate

care;
needs;
growth

Signs that the parents are accomplishing these tasks may be noted by the observant nurse. The first and second tasks, which take place at the time of delivery, involve signs of anticipatory grief and depression. These are healthy responses, which will be observed until there is reassurance that the baby will live. The third and fourth tasks are accomplished after the mother goes home and while the baby is still in the hospital. When the parents really can see signs that the baby is going to live (it gains weight, starts to take a bottle), they can begin to prepare for its homecoming. The fourth task is accomplished by the input of information through medical or nursing intervention, reading of books, and talking to other parents who have had premature infants.

If these tasks are accomplished, the parents are able to see their baby as normal, move out to give normal care, and believe in their ability to meet the needs of this infant. Once these tasks are accomplished, the family may move into a state of equilibrium and health.

Let us now discuss some of the characteristics of the premature infant.

In contrast with the length of the normal newborn infant, which is about _____ inches, the premature is about *18 inches long or less*. We already have discussed the weight, which is under _____ grams or _____ pounds. The neck and extremities are shorter than those of a full-term infant, and the eyes and tongue seem prominent. The circumference of the *chest is under 11½ inches*. Instead of being the active infant with a strong cry usually seen at term, *these babies are weak and sluggish, and often appear drowsy*. Premature babies have *red, wrinkled skin* because of the *lack of adipose tissues*; there may be much lanugo and limited amount of vernix on the skin. The body temperature is difficult to maintain.

20;

2,500; 5½

The chest circumference of a normal newborn is about 13 inches while that of a premature infant is under _____.

⇩

$11\frac{1}{2}$ inches

These babies appear _____ , _____ , and drowsy.

weak; inactive

Their skin is red and wrinkled because of a lack of subcutaneous _____. There is little vernix covering the skin, but the silky hair called _____ is present.

fat;

lanugo

These babies have *respiratory* difficulties. The more premature the infant, the less the respiratory system has had the opportunity to develop. The respiratory muscles are weak, there has been little surfactant, circulation through the lungs is poor, and the nasal passages are narrow and extremely susceptible to injury. These infants often succumb to respiratory distress syndrome within the first few hours or days after birth. (We will discuss this at length in Unit VII, Chapter Four.) Typically, periods of apnea, cyanosis, and irregular respirations may be present, and cough reflexes may be absent.

Because of the premature state, the respiratory system is _____, and this situation causes respiratory difficulties.

underdeveloped

The nurse may observe periods of _____,

apnea;

_____, and an _____ pattern of respirations.

cyanosis; irregular

The respiratory system reflex that may be absent is the _____ reflex.

cough

There also are alterations in the *circulatory system* in the premature neonate as compared with that of the normal full-term newborn. The heart is large, but the heart action may be slow. There is poor peripheral circulation, and the walls of the blood vessels are weak. This complication, combined with the problem of a decrease in clotting factors, makes bleeding, especially intracranial hemorrhage, an ever-present threat. These infants also have low gammaglobulin levels, making them especially susceptible to infection.

Some of the alterations in the circulatory system are concerned with the fact that the heart is _____ and the heart action _____.

enlarged;

slow

Bleeding always is a threat, and these babies must be handled very little and very carefully because of the decreased _____

factors and the weakness of the walls of the _____ vessels.

> clotting;
> blood

    Asepsis is extremely important because these babies are more

prone to _____ due to the low levels of

_____.

> infection;
> gammaglobulin

    These babies pose a feeding problem because they have weak
sucking and swallowing reflexes and become exhausted easily. They
also seem to regurgitate frequently and must be watched for aspiration.
Prematures have poorly developed gastric mucosa and absorb fat
poorly, and they also may exhibit problems with constipation because
the muscles of the bowel are weak.

    Digestive problems arise from the fact that the babies have poor

_____ and _____ reflexes and become

_____ easily during feeding.

> sucking; swallowing;
> exhausted

    These babies have difficulty with defecation because the muscles
of the bowel are _____.

> weak

    Unlike the normal full-term infant, prematures often have *oliguria*
and an *increase in interstitial fluid*. There is incomplete formation of
the tubules of the kidney, and the babies have an increased tendency
to become acidotic.

    Prematures often have a decrease in the amount of _____

excreted, have underdeveloped _____, and

must be watched carefully so that _____ can be treated

should it occur.

> urine;
> kidneys;
> acidosis

    The development of the *neurological system* will depend upon the
extent of the prematurity. External stimulation results in weak, jerky
movements by the infant. The Moro, Babinski, and tonic neck reflexes
are present.

    The reflexes that are present in the normal full-term neonate and

in the premature infant are the _____, _____,

and _____.

> Moro; Babinski;
> tonic neck

Let us now discuss the nursing care of the premature neonate. Care is directed to *maintaining and improving respirations, body heat, and nutrition*; to *preventing infection*; and to *providing emotional support*, in other words, delivering "tender loving care."

In the delivery room, the nurse must be alert to any respiratory depression and to the need for resuscitative measures. It also is the nurse's responsibility to make sure that the infant is immediately placed in a warm environment so that its body heat is conserved. The pediatrician should examine the infant before it is removed from the delivery room, and the premature nursery should be alerted about the new admission.

Nursing responsibility in the delivery room concerning the needs of a newborn premature infant includes the infant's needs for maintenance of _____ and body _____.

It also is the responsibility of the nurse to have the baby seen by a _____ before transfer to the nursery and to alert the premature _____ to the imminent birth of a premature infant.

respirations; heat

pediatrician;

nursery staff

When the premature infant is admitted to the high-risk nursery, it should be placed in an incubator. This equipment is necessary for several reasons. Because of its large surface area in comparison to body mass, the infant has an especially large surface from which to lose heat. In addition, these babies have little subcutaneous fat and weak muscular movements, making temperature stabilization difficult. We already have mentioned their poor respiratory function and their susceptibility to injury and infection. The incubator provides an environment in which care can be given safely to the infant and oxygen, heat, and humidity levels can be maintained.

Some premature centers have found that by introducing sound, such as that of waves rhythmically and gently breaking on a shore, and gentle, continuous motion within the incubator, an intrauterine-like environment is replicated. Some studies have shown that the infants in these incubators rest and sleep better and gain weight faster. Further studies to validate these results are being conducted.

The premature infant has poor body heat maintenance because it has a large surface area from which to lose _____.

Shivering and body movements do not help increase body heat

heat

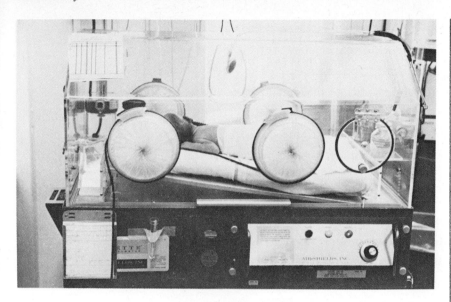

Infant in incubator. (*From Comprehensive Pediatric Nursing by G. Scipien et al. Copyright © 1975 McGraw-Hill Book Company. Used with the permission of McGraw-Hill Book Company.*)

because _____ movements are weak, and heat is not
maintained because there are small deposits of _____
_____.

muscular;

subcutaneous

fat

In order to remedy the above situation and to provide a
controlled oxygen and humidity environment, these babies are placed
in _____.

incubators

The nurse must be ever alert to the status of the baby's respirations, temperature, color, and activity. While we are speaking about
the administration of oxygen, it is important to mention *retrolental
fibroplasia*. This is a condition precipitated by too high concentrations
of oxygen, and results in blindness. Too much oxygen over a prolonged
period of time at too high a concentration can cause retinal detachment
in the immature eyes of the neonate. When this occurs, scar tissue
forms behind the lens, causing irreversible blindness. It therefore is
essential that oxygen be administered only when there is a clinical
indication for its use and, when possible, kept below 40 percent.

The nurse, in observations of the premature infant, must be
aware of changes in status and is especially concerned about the
baby's _____, _____, _____,
and _____. The nurse also must recognize the
importance of utilizing oxygen only when _____ by

respirations; color; temperature;

activity

indicated;

symptomology, because the result of too _____ oxygen

over too _____ a period can cause retrolental

fibroplasia, which is a cause of _____. The best

percentage of oxygen to use when symptoms do not demand more is

_____ percent.

much;

long

blindness;

40

Nutrition and the provision of fluids are of extreme concern in
the care of the premature infant. In addition to the previously
mentioned characteristics of the digestive system, namely, poor
_____ and _____ reflexes, a tendency to
_____, and a sluggish bowel, these babies have a very
small stomach capacity. They also have decreased storage of minerals,
vitamins, and glycogen; have difficulty in fat absorption; and need
increased amounts of protein, calcium, and phosphorus, since these
are stored late in the gestational period.

sucking; swallowing;

vomit

Premature infants lose between 10 and 15 percent of their birth
weight, the lowest level being reached between the fourth and eighth
days after birth. Depending upon how mature they are and how successfully they are hydrated, they should regain this loss in one to three
weeks. It is essential that the staff recognize this and not get discouraged
when their careful care is not immediately evident on the weighing
scale.

Feeding is a problem because of the small _____
capacity of these babies and their need for large amounts of vitamins,
the essential nutrient _____, and the minerals
_____ and _____, which usually are stored
late in pregnancy.

stomach;

protein;

calcium; phosphorous

The weight loss sustained by premies usually is between
_____ and _____ percent; they usually reach the lowest level
of weight between the _____ and _____
days after birth. Birth weight usually is regained sometime
between the _____ and _____ weeks
after birth.

10; 15;

fourth; eighth;

first; third

Because of the small stomach capacity, these babies are given
small, frequent feedings. The amount of feeding will depend upon the

baby's ability to handle it. The nurse must observe the infant for signs of distress due to overfeeding, such as overdistended stomach; respiratory distress, such as dyspnea and cyanosis; and vomiting.

When feeding prematures, the nurse must be aware of the need to give _____, _____ feedings; must be alert to the possibility of distress after the feeding; and must observe the baby for signs of distress, such as a _____ stomach, and respiratory distress, such as _____ of breath and cyanosis.

small; frequent;

distended;

shortness

The babies are fed according to their ability to handle the feeding method. That is, they may be gavaged (tube-fed), fed with a medicine dropper, or bottle-fed with a premature nipple. Many specialists feel that breast milk, because of its easy digestibility and nutritional value, is the best form of feeding for these babies. On this recommendation, some institutions are starting breast milk banks. Others feel that skimmed cow's milk, a prepared formula, or an evaporated milk formula is tolerated just as well. Therefore, the type of feeding offered depends upon the orientation of the pediatrician in charge of the care of the premature infant.

When the babies are very small, cannot suck well, and are easily fatigued, they usually are fed through a tube inserted into their stomachs. This type of feeding is called a _____ feeding. As the babies get stronger they first are fed with a _____ dropper, than graduated to an infant _____.

gavage;

medicine; bottle

The actual feedings may be of various types. After the first few feedings of glucose and water, the baby may be given small, _____ feedings of _____ milk or formulas made from _____ cow's milk, synthetic milk, or _____ milk.

frequent; breast;

skimmed;

evaporated

You remember that the immaturity of the premature infant's organs and its low gammaglobulin level, capillary fragility, and easily traumatized skin make the baby highly susceptible to infection. It is essential to handle these babies very little and very gently when caring for them. These babies seem to acquire upper respiratory infections very easily. Therefore, a staff member who is suffering from an upper respiratory infection must not care for these high-risk infants. Other nursing personnel, who may transmit organisms from the nasopharynx or skin, must be made aware of the need for strict aseptic technique. The safety and well-being of a premature infant depend upon the reliability of those who care for it.

Although little handling of premature infants is recommended, they need human contact and tender loving care for their emotional development. This need can be met through stroking, hair combing, and gentle touching through the portholes of the incubator. Mobiles or other stimulation can be provided when the infants are ready for it.

Premature infants are especially susceptible to infection because of the _____ of their organs, the _____ of their capillaries, the easily abrased _____, and the low levels of _____, which contains antibodies.

immaturity; fragility; skin; gammaglobulin

In order to help prevent infection, in addition to handling these infants gently and infrequently, staff must use extreme techniques of _____.

asepsis

Persons caring for these infants also must remember that these babies need _____ contact for their emotional development.

human

Do not forget the importance of including the parents in the care of these babies. The sooner the parents can begin participating in their baby's care, the better for the baby and its parents.

In helping the mother to accomplish the first two tasks while in the hospital, it is essential for the nurse to recognize signs of normal grief and anticipatory separation. Grief and mourning often begin before the actual loss takes place. The mother may experience feelings that she refers to as "being helpless," sad, and lonely. She may express anger and guilt. There may be times when her feelings express themselves in a physical way, such as in difficulty in sleeping, anorexia, tightness in the throat, or weakness. It is said that "grief is analogous to pain; it is a subjective symptom."[3] The nurse also may be aware that these "symptoms" are shown after visitors, who have expressed feelings of sympathy, leave the mother's room, eliciting on the part of the mother wishes that visitors would stay away or expression of anger and hostility.

In order for the nurse to help the mother to reach a level of functional equilibrium, the nurse must accurately assess the mother's behavior. The nurse also must have information about the manner in which this particular family copes with stress and the meaning of loss to them and must support them in their own familiar adaptive mechanisms. The parents must be allowed to express their feelings freely; they must be given accurate information about the condition of their child so that they lose the feeling of isolation; and the "conspiracy of silence" must be interrupted.

It is essential that the nurses also examine their own feelings about death and particularly about the dying child. If not evaluated and handled, the nurse's needs may take precedence over the needs of the family. It also is important for the nurse to set realistic goals for nursing intervention.

Let us look at the way a particular mother reacts to the birth of a premature baby.

You have been assigned to care for Ruth Brenner, who gave birth to a 3-pound baby girl born at 33 weeks of gestation. You have checked to see how the baby is doing and have found out that it is receiving gavage feedings, is in an incubator, and now is experiencing respiratory distress. When you enter the room, Ruth says, "Did you see her? She's so skinny and little, I'm sure she won't make it. If she does, she'll never be right, so maybe it's better that way. I knew I shouldn't have moved to the new house until after the baby came, all that work and aggravation. . . ."

You recognize that Ruth's reaction is described best by which of the statements below?

A. Ruth has no information about the condition of the baby; this situation explains her high level of anxiety.

Go to page 454 top.

B. Ruth has had some experience with the birth of premature infants and recognizes the potential hazard that prematurity presents.

Go to page 455 bottom.

C. Ruth is beginning to show evidence of coping with the disequilibrium caused by the birth of a premature infant.

Go to page 456 top.

If you chose *A*, "Ruth has no information . . . ," you are incorrect. You have not verified whether or not information has been given to her. Rather, you have jumped to the conclusion that this mother is a "victim" of silence. This kind of assessment may inhibit you from appropriate intervention. You have not been able to identify the meaning of the mother's words.

Return to page 442. Review the material and choose another answer from page 453.

———————————————

Excellent! You have shown great acceptance of the mother's feelings by your choice of *B*. You have allowed the mother to ventilate her feelings without intruding or judging her. In addition, you have recognized her need for current, realistic information. Your checking on the condition of the baby and giving the mother the information about the baby's condition shows the mother that you really care about her and understand what she is going through. Your reassurance that you will have the doctor let her know more fully about the baby's condition also is reassuring and therapeutic. Well done.

Advance to page 458 and take the post-test.

Very poor. Your choice of *C* gives evidence to the mother that you are completely unaware of her needs. You did not recognize or hear what she was asking of you. Rather, you changed the subject from the area of stress without reducing its effects in any way or giving the mother anything with which to handle it. You also did not recognize that her inability to eat breakfast may have been a normal manifestation of the effect of the stressor and may have called for a different response. You have been most untherapeutic.

Return to page 445. Review the material and choose another response from page 456.

No. You chose *B*, "Ruth has had some experience . . ."; how do you know this? You are jumping to conclusions and hearing only the superficial meaning of the mother's words.

Review the material on page 442, listen to the mother again, and try to evaluate, on the basis of your understanding of grief and mourning, what mechanism is involved. Then choose another response from page 453.

Good. You chose *C*, "Ruth is beginning to show evidence. . . ." You have recognized that normal adaptation is occurring. You are tuned in to the fact that anticipatory separation, grief, and feelings of guilt are part of this adaptive mechanism. Knowing this, what is your next response in this situation?

A.   "Ruth, I have just seen your baby and she really is doing great. She held her morning feeding down, and the nursery staff is very pleased with her condition. I'm sure she will be OK."   Go to page 457.

B.   "It really must be hard not to know exactly what is happening with the baby. I can understand how upset and frightened you must be. I checked with the nursery before coming in and found that the baby did retain her feeding this morning and that her breathing is much better. I will make sure Dr. Dann speaks to you after he sees her this morning."   Go to page 454 bottom.

C.   "Ruth, you know all of this anxiety isn't good for you now. You have to rest and regain your strength; your husband needs you now. Let the doctors take care of the baby, and we will concentrate on getting you strong enough to go home. Now eat your breakfast, and I'll be back in a little while to help you get washed."   Go to page 455 top.

Not good; your choice of *A* shows that you still are not aware of the appropriate nursing intervention. You have moved in to "make the mother feel better." Your statement gives the impression that all is well. You have given the mother hopes that may be unrealistically high at this time, and you also have made it impossible for her to express any more fears to you.

Return to page 445. Review the entire situation, and evaluate the needs of the mother in light of the fact that your needs seem to have taken precedence. Deal with your own feelings, then try again to intervene on the mother's behalf. Choose another response from page 456.

POST-TEST Indicate whether each statement is true or false by circling the appropriate letter. Then turn to page 460 and see how well you have done.

1. Parents adapt easily to the birth of a premature infant.   T   F

2. Prematurity is defined according to neurological status and gestation.   T   F

3. The mother's grief, sorrow, and separation from the child during her hospital stay should alert the nurse to the need for immediate intervention to establish a close mothering role.   T   F

4. A premature infant has difficulty maintaining body temperature because of his weak muscular movements.   T   F

5. It is not necessary initially to place all premature infants in an incubator.   T   F

6. Premature infants are prone to respiratory distress.   T   F

7. If handled correctly, the premature infant should offer no special feeding problem.   T   F

8. Neurologic responses will depend on the maturity of the infant.   T   F

9. A premature infant, unlike a full-term newborn, needs additional protein in its diet.   T   F

10. A very small premature infant can be fed easily with a bottle as long as it has a premature nipple.   T   F

11. Infection is not a priority problem with the premature infant.   T   F

12. An infant in an incubator should never be given a concentration of oxygen higher than 40 percent.   T   F

In the specific areas with which you had difficulty, return to the material and review.

REFERENCES
1. Sheldon Korones: *High-Risk Newborn Infants*, C. V. Mosby Co., St. Louis, Mo., 1976, p. 75.
2. David Kaplan and Edward Mason, "Maternal Reaction to Premature Birth Viewed as an Acute Emotional Disorder," in Howard Parad (ed.): *Crisis Intervention,* Family Service Association of America, New York, 1965, pp. 124–126.
3. Carolyn E. Carlson, "Grief and Mourning," in *Behavioral Concepts and Nursing Intervention,* coordinated by Carolyn E. Carlson, J. B. Lippincott Co., Philadelphia, 1970, pp. 96–112.

BIBLIOGRAPHY

Aquilera, Donna, Janice M. Messick, and Marlene S. Farrell: *Crisis Intervention: Theory and Methodology*, C. V. Mosby Co., St. Louis, Mo. 1970.

Avery, Gordon: *Neonatology, Pathophysiology and Management of the Newborn,* J. B. Lippincott Co., Philadelphia, 1975.

Babson, S. Gorham and Ralph C. Benson: *Management of Hi-Risk Pregnancy and Intensive Care of the Neonate*, 2d ed., C. V. Mosby Co., St. Louis, Mo., 1971.

Barnett, C., et al., "Neonatal Separation: The Maternal Side of Interactional Deprivation," *Pediatrics*, pp. 45 and 197.

Chase, Helen and Mary E. Byrnes, "Trends in Prematurity: United States 1959–1967," *American Journal of Public Health*, Vol. 60, No. 10, pp. 1967–1983, Oct. 1970.

Christensen, Ann, "Coping with the Crisis of a Premature Birth: One Couple's Story," *Maternal Child Nursing*, Vol. 2, pp. 33–37, Jan.–Feb. 1977.

Cornblath, Marvin, "Diagnosing and Treating Neonatal Hypoglycemia," *Contemporary Ob/Gyn*, Vol. 8, pp. 95–99, Sept. 1976.

Crosse, V. Mary: *The Premature Baby and Other Babies with Low Birth Weight*, Little, Brown, Boston, 1966.

DuBois, Don, "Indications of an Unhealthy Relationship Between Parents and Premature Infant," *Nursing Digest*, Vol. 4., pp. 56–59, Fall 1976.

Evans, Marian, "Adaptation of the Infant at Birth and Intervention Techniques for Distressed Neonate," *Journal of Nurse Midwifery*, Vol. 20, No. 7, pp. 18–28, Winter 1975.

Kopf, Rita and Elizabeth Linder McFadden, "Nursing Intervention in the Crisis of Newborn Illness," *Journal of Nurse Midwifery*, Vol. 18, No. 1, pp. 11–19, Spring 1973.

McLean, Frances, "Assessing Gestational Age," *Canadian Nurse*, Vol. 68, pp. 23–26, March 1972.

Marlow, Dorothy: *Textbook of Pediatric Nursing*, W. B. Saunders Co., Philadelphia, 1977.

Moore, Mary Lou: *The Newborn and the Nurse*, W. B. Saunders Co., Philadelphia, 1972.

Schaffer, Alexander and Mary Ellen Avery: *Diseases of the Newborn*, W. B. Saunders Co., Philadelphia, 1977.

Warrick, Louise, "Family-Centered Care in a Premature Nursery," *American Journal of Nursing*, Vol. 71, No. 11, pp. 2134–2138, Nov. 1971.

PRETEST ANSWERS

1. Gestation; neurological maturity   2. Emergency   3. Dead   4. a. Accept the possible loss of a child; b. accept her feelings of failure; c. after leaving the baby in the hospital, be able to reidentify with the infant and begin to define her maternal role; d. be realistic in her view of the baby as normal and accept its special needs and growth patterns   5. 2,500   6. 18   7. Activity, weak; cry, weak; color, red   8. Immature; respiratory distress   9. a. Poor clotting mechanism; b. weak walls of the blood vessels   10. Sucking; swallowing   11. Moro; tonic neck; Babinski   12. Gavage; medicine dropper; bottle   13. a. Breast milk fortified with protein; b. skim milk formula; c. synthetic formula; d. evaporated milk formula   14. Calcium; phosphorous; protein; fat; vitamins   15. Controlled oxygen; heat; humidity; an aseptic environment   16. Too high a concentration of oxygen for too long; blindness

POST-TEST ANSWERS

1. F   2. T   3. F   4. T   5. F   6. T   7. F   8. T   9. T
10. F   11. F   12. T

CHAPTER THREE

POSTMATURITY AND INTRAUTERINE GROWTH RETARDATION

OBJECTIVES *Define postmaturity.*

Identify the physical characteristics of a postmature infant.

Identify five tests done on amniotic fluid to determine fetal maturity.

Define intrauterine growth retardation.

Identify the characteristics of intrauterine growth retardation.

Identify nursing intervention.

GLOSSARY *Postmature newborn:* A neonate born more than two weeks after the normal gestational time

PRETEST   In the spaces provided, fill in the word or words that best complete(s) the statements. Then turn to page 473 and check your answers.

1. A fetus is considered postmature if it is still undelivered _____ or more weeks after the EDC.

2. Four physical characteristics of the postmature infant are a. _____ _____, b. _____, c. _____, and d. _____ _____.

3. A major hazard of postmaturity to the fetus is _____.

4. After birth the postmature neonate must be observed for the following three complications: a. _____, b. _____, and c. _____.

5. A small-for-gestational-age infant is one who is _____ _____ _____.

6. SGA may be due to _____, _____, _____ _____, or _____.

7. SGA is found more often among mothers who during pregnancy have a. _____, b. _____, c. _____, d. _____, or are e. _____ or f. _____.

⬇

When delivery occurs two or more weeks after term, so that the gestational time is 42 weeks or longer, the infant is considered *postmature*. The factors that cause postmaturity are unknown, but the fetus is at risk in utero because of placental dysfunction. The circulation through the placenta becomes diminished; therefore, all the nutrients and oxygen are exchanged in smaller amounts. The characteristics of the postmature infant are low birth weight; absence of lanugo and vernix; much scalp hair; long nails; pale, desquamated skin; and alertness. There is a higher incidence of stillbirths when the fetus is postmature. During labor the postmature fetus is more susceptible to stress than a normal term baby is. Often there is neonatal respiratory distress at delivery time. Other problems encountered are hypoglycemia, pneumonia, and dehydration.

Postmaturity occurs when the gestational time is _____ _____.

42
weeks or longer

The fetus is at risk because of _____ _____.

placental
dysfunction

A physical characteristic of the postmature infant is an absence of _____ and vernix.

lanugo

The skin is _____ ___ _____ in color and appears _____.

pale;
desquamated

The infant has a lot of scalp hair, and his nails are _____.

long

Some people think it is advantageous to induce labor by three weeks after term if the maturity of the fetus has been determined. Others feel that the less intervention, the better the prognosis. The exact gestational time is difficult to determine. The tests available usually can only estimate maturity; they are not precise.

The test for integumentary system maturity is based on the nile blue stain of _____ cells.

fat

The test for pulmonary system maturity is an _____ ratio.

L/S

Bilirubin level tests are done because by term the bilirubin levels are _____ or entirely _____.

very low; absent

Maternal urinary estriol levels indicate the functioning of the fetoplacental unit. If these levels drop significantly, it is thought that the fetus should be delivered since it may be in jeopardy.

Other tests done to determine fetal maturity are amniotic fluid creatinine levels. If the creatinine, which is excreted in the urine of the fetus, is over 1.8 per 100 milliliters in the absence of maternal toxemia, it is felt that the fetus has reached the gestational age of about 36 weeks.

By measuring the biparietal diameters of the fetal skull through ultrasound visualization, fetal maturity can be also estimated.

Some institutions are now using a stress test, also called the "oxytocin challenge test" (OCT), to determine placental functioning. This is actually a trial labor, stimulated by intravenous oxytocin, diluted 5 units of Pitocin in 500 cubic centimeters of 5 percent dextrose and water. The fetal heart rate is monitored for reaction to mild uterine contractions. If the fetus demonstrates a late deceleration in response to two uterine contractions, vaginal delivery is not considered to be safe for the fetus, and elective cesarean section is indicated when fetal maturity or fetal jeopardy is determined.

As the time for delivery approaches and the tasks of the third trimester are completed, the mother packs her suitcase and truly becomes a "lady-in-waiting." As the delivery date draws closer, she primes herself for it. She is tired of being pregnant and longs for her clumsiness and distorted appearance to be things of the past. The doctor has given her an expected "due date" and has cautioned her that it is, in fact, only an estimate, but she really believes it to be the date. As the date comes and goes and she is still pregnant, she begins to wonder if everything is all right. Well-meaning friends and neighbors call and ask if she has seen the doctor. The tension, irritability, and fears of both parents grow. The nurse must recognize the feelings that are present and must be aware of the crisis that is being precipitated. The nurse should carefully explore the parents' adaptive mechanisms and the effectiveness of these mechanisms.

The infant is considered to be small for gestational age (SGA) or to be the victim of intrauterine growth retardation if it is full-term, that is, born between the _____ and   thirty-seventh;

_____ week of gestation; ex-   fortieth
hibits full-term neurological behavior; but weighs under 2,500 grams. These babies have many problems that demand careful nursing observations and continuous measurements of status.

First, let us look at some of the reasons a full-term baby might have a low birth weight. These causes may be divided into (1) maternal factors, such as hypertensive or respiratory disorders or anemia that interfere with transfer of nutrients to the fetus; infections; malnutrition; multiparity; or chemical abuse, such as drug or alcohol abuse or heavy cigarette smoking; (2) environmental stressors, such as radiation or residence in high altitudes that limit oxygen consumption; (3) placental problems; and (4) fetal stressors, such as multiple pregnancy, in which the internal environment is crowded, or chromosomal aberrations.

"SGA" means that a baby is full-term but the amount of physical development is _____.

below normal

Maternal stressors that might cause SGA infants are those that interfere with the transfer of _____ or _____, infections, and _____ abuse.

oxygen; nutrients; chemical

External environmental stressors thought to predispose to SGA are _____ and residence in _____ _____.

radiation; high altitudes

Twins are more susceptible to being SGA because of intrauterine _____.

crowding

The SGA neonate will appear to be alert but will look emaciated. The morbidity in this newborn results from malnourishment in utero; the prognosis depends upon how greatly growth was retarded and upon whether or not there are congenital malformations. In the nursery this baby should be observed for signs of hypoglycemia caused by having few energy stores for metabolic activity and for lack of body insulation due to having little subcutaneous tissue. Other nursing observations would be directed toward the detection of asphyxia, hypothermia, and signs of irritability and pain, for example, crying or other evidence that the infant may be in pain. Laboratory reports should also be carefully noted.

The infant of the diabetic mother is considered to be large for gestational age (LGA). This infant's development is not at the expected level for gestational age.

Once the mother has reached term and delivery is completed, the parents are concerned about the condition of their baby. "Is it normal?" usually is the first question asked of the nurse as the baby is placed in the warmer. If the infant is postmature or SGA he often is placed in an intensive care area of the nursery. Thus the fear of the parents concerning the well-being of their child is heightened. The families need much information and support from the nurse at this time.

Now, let us see how you would respond to a woman you might meet in the hospital.

Helen Rodriguez is admitted to the labor room. While you are doing the admission interview, she tells you that the baby is three weeks overdue and the doctor is going to induce her labor. You ask her if she knows what that means. She answers, "Yes, my sister had it done. She told me that the doctor puts medicine in your arm; then very strong pains start and last until the baby comes." Helen watches you closely as she says, "I feel the baby moving, so it's all right. How come the doctor wants to bring it on? I know that the baby comes when it is ready and the longer it stays in, the bigger and stronger it gets."

From this conversation you identify several areas of concern. Which of the following statements would be nursing intervention based on the primary stressor?

A. "You have the general idea of how labor is induced. Maybe I can clarify a few points for you."

Go to page 467 bottom.

B. "It's good that you feel the baby moving; however, if it waits too long to get born, sometimes your body is no longer able to feed it and it begins to lose weight."

Go to page 470.

C. "Everybody is different. The contractions aren't always so strong. But don't worry: if you are uncomfortable, the doctor will order medication to help with the pain."

Go to page 471.

If you chose *B*, "How carefully the baby will be observed," you did not use the problem-solving approach effectively. Review the initial interview on page 465, the primary stressor, and your immediate intervention. Then reread the situation on page 470. Identify the information already given, and then identify the primary stressor at this time.

Return to page 470 and choose another response.

If you chose *A*, "You have the general idea . . . ," you have not selected the primary area of stress for your immediate intervention. Although you have recognized the mother's fear and acknowledged the information she has, your assessment is not correct.

Return to page 465. Reread the situation, identify the primary stressor, and choose another response.

If you chose C, you completely missed the boat. Reread the situations on pp. 465 and 470 using the problem-solving approach. Identify the primary stress at this precise moment. Later you will give the information concerning the monitoring device . . . but first things come first. Sometimes by giving information too soon all you do is introduce another unexpected stressor before the family has had time to deal with the current crisis situation.

Return to page 470 and choose another response.

If you chose A, "How the induction is done," you are correct. Stress is increased by the unknown. When a family is helped to see the reality of a situation, they are given something factual to deal with instead of their fantasies. They then can draw upon resources used in previous similar situations. If the stress at this time is too strong to be handled by the family's resources, you will have to identify how you will change your role in order to help the family.

Advance to page 472 and take the post-test.

Good. In your choice of *B*, "It's good that you feel the baby moving . . . ," you have correctly assessed that Helen's primary concern is fear for the baby. You have listened to what she has said and have observed her nonverbal communication. You were correct in reassuring her that her evaluation of fetal movements was meaningful, and you also have added the information that she needed to be reassured that the induction will be done as further protection for the well-being of the baby.

As you take Helen's vital signs, you explain the admission procedure and the need for a vulval shave and an enema. After these procedures have been completed, Joe, Helen's husband, comes into the labor room to be with Helen during the labor and delivery. In setting your priorities, which of the following areas should you first discuss with the Rodriguezes to reduce areas of stress?

<ul>
<li>A.   How the induction is done.   Go to page 469.</li>
<li>B.   How carefully the baby will be observed during the procedure.   Go to page 467 top.</li>
<li>C.   How a monitoring device will monitor both the mother and the baby during the procedure.   Go to page 468.</li>
</ul>

If you chose C, you were unable to identify Helen's primary concern. You were aware that she was afraid of pain, but you did not hear what else she was saying to you or identify the meaning of her nonverbal communication.

Return to page 465. Reread the situation, listen to and observe Helen, and choose another response.

POST-TEST   Indicate whether each statement is true or false by circling the appropriate letter. Then turn to page 473 and see how well you have done.

1. If a fetus is born three weeks after the EDC, it is considered to be postmature.   T   F

2. The postmature infant has short nails, much vernix, and lethargy.   T   F

3. Stillbirth is a complication of postmaturity.   T   F

4. SGA and prematurity are the same.   T   F

5. Placental size may be a factor that contributes to SGA   T   F

6. Multiparity with or without toxemia may be a factor that contributes to SGA infants.   T   F

7. In the newborn nursery, the SGA infant must be observed for hypoglycemia and malformations.   T   F

In the specific areas with which you had difficulty, return to the material and review.

BIBLIOGRAPHY   Avery, Gordon: *Diseases of the Newborn*, J. B. Lippincott Co., Philadelphia, 1975, pp. 51–58.

Cetrulo, Curtis, "Minimizing the Risks of Twin Delivery," *Contemporary Ob/Gyn*, Vol. 9, pp. 47–51, Feb. 1977.

Clark, Ann, and Dyanne O. Alfonso: *Childbearing: A Nursing Perspective*, F. A. Davis Co., Philadelphia, 1976, pp. 697–704.

Clausen, Jay, Margaret Flook, and Bonnie Ford: *Maternity Nursing Today*, 2d ed., McGraw-Hill Book Co., 1977, pp. 831–836.

Cornblath, Marvin, "Diagnosing and Treating Neonatal Hypoglycemia," *Contemporary Ob/Gyn*, Vol. 8, pp. 95–99, Sept. 1976.

Crosse, V. Mary: *The Premature Baby and Other Babies with Low Birth Weight*, Little, Brown, Boston, 1966.

Doran, T. A., et. al., "Amniotic Fluid Tests for Fetal Maturity in Normal and Abnormal Pregnancies," *American Journal of Obstetrics and Gynecology*, Vol. 125, No. 5, pp. 591–592, July 1976.

Houlton, M. C. C., "Divergent Biparietal Diameter Growth Rates in Twin Pregnancies," *Obstetrics and Gynecology*, Vol. 49, No. 51, p. 544, May 1977.

Kitay, David, "Bleeding Disorders in Pregnancy," *Contemporary Ob/Gyn*, Vol. 7, pp. 86–94, Jan. 1976.

Klaus, Marshall and John Kennell, "Mothers Separated from Their Newborn Infants," *Pediatric Clinics of North America*, Vol. 17, No. 4, p. 1015, Nov. 1970.

Korones, Sheldon: *High-Risk Newborn Infants*, C. V. Mosby Co., St. Louis, Mo., 1976, pp. 85–98.

Marlow, Dorothy R.: *Textbook of Pediatric Nursing*, 3d ed., W. B. Saunders Co., Philadelphia, 1977.

Nelson, Waldo, Victor Vaughn, and James McKay: *Textbook of Pediatrics*, 9th ed., W. B. Saunders Co., Philadelphia, 1975.

Scipien, Gladys, et al.: *Comprehensive Pediatric Nursing*, McGraw-Hill Book Co., 1975, pp. 316–318.

Trierweiler, Michael, "Baseline Fetal Heart Rate Characteristic as an Indicator of Fetal Status During Antepartal Period," *American Journal of Obstetrics and Gynecology*, Vol. 125, No. 5, p. 622, July 1, 1976.

Whetham, J. C., et al., "Assessment of Intrauterine Growth Retardation by Diagnostic Ultrasound," *American Journal of Obstetrics and Gynecology*, Vol. 125, No. 5, July 1, 1976.

PRETEST ANSWERS   1. Two   2. Any four of these: long nails; absence of vernix; absence of lanugo; alertness; pale skin; much scalp hair; peeling skin; low weight   3. Stillbirth   4. Any three of these: respiratory distress; hypoglycemia; pneumonia; dehydration   5. Less developed than the normal range for the gestational age   6. Fetal, maternal, internal, and/or external environmental factors   7. a. Hypertensive problems; b. respiratory problems; c. had six or more pregnancies; d. malnutrition; e. young; f. chemical abusers

POST-TEST ANSWERS   1. T   2. F   3. T   4. F   5. T   6. T   7. T

CHAPTER FOUR

RESPIRATORY DISTRESS SYNDROME

OBJECTIVES *Identify the major characteristics of respiratory distress syndrome.*

Identify the factors that predispose to the development of respiratory distress.

Identify the significant stressor that produces some of the changes found in respiratory distress.

Identify the nursing intervention with the newborn who has respiratory distress.

GLOSSARY *Atelectasis:* Decreased expansion of the lungs
Hyaline membrane: A thin covering composed of necrotic cells

PRETEST In the spaces provided, fill in the word or words that best complete(s) the statements. Then turn to page 481 and check your answers.

1. Another term for "respiratory distress syndrome" is _____ _____.

2. The neonatal population that seems most susceptible to this condition is composed of babies of mothers who a. _____;

    b. _____;

    c. _____;

    and d. _____.

3. A common characteristic of respiratory distress syndrome is _____ _____.

4. The most common finding in infants with respiratory distress syndrome is _____.

5. Respiratory symptoms that may develop are _____ _____, _____ _____, _____, _____ _____, _____, and _____.

6. Intervention is concerned primarily with the treatment of the _____.

7. The nurse is concerned with the care of both the _____ and the _____.

Respiratory distress syndrome (RDS) describes an acute type of respiratory distress found at birth or shortly following it. This syndrome previously was termed "hyaline membrane disease" because, at autopsy, a thin membrane composed of necrotic cells was found to be lining the alveoli and the bronchioles. The conditions that predispose to the development of respiratory distress syndrome are prematurity, maternal diabetes, maternal bleeding, cesarean section, and ruptured membranes less than 12 hours before birth. The mortality rate is high.

Respiratory distress syndrome is _____ _____.

an acute type
of respiratory distress

Factors that predispose toward the development of this condition include _____, _____ _____, _____ , _____ , and _____ _____ _____.

prematurity; maternal
bleeding; maternal diabetes;
cesarean section; ruptured
membranes less than 12 hours
before birth

The cause of respiratory distress syndrome is unknown, but the stressor that is operating is a *deficiency of surfactant*. This deficiency results in an inadequate expansion of the lungs, producing *atelectasis*, the most significant characteristic of respiratory distress syndrome. As a result of this decreased surfactant, there is poor elasticity of the lung tissue, which does not respond effectively to the forces of inspiration and expiration. Another stressor that operates is *asphyxia*, present either intrauterinely or after delivery. The asphyxia causes vasoconstriction of the pulmonary capillaries due to increasing CO_2 and decreasing O_2 supply. This results in a decrease in the blood pH, and neonatal cooling during resuscitation efforts further decreases the circulation in the alveoli, leading to further atelectasis of the lungs. It is also possible that the stress of the acidotic condition increases the activity of the sympathetic nervous system, producing the symptoms associated with this nonhealth state. The infant must use more energy to breathe than the healthy infant does.

The factor that produces respiratory distress syndrome is _____.

unknown

A stressor that contributes to respiratory distress is a decreased amount of _____.

surfactant

Upon examination of the infant with respiratory distress syndrome, a characteristic finding is _____.

atelectasis

A stressor that produces further atelectasis is _____. | asphyxia

In order to breathe, the infant must expend _____ | greater

_____. | energy than normal

Most infants who exhibit signs of respiratory difficulty do so at the time of birth or within the first few hours of life. If there are no signs of respiratory distress syndrome before the first eight hours of life, but signs occur later, then another type of health interruption is operating. In RDS, the most common clinical sign the infant shows is an *increased respiratory rate*, usually 60 or more respirations a minute. At times the only behavior seen clinically which indicates the respiratory difficulty is an *expiratory grunt*. The expiratory grunt is an adaptive mechanism that attempts to increase the residual capacity of the lungs and thus raise the pO_2 level in the arterioles.

The most frequent clinical sign of respiratory distress is

_____. | an increased respiratory rate

The oxygen saturation of the arterial blood is raised by the

infant's _____. | expiratory grunt

Another respiratory movement that attempts to increase the amount of air entering the lungs is *chest retraction*, which is the in-pulling of the chest between the ribs or at the lower margin of the sternum during an inspiration as the diaphragm and respiratory muscles work to draw air into the lungs.

Nasal flaring is another indication of poor oxygenation.

If you observe that the infant's chest is pulled in during

inspiration, this action is termed _____. | chest retraction

Another indication that the infant is taking in an inadequate

amount of oxygen is _____. | nasal flaring

The newborn may experience periods of *apnea* during the first 24 hours. If this occurs, it is indicative of a crisis state. It is common to find *cyanosis* when the infant is in the room environment, but if the condition persists when the infant is placed in a high-oxygen environment, a poor prognosis is indicated.

Those signs of respiratory distress which are associated with

crisis are _____ and _____. | apnea; cyanosis in oxygen

In respiratory distress syndrome, the infant does not move about and the muscle tone is *flaccid*. The skin of the infant is pale because of vasoconstriction of the *peripheral circulation*. These two findings demonstrate that the infant's resources, energy, and circulation are being directed to the primary organs—the heart, lungs, and brain—as the infant attempts to modify the stressor through respiratory effort and altered circulatory functioning.

The *temperature* of the infant usually is decreased, and it needs to be stabilized by a controlled environment. *Edema* often is present in the premature infant, but the edema seen when the infant has respiratory distress syndrome is pitting, especially in the hands and feet. The edema is seen within the first 24 hours and subsides by the fifth day as circulatory function improves and the infant becomes more active. Retractions may persist for 72 hours before they begin to subside, while the increased respiratory rate usually continues until the infant becomes more active.

Protective mechanisms that attempt to modify the strength of the stressor result in two findings: _____ and _____.

flaccid muscles;
pale skin

Along with these symptoms, one also can observe _____ _____ and find _____.

pitting
edema; a decreased temperature

The nurse and the delivery room staff should be alert to signs of respiratory difficulty, especially if there is a history that would predispose the infant to develop RDS. Since infants who have RDS often display signs of respiratory difficulty at birth or need resuscitation measures, parents usually are aware that their infant is in difficulty. It is not possible to reassure them that all will be well, but it is important to inform them of the baby's current status and the measures that are being taken to assist the infant. The treatment measures are directed to the symptomatology and to promoting the functioning of the respiratory system, thereby, if possible, correcting the existing hypoxia.

The infant is under intensive care and constant observation. He is placed in an incubator with an oxygen-rich environment (in which the oxygen preferably is below 40 percent so that there is no danger of retrolental fibroplasia but above this if cyanosis is present). Humidity is supplied to assist in maintaining good respiratory function. The environment is warmed to 95°F since the infant's temperature is _____ and acidosis does not develop as readily when the infant's temperature is normal.

decreased

You may also find that in some instances external negative pressure to the infant's body is being administered with a small body-tank-like respirator or positive pressure is being administered with a mask or endotracheal tube. These methods are considered extremely helpful in combating the hypoperfusion.

In order to increase the blood volume of the infant and increase the level of oxygen available to the cells, transfusions with adult hemoglobin seem to be helpful.

Good nutrition through intravenous therapy is started rapidly, and the environmental temperature is regulated carefully. Remember that changes in body temperature cause changes in oxygen, metabolic, and ventilation needs.

Frequent assessment of the infant's level of oxygenation is carried out through monitoring of blood gases using samples of blood taken from an arterial line, and the level of oxygen is adjusted accordingly. Acidosis is assessed using blood samples from a central venous line, and sodium bicarbonate is given to correct the pH of the blood. The infant is supplied with fluids and electrolytes by intravenous therapy.

The treatment of RDS is related to the _____.   symptoms

The infant is placed in an environment that is _____   high in

_____, ___ ____ ___, and _____.   oxygen; humid; warm

If the infant is severely retracting, then _____   ventilation

_____.   is assisted

Acidosis is assessed through _____   blood sampling

_____ and corrected with   from the venous line;

_____.   sodium bicarbonate

Parents often are overwhelmed by all the equipment and find it difficult to relate to their child. The nurse can help the parents begin to feel comfortable with all the various pieces of apparatus by explaining what they are and what they do. Frequently when the prognosis of the child is guarded, the parents have difficulty identifying with the infant since they may lose it and, in a sense, they may lose their investment of feeling as well. When the condition of the infant stabilizes and improves, then the parents often feel more comfortable in relating to the child. It is important for the parents to begin the parental roles as soon as possible, for this task is more difficult if it is not begun within the normal first two or three days after birth. Removal of the infant to a larger hospital center for intensive care can create a difficult problem for the parents, and they will need much support when they are reunited with their child.

POST-TEST   Indicate whether each statement is true or false by circling the appropriate letter. Then turn to page 481 and see how well you have done.

1. Respiratory distress syndrome always is fatal.   T   F

2. The initial symptom of RDS usually is an increased respiratory rate.   T   F

3. The infant with RDS usually has an elevated temperature.   T   F

4. The nurse must be alert for signs of cyanosis and increased respirations.   T   F

5. The baby with RDS shows signs of increased oxygenation.   T   F

6. The baby with RDS is placed in an incubator with a controlled environment.   T   F

7. The infant with RDS will show symptoms of alkalosis.   T   F

8. Periods of apnea indicate a crisis state.   T   F

9. Parents may have difficulty relating to their child.   T   F

In the specific areas with which you had difficulty, return to the material and review.

BIBLIOGRAPHY Avery, Gordon: *Neonatalogy, Pathophysiology and Management of the Newborn*, J. B. Lippincott Co., Philadelphia, 1975, pp. 225–230.

Korones, Sheldon B.: *High-Risk Newborn Infants*, C. V. Mosby Co., St. Louis, Mo., 1976.

Kumpe, Mary and Leonard Kleinman, "Care of the Infant with Respiratory Distress Syndrome," *Nursing Clinics of North America*, Vol. 6, pp. 25–37, March 1971.

McCleary, E., "All-out Care for Newborns in Trouble," *Family Health*, July 1972.

McNall, Leota and Janet Galeener: *Current Practices in Obstetric and Gynecologic Nursing*, C. V. Mosby Co., St. Louis, Mo., 1976, pp. 125–142.

Marlow, Dorothy: *Textbook of Pediatric Nursing*, W. B. Saunders Co., Philadelphia, 1977, pp. 203–205.

Moore, Mary Lou: *The Newborn and the Nurse*, W. B. Saunders Co., Philadelphia, 1972.

Nelson, Nicholas, "On the Etiology of Hyaline Membrane Disease," *Pediatric Clinics of North America*, Vol. 17, p. 943, Nov. 1970.

———, Vaughan, V. and James R. McKay: *Textbook of Pediatrics*, 10th ed., W. B. Saunders Co., Philadelphia, 1975.

Rhodes, Phillip, Robert Hall, and Stanley Hellerstein, "The Effects of Single Infusions of Hypertoxic Sodium Bicarbonate on Body Composition in Neonates with Acidosis," *Journal of Pediatrics*, Vol. 90, No. 5, pp. 789–795.

Shaffer, Alexander and Mary Ellen Avery: *Diseases of the Newborn*, W. B. Saunders Co., Philadelphia, 1977, pp. 134–141.

Stein, Leo, "Therapy of the Respiratory Distress Syndrome," *Pediatric Clinics of North America*, Vol. 19, pp. 221–240, Feb. 1972.

Williams, Joann and Jean Lancaster, "Thermoregulation in the Newborn," *Maternal Child Nursing*, Vol. 1, pp. 355–360, Nov.–Dec. 1976.

PRETEST ANSWERS

1. Hyaline membrane disease   2. a. Have diabetes; b. have had a cesarean section; c. have given birth prematurely; d. have had antenatal vaginal bleeding   3. Atelectasis   4. A decreased amount of surfactant   5. Grunting on expiration; periods of apnea; cyanosis; rapid, shallow respirations; retractions; nasal flaring   6. Symptoms   7. Baby; parents

POST-TEST ANSWERS

1. F   2. T   3. F   4. T   5. F   6. T   7. F   8. T   9. T

CHAPTER FIVE
BIRTH INJURIES

OBJECTIVES　*Identify the manifestations of brachial palsy in the neonate.*

Identify a factor that may predispose to brachial palsy.

Identify the differences between cephalohematoma and caput succedaneum.

Identify the factors that may predispose to a cephalohematoma.

Identify the manifestations of an intracranial hemorrhage in the neonate.

Identify the factors that may predispose to an intracranial hemorrhage.

Identify the nursing intervention for each of the above conditions.

GLOSSARY　*Abduction:* The act of moving a part away from the body
Adduction: The act of moving a part toward the body
Brachial palsy: Paralysis due to injury to the brachial plexus
Brachial plexus: The network of nerves found in the neck, shoulder, and arm
Caput succedaneum: A soft swelling on the head of the neonate due to edema of the soft scalp tissues which crosses the suture lines
Cephalohematoma: A defined swelling on the head of the neonate due to bleeding under the periosteum of one or more skull bones which does not cross the suture lines
Contracture: Shortening of muscle fibers due to disuse

Erbs-Duchenne paralysis: Inability to move the upper arm due to the injury of the fifth and sixth cervical nerves

Flexion: The act of causing a joint to bend

Gavage feeding: Passage of a tube into the stomach for the purpose of introducing food

Sequelae: Aftereffects of an injury or illness

PRETEST In the spaces provided, fill in the word or words that best complete(s) the statements. Then turn to page 493 and check your answers.

1. Brachial palsy may be a result of _____

   _____

   _____ .

2. Symptoms of brachial palsy include a. _____

   _____ ,

   b. _____ , c. _____

   _____ ,

   d. _____

   _____ , e. _____

   _____ , and f. _____ .

3. Cephalohematoma is _____

   _____

   _____

   _____ .

4. Caput succedaneum is _____

   _____

   _____

   _____

   _____ .

5. Comparing the prognosis of cephalohematoma and caput succedaneum and the length of time they persist, _____

   _____

   _____ ; _____

   _____

   _____ ; _____

   _____

   _____ .

6. Symptoms of intracranial hemorrhage are _____ ,

   _____ , _____ ,

   _____ , _____ , and _____

   _____ .

7. Intracranial hemorrhage may be of several types: _____,
   _____, or _____.

8. Care of the infant with an intracranial hemorrhage includes
   a. _____, b. _____
   _____, c. _____
   _____, d. _____
   _____, e. _____,
   f. _____, and g. _____.

We have discussed the management of labor and the cardinal movements of the fetus during the birth process. You also have become familiar with some of the interruptions of the normal process of labor, such as dystocia. When these interruptions occur, the equilibrium of the mother, and in many instances that of the neonate, is disrupted. The nurse must be aware of the signs and symptoms signaling disruptions of the neonate's homeodynamic state and the effect these interruptions of the neonate's health status will have on the parents.

It is essential for the nursery nurse to be very familiar with the prenatal and intranatal history of the mother; only then will you be able to identify the infant who needs to be specially observed during the first few days after birth. Without this information your observations may be intuitive rather than based on objective data. You also must recognize the nursing care measures that must be instituted in the nursery; the teaching, guidance, and reassurance that will be needed by the parents; and, in some cases, the referrals that should be made.

Let us discuss some of the injuries to the neonate which can occur as a result of interruptions of the normal processes of parturition.

Brachial palsy is an injury of the brachial plexus, the network of nerves that are found in the neck, shoulder, and arm. The main sign of this injury is an *unequal Moro reflex*. That is, on the affected side, the Moro response is absent. Other symptoms of a brachial injury depend upon the amount of nerve paralysis and the muscles affected by this paralysis.

The network of nerves found in the neck, shoulder, and arm is known as the _____ plexus.

brachial

If the nurse doing a newborn nursery evaluation observes a missing Moro reflex on one side of the infant, further evaluation of the baby is necessary to see if there is an injury to the brachial plexus. This injury is known as _____ palsy.

brachial

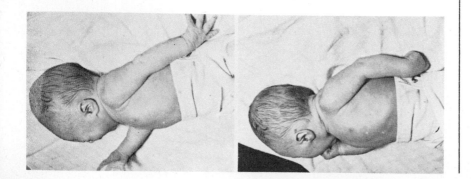

Brachial palsy of the left arm (asymmetric Moro reflex). *(From Nelson Textbook of Pediatrics, 10th ed., by V. Vaughan and R. J. McKay, Copyright © 1975 W. B. Saunders Company. Used with the permissions of W. B. Saunders Company and V. Vaughan.)*

The extent of the injury depends upon the _____   nerves
that are affected.

Brachial palsy usually is caused by tension placed on the brachial
plexus when traction is applied to the head during a vertex, breech,
or forceps delivery.

The prognosis depends upon how severely the nerves are injured.
If lacerations of the nerves were not incurred and stretching and edema
are the only causes of the symptoms, recovery usually occurs within
a few months. With a more severe injury, there may be residual effects
such as permanent paralysis and loss of sensation in the arm. If the
nerves have been lacerated, neuroplasty in three to six months may
provide for partial recovery.

Brachial palsy usually is caused during the _____   second;
stage of labor by the application of _____ to the head   traction
of the baby.

The prognosis usually is favorable, but it depends upon the
extent of the _____ injury.   nerve

When the injury involves only the fifth and sixth cervical nerves,
causing paralysis only to the upper arm, it is called *Erbs-Duchenne
paralysis*.

Erbs-Duchenne paralysis is a type of _____   brachial
palsy.

It usually affects only the _____ arm since the   upper;
nerves affected are the cervical _____ and _____.   fifth; sixth

Another symptom that may be observed by the nurse is a flaccid
arm in an adduction. The arm also will be rotated inward with the
forearm pronated. As the nurse observes the baby for movement, it
will be noticed that the infant is unable to raise the arm on the affected
side.

The nurse, upon noticing an infant who is unable to elevate one
arm, will check to see if that arm also is rotated _____   inward;
with the forearm pointed _____.   downward

The nurse also will notice that the arm is _____.   adducted

The treatment is geared mainly toward restoration of normal movement for the infant. If the nerves are injured merely by edema, restoration can be accomplished by immobilizing the arm with the elbow flexed and the arm elevated, with external rotation and abduction provided. The nurse may put the arm into a sling or elevate it by applying a restraint around the wrist and tying it to the head and top of the crib. The mother must be taught how to exercise the arm to prevent the formation of contractures. When the infant goes home and removal from the crib becomes necessary, a splint may be applied.

The nurse must show the mother how to keep the arm in the proper position by applying a wrist tie to the head of the bed. This will keep the arm in the necessary _____ position. It also is necessary to keep the elbow _____ and the forearm _____ and _____ rotated.

elevated;

flexed;

abducted; externally

The parents must be taught the proper method of _____ the arm to prevent contractures.

exercising

Caput succedaneum is a soft swelling on the head of the neonate due to edema of soft scalp tissues. This area of swelling crosses the suture line. The shape of the head is slightly distorted as a result. Caput succedaneum is caused by the pressure of the undilated portion of the cervix on the soft tissues of the scalp of the fetus. This swelling disappears during the first several days after birth. The parents may be concerned and may be afraid to ask why their baby's head is so soft in one spot and is misshapen. It is a good idea for the nurse to show this area to the mother during one of the early mother-baby interactions, explain what it is and how it came about, and offer the reassurance that it appears very frequently, goes away, and has no effects on the baby.

Caput succedaneum is an _____ area on the _____ of the neonate's head. This soft swelling disappears _____ without any residual _____.

edematous;

scalp

spontaneously; effects

A cephalohematoma, which also is evidenced by a swelling on the head of the neonate, actually is caused by bleeding due to the rupture of small blood vessels. This bleeding causes a hematoma or small, circumscribed collection of blood to occur under the periosteum of the cranium. It may occur either under a single cranial bone or under several cranial bones, but it does not extend into or beyond the sutures.

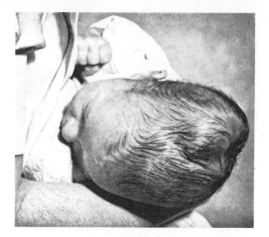

The cephalohematoma usually is due to injury to the cranium during the birth process caused either by the pressure of the head against the mother's pelvic bones or by forceps used to effect the delivery.

Bleeding under the periosteum of one or more cranial bones of the neonate is called _____.

It is caused by a cranial _____ during the birth process and is due to the use of _____ or to the _____ caused by the head of the fetus rubbing on the mother's pelvic _____.

A cephalohematoma may take several weeks to be absorbed, unlike the caput succedaneum, which takes _____ _____, but like the caput succedaneum it will cause no residual effects.

cephalohematoma

injury;

forceps;

pressure;

bones

several

days

Another, more complicated injury to the head of the fetus is an *intracranial hemorrhage*. This bleeding can occur in the ventricles, the subarachnoid space or the subdural spaces. Intracranial hemorrhage is a severe complication of the central nervous system usually caused by injury due to a long and difficult labor, fetal anoxia, or an instrument delivery. The premature infant is particularly susceptible to this complication because its blood vessels are most susceptible to injury, and since the clotting mechanism of the premature infant is immature, bleeding may be extensive.

Symptoms of intracranial hemorrhage may not be observed for several days after birth and may be similar to those of other conditions, such as cardiac or respiratory problems, present in the premature infant.

Often the first sign observed is the characteristic sharp, shrill, high-pitched cry associated with cerebral irritation. Other symptoms are lethargy, attacks of cyanosis, difficulty in sucking, and forceful vomiting. In addition, the nurse should be alert for either very slow or rapid breathing with or without grunting, twitching of the lower jaw, or true convulsive movements. Bulging of the fontanels also may be felt. Any of these symptoms should be reported immediately and carefully recorded.

The nurse in the newborn nursery who is aware of a difficult delivery or fetal distress during labor should be alert for the symptoms of _____ hemorrhage.

intracranial

The respiratory symptoms that might be evidenced by the full-term or premature infant who has an intracranial hemorrhage are _____ and _____ or _____ breathing with or without a _____ sound.

cyanosis; slow; rapid; grunting

Sucking for these babies is _____, and the babies may show signs of twitching or _____.

difficult; convulsions

Cerebral irritation also may give rise to a characteristic _____, _____, _____ cry. Due to the bleeding, the fontanels may _____.

sharp; shrill; high-pitched; bulge

These babies often are placed in isolettes so that heat, oxygen, and humidity can be controlled. Also they are kept quiet by minimal handling and occasionally are given sedation to help keep the bleeding to a minimum and to decrease the possibility of convulsions. Because they may convulse and because their sucking ability is poor, they are fed initially by gavage or nourished intravenously and are gradually introduced to bottle feeding with a soft nipple. It is essential that they not be placed in Trendelenberg position but rather have their heads slightly elevated to alleviate some of the intracranial pressure.

Treatment includes intravenous or _____ _____ feeding and control of convulsions by the administration of _____.

gavage tube; sedation

Because of the possibility of shock, cyanosis, or other associated problems, warmth, humidity, and oxygen are provided by placing these babies in _____.

isolettes

The pressure caused by the bleeding precludes these babies' being put into _____ position.

⬇

Trendelenberg

The prognosis for these babies is grave although there may be complete recovery. Death may occur if the hemorrhage is severe, or there may be residual effects such as mental retardation or one of the cerebral palsies.

The parents must be told of this condition as soon as it is identified. The parents of necessity are separated from their child; thus a new stressor is introduced. In addition, they cannot be given the reassurance of complete recovery or, for that matter, any recovery at all. How they handle this loss of equilibrium depends upon their previous experiences and relationships with one another as well as what this child meant to them.

One or both parents may find themselves in the supportive role. This may be a new role-sharing event for this family, and it may be difficult because of its unfamiliarity. The usually supportive member may withdraw and be totally unable to cope. The normal mechanisms of becoming a family are being interrupted, and the possibility of permanent loss is ever present.

It is up to the staff to keep both parents well informed about the condition of their child. Reports should state only what is happening now, without offering false hopes or reassurances. The nurse must observe the ability of the family to deal with the crisis and intervene when their adaptive mechanisms no longer meet the needs of the situation. The nurse should be available to the parents in order to clarify reality and allow them to ask questions and vent feelings. They must be encouraged to see their child and not to start the grieving of permanent separation until it is evident that the child will die; otherwise they may find it difficult to accept a healthy or handicapped child at a later date.

POST-TEST Indicate whether each statement is true or false by circling the appropriate letter. Then turn to page 493 and see how well you have done.

1. The nurse in the nursery must be well informed only about the infants under her care. T F

2. Erbs-Duchenne paralysis involves the upper arm. T F

3. The nerves usually involved are the facial fifth and sixth. T F

4. In treating the baby with brachial palsy, one elevates the arm and flexes the elbow. T F

5. In brachial palsy, one of the first signs picked up by the admitting nurse is an unequal Moro reflex. T F

6. Brachial palsy usually has a good prognosis. T F

7. Caput succedaneum is bleeding under the periosteum of one or more cranial bones. T F

8. Caput succedaneum and cephalohematoma both resolve with no residual damage. T F

9. Intracranial hemorrhage always is fatal in utero. T F

10. A shrill, high-pitched cry is a common symptom of intracranial hemorrhage. T F

11. An infant with intracranial hemorrhage should be started on an enriched bottle feeding as soon as possible. T F

12. Babies with intracranial hemorrhage rarely show signs of respiratory distress. T F

13. Babies with intracranial hemorrhage should not be denied breast feeding. T F

14. If a baby recovers from intracranial hemorrhage, he may be free from residual damage. T F

In the specific areas with which you had difficulty, return to the material and review.

BIBLIOGRAPHY Korones, Sheldon B.: *High-Risk Newborn Infants*, C. V. Mosby Co., St. Louis, Mo., 1972.

Pritchard, Jack and Paul MacDonald: *Williams Obstetrics*, 15th ed., Appleton-Century-Crofts, New York, 1976.

Roberts, Florence Bright: *Perinatal Nursing*, McGraw-Hill Book Co., New York, 1977.

Vaughan, V. and R. James McKay: *Nelson Textbook of Pediatrics*, 10th ed., W. B. Saunders Co., Philadelphia, 1975.

PRETEST ANSWERS

1. Unequal traction on the head of the infant during delivery   2. a. Missing Moro reflex on one side; b. arm limp; c. adduction of arm on affected side; d. inability of the infant to raise affected arm; e. inward rotation of the arm; f. pronated forearm   3. Bleeding under the periosteum of one or more cranial bones   4. A soft swelling on the head of the neonate caused by injury to the soft scalp tissues   5. Both cure spontaneously with no residual effects; caput succedaneum lasts two to three days; and cephalohematoma lasts several weeks   6. Lethargy; cyanosis; difficulty in sucking; twitching; convulsions; shrill, high-pitched cry   7. Subarachnoid; ventricular; subdural   8. a. Placement in an incubator; b. control of humidity; c. administration of heat and oxygen; d. intravenous or gavage feeding; e. little handling; f. elevation of head; g. sedation

POST-TEST ANSWERS

1. F   2. T   3. F   4. T   5. T   6. T   7. F   8. T   9. F
10. T   11. F   12. F   13. F   14. T

CHAPTER SIX

INFECTIONS IN THE NEONATE

OBJECTIVES *Identify the meaning of infection to the neonate.*

Identify the meaning of neonatal morbidity to the parents.

Identify the causative agent of thrush.

Identify manifestations of thrush.

Identify the causative agent of ophthalmia neonatorum.

Identify the course of the infection.

Identify the causative agent of congenital syphilis.

Identify the manifestations of congenital syphilis.

Identify the causative agent of impetigo of the newborn.

Identify manifestations of impetigo of the newborn.

Identify nursing intervention when the neonate develops infection.

GLOSSARY *Congenital syphilis:* Infection caused by *Treponema pallidum*, transmitted from an infected mother through the placenta to a fetus in utero
Gammaglobulins: Parts of the blood which contain antibodies
Hepatomegaly: Enlarged liver
Impetigo: Contagious skin infection caused by a staphylococcus or a streptococcus

Macular rash: A skin rash that resembles blotches

Ophthalmia neonatorum: Eye infection caused by a gonococcus

Osteochondritis: Inflammation of cartilage

Papular rash: A skin rash that has small elevated areas

Periostitis: Inflammation of the membranous covering of bones

Phagocytosis: The surrounding engulfing of foreign matter such as organisms

Splenomegaly: Enlarged spleen

Thrush: An oral infection caused by *Candida albicans*

Topical application: Application directly to the affected area

PRETEST   In the spaces provided, fill in the word or words that best complete(s) the statements. Then turn to page 507 and check your answers.

1. The most common cause of morbidity in the neonate is _____ .

2. Thrush is _____
    _____ .

3. The organism causing thrush often is found in the mother's _____ .

4. Thrush is identified by the presence of _____
    _____ .

5. Thrush is treated by _____
    _____ or _____ .

6. Ophthalmia neonatorum is transmitted to the neonate during
    _____
    _____ .

7. Ophthalmia neonatorum is caused by a _____ .

8. Ophthalmia neonatorum is treated by _____
    _____ .

9. Congenital syphilis is transmitted to the fetus from the mother through the
    _____ .

10. The fetus acquires congenital syphilis symptoms after the _____
    month of gestation because of _____
    _____ .

11. Some symptoms of congenital syphilis include _____
    _____
    _____
    _____ , _____
    _____ ,
    _____ , _____ , and _____ .

12. Congenital syphilis is treated with _____ ,
    _____ , or _____ .

13. Impetigo of the newborn is _____

    _____.

14. The organism causing impetigo is a _____

    or a _____.

15. Symptoms of impetigo are _____

    _____

    _____.

16. Impetigo is transmitted through _____

    _____.

17. Impetigo is treated by _____,

    _____, and _____

    _____.

18. The primary stressor for the mother when the neonate has an infection is

    the _____.

Infection in the newborn is the most common cause of a nonhealth state or morbidity within the first few weeks of life. The infection may be due to many factors: the normal neonate is particularly susceptible to bacterial and viral infections, and the premature infant is even more highly susceptible. Although the newborn has some immunity passed from the mother, by placental transfer and by breast milk, the infant has not been exposed to the organisms that provide antigenic stimulation to increase the levels of the newborn's own antibodies. In addition, there is thought to be a macrophage deficiency and the levels of IgA and IgM are low.

The neonate may become infected from the environment, either intrauterine or extrauterine. In utero, many infections, such as syphilis, measles, and chicken pox, may be passed on to the fetus; during the birth process, the infant may acquire gonorrhea, monilia, or herpes simplex from the mother's vagina. After birth, the infant is highly susceptible to infections present in the nasopharynxes and on the hands of the personnel caring for him.

It is essential, therefore, that all persons coming in contact with the newborn in the labor room, delivery room, or nursery not be carriers of infectious organisms. In addition, a baby born to a mother whose membranes ruptured over 24 hours before delivery should be isolated and carefully observed for signs of infection. Nursing personnel should be fully aware of the behavior and appearance of the baby.

Symptoms of infection in the newborn are obscure. Often there is no temperature rise, cough, or obvious inflammation. Symptoms presented, such as lethargy, poor feeding, occasional vomiting, some respiratory irregularities, diarrhea, and icterus after the third day are present in conditions other than infection. Sometimes there really is no definite reason to suspect illness, yet the nursery nurse knows that something is not right. Should the nurse have this reaction, the baby should be put into an isolation nursery until a state of health can be differentiated from one of nonhealth.

This sudden removal of the infant from the regular nursery will cause the parents a great deal of concern. It is essential that they be told the reason for the transfer as soon as it is effected and be kept aware of treatment and progress.

The meninges of the newborn are particularly susceptible to infection because the blood-brain barrier is ineffective. One of the most feared consequences of neonatal infection is meningitis. Septicemia is another very serious condition resulting from an infection in the newborn.

Prevention and early diagnosis are the best measures for restoring and maintaining the health state which are available to us; it is essential to utilize both to their maximum potentials.

Although the neonate has some active and passive immunity

passed to it through the placenta from the mother, the baby is more prone to infection because the levels of immunoglobins are _____.

low

A neonate with any infection is considered a high-risk candidate, for that infection may progress to _____ or _____.

meningitis; septicemia

The two best methods of keeping and/or restoring the health state of the neonate are _____ and _____ _____.

prevention; early detection

We will discuss thrush, gonococcal infection, congenital syphilis, and impetigo in detail. It should be remembered, however, that the newborn is highly susceptible to pneumonia, diarrhea, and, as previously stated, septicemia and meningitis.

Thrush, an oral infection caused by maternal moniliasis, is acquired from the vagina of the mother during parturition. The organism invades the mucus membranes of the mouth and the perianal areas of the body. Thrush is characterized by white patches somewhat resembling milk curds. The fungus causing this infection is *Candida albicans*, and it is easily spread throughout a nursery if strict aseptic technique is not observed. Now that infants are going home within the first few days after birth, a nursery nurse may never see the symptoms of the infection since they usually are not observable until after the fifth day after birth. Thus, it is essential that the parents be given guidance regarding its symptomology.

Thrush is caused by the organism called _____ _____.

Candida albicans

It is a yeast _____ found in the _____ of the mother and transmitted to the baby during _____.

fungus; vagina; delivery

The fungus invades the _____ membrane of the baby's mouth and also may infect the _____ area.

mucus; perianal

The infection usually does not show symptoms until after _____ days following birth.

five

The infection is seen in the mouth and perianal area as white _____ like patches.

curd

The parents should be told also that if they are not sure if the baby truly has an infection or just some partially digested milk in its mouth, they might try to wipe the patch away gently. Thrush patches do not wipe away easily and, when removed, often leave a small area of bleeding. Another means of determining the presence of thrush is to give the baby water; milk curds will be washed away. Should the parents or nurse suspect thrush, it should be reported to the physician immediately. Feeding utensils should be sterilized carefully and the patches treated topically with mycostatin or 1 percent gentian violet. When using mycostatin, administer it slowly with a dropper so that the tongue is bathed with the medication before the baby swallows it. If the physician orders gentian violet, remind the mother that after the application, she should put a bib with a plastic backing on the baby. The baby will salivate and drool this deep purple stain onto his clothing, and it does not wash out. Also remind the parents that the baby's mouth will appear deep purple. This treatment will effect a complete cure fairly rapidly.

When the patches of thrush are wiped, they will leave _____   bleeding

lesions in the mouth.

If the infant is diagnosed as having thrush, bottle and feeding

nipples, feeding spoons, and dishes should be _____.   sterilized

The medication that may be used in the treatment of this

infection is either _____   1 percent gentian violet;

or _____.   mycostatin

Ophthalmia neonatorum, or gonorrheal ophthalmia, long has been considered extinct in this country. However, with the present epidemic of venereal infections and the upsurge in home and communal deliveries, it needs to be discussed. Gonorrhea often goes undetected in the female, thus making her baby a possible victim of this blinding disease. All women who have their babies outside of a hospital or clinic must be informed that as a prophylactic measure, their baby's eyes must be treated immediately after birth with either 1 percent silver nitrate immediately followed by a distilled saline water irrigation, or an antibiotic opthalmic ointment.

It is essential that all maternity and community nurses be aware of the symptoms of ophthalmia neonatorum because prompt diagnosis and treatment will prevent the extreme result of blindness.

The symptoms of gonnorrheal conjunctivitis (gonorrheal ophthalmia) usually do not appear until after the first 48 hours following birth. The first noticeable symptom is reddened, swollen eyelids, and the eyes secrete a serosanguinous discharge that changes within a day to a thick, greenish, purulent material. The conjunctiva appears edematous and reddened. If treatment is not started immediately, the lids become so swollen that they cannot be opened, and the corneas become opaque, ulcerated, and liable to perforate and collapse, causing blindness.

Ophthalmia neonatorum also is known as _____ | gonorrheal;

ophthalmia. It is contracted by the baby from the _____. | mother;

If the infant's eyes are treated prophylactically with either

_____ | 1 percent silver nitrate;

or an _____ ointment, the child | antibiotic;

usually is protected from infection. The first symptoms of the infection

appear after the first _____ hours following birth and start with | 48;

_____ and _____ eyelids. | red; swollen

The discharge changes as the infection progresses. It starts as a

_____ discharge and changes to a thick, | serosanguinous;

_____, purulent one. | greenish

The conjunctiva becomes inflamed, the corneas become

_____, and ulcerations form on the _____, | opaque; corneas;

causing _____ and blindness. | perforation

Therapy effects a cure within 24 hours. The most common therapeutic agent is intramuscular aqueous penicillin.

Congenital syphilis, or syphilis transmitted to the fetus while in utero, would not occur if every pregnant woman received good prenatal care with a serologic study done both before and late in pregnancy. Unfortunately there is a rising incidence of congenital syphilis.

Congenital syphilis can result in abortion or stillbirth or an infant who at birth presents no symptoms. The fetal response to the spirochete *Treponema pallidum* depends on the gestational age. Before the sixteenth week of gestation, the inflammatory and antibody responses are not present so that no abortion or symptomatology occurs. It is between the sixteenth and twentieth weeks, as the antibody and inflammatory responses develop, that the symptoms arise and abortions can occur.

The effect of the *Treponema pallidum* on the fetus is determined

by _____. | the gestational age of the fetus

Symptoms of congenital syphilis can occur once _____ | antibody

_____ are developed. | and inflammatory responses

If an infant is born with syphilis transmitted to it while in utero,

the baby is said to have _____. | congenital syphilis

The medical staff can prevent this by examining the prepregnant

woman's blood for proof of _____and treating her | infection;

_____ with penicillin. | before pregnancy

A child born with syphilis may show signs immediately or not for several weeks or months. The child will show some of the symptoms of secondary syphilis. These may be *snuffles*, a very irritating rhinitis that often causes excoriation of the upper lip; a coppery maculopapular rash of the palms and soles of the feet, the back, and the buttocks; and a rash and lesions around the mouth, anus, and genitals. The child may show evidence of pseudoparalysis. This immobility of the extremities is due to pain caused by inflammation of the periosteum of the long bones.

A more extensive examination of the child may reveal osteochondritis and hepatomegaly and/or splenomegaly. Blood studies will show evidence of anemia. Blood serology tests may or may not show positive reactions before six months of age and therefore are not as reliable during this period as they are in later life. However, the spirochete often can be seen in slides made from the exudate in the lesions.

If a nurse observes an infant in the nursery or well-baby clinic with an irritating nasal discharge, this should be reported immediately. It is possible that this symptom, called _____, might be indicative of a _____ infection. Further observations of the baby's skin, especially the palms of the hands and soles of the feet, may reveal a coppery _____ rash.

"snuffles";
syphilitic;

maculopapular

In addition, it is important to examine the baby's _____ and around the _____ areas for lesions.

mouth;
anal and genital

The baby's inability to move its extremities is not a true _____ but is due to the _____ caused by inflammation.

paralysis; pain

Three types of laboratory diagnostic measures used for more differential diagnosis are _____, _____, and _____.

blood; x-ray;
slide studies of exudate
from lesions

Slide studies done before the child is _____ months old are not reliable.

six

Treatment by penicillin, tetracycline, or erythromycin should result in a swift and complete cure. It is essential that the mother be treated also and that any sexual contacts that she may have had undergo treatment as well. It is the responsibility of every nurse and doctor to report any cases of venereal disease of which they are aware. The health department must follow all leads concerning direct and indirect contacts to prevent further spread of this condition.

It is necessary to reassure the mother that she will not be prosecuted or stigmatized in any way for having this infection. If the mother is under age, it also may be necessary to reassure her that her parents will not be told and that treatment can be given to her without their permission.

The drugs of choice in the treatment of syphilis are _____,   penicillin;

_____, or _____.   erythromycin; tetracycline

When caring for an infant with congenital syphilis, the nurse must follow extreme aseptic measures. The use of gloves is recommended because the organisms are found in the infant's skin and mucus membrane lesions. Although the organism has a short life-span when removed from the host, it can and does penetrate minute breaks in the skin or mucus membranes of another person (infant, parent, or staff member).

The ill child may have feeding problems. The painful effect of the snuffles, the constant irritation produced by the mucoid material running from the nose, and the painful lesions make it difficult for the child to suck. The nares should be cleared gently before feeding and the skin protected by a soothing ointment to alleviate some of the painful excoriation. It should be remembered that the child may be in severe pain due to the inflammation of the periosteum of the

_____ bones and therefore should be handled very gently,   long

with support given to the extremities.

Congenital syphilis may be transmitted actively through the

_____ found in the lesions of the _____   spirochete; mouth;

and anal area as well as from the _____ exudate.   nasal

Because of the oral pain and the constant rhinitis, the child may

have difficulty in _____.   sucking

The _____ must be carefully supported when the   extremities

child is moved or held.

Obviously, a child born with congenital syphilis presents many medical problems that require adept and careful nursing care. Likewise, nursing intervention measures should be geared toward meeting the many emotional needs, such as feelings of guilt, anger, and isolation from each other, which the parents may have at this time.

Syphilis always has carried much social stigma with it. Thus, it is essential that you identify your feelings about this disease and if necessary get help in dealing with them. For example, if your approach to the parents is either overtly or covertly judgmental, you will be unable to help them to discuss and come to terms with their anger. You may find that the appropriate nursing intervention for this family is a social service referral. Remember, the nurse may call upon other members of the health team when indicated to help restore a measure of homeodynamics to the family system.

Impetigo of the newborn is a skin infection that can be caused by either a streptococcus or a staphylococcus. At one time, it was one of the most feared infections of newborn nurseries because it spread rapidly. Bathing in Phisohex seemed to make this infection almost extinct. However, with the disuse of Phisohex in nurseries, due to the recent research and the fear of damage to the neonate, the nurse again must be alert to symptoms of impetigo and recognize her responsibilities in preventing this disease from occurring and/or spreading.

The infection is manifested by the eruption of small red papules, which usually are found in places, such as the groin, axilla, and neck, where moist surfaces meet. The fluid in the vesicles soon becomes purulent, and the papule has a reddened area surrounding it. These early red elevations are not to be confused with the normal skin eruptions found on the newborn, and when unsure of their nature, it is wise to transfer the infant into an isolation nursery as a precautionary measure until a more definitive diagnosis can be made.

Impetigo is a neonatal infection of the _____.

    skin

The causative organism can be either _____

or _____.

    a streptococcus;

    a staphylococcus

The first lesions usually are found in creases and places where _____ surfaces meet. The lesions are filled with a _____ exudate, through which the infection is transmitted. Therefore, an infant suspected of having impetigo should be _____ immediately.

    moist;

    purulent;

    isolated

The treatment for impetigo is to remove the crusts that form on the vesicles as they rupture and then to expose the area to a heat lamp. Some physicians may order hexachlorophene baths followed by the application of bacitracin or neomycin ointment. The prognosis for complete recovery without scarring is excellent.

Because of the highly contagious nature of impetigo, strict isolation measures should be instituted and carried out. As previously stated, the baby is placed in isolation, and thus is separated from the mother at a point when the crucial postpartum "taking-in, taking-hold" phase is to begin. The mother may exhibit anger and may blame the hospital, doctor, or nursing staff for the baby's infection. Of necessity, careful explanations should be given to both parents as to the reasons for the separation as well as the nature of the infectious process. Since the father also may be experiencing frustration and anger, he should be allowed to express his feelings and should be supported throughout this difficult experience.

The treatment for impetigo is to denude the _____

from the lesions and then expose the area to _____.

Medicinal ointments such as _____ and _____

may be ordered as well as _____ baths.

Separation of mother and infant adds an unexpected

_____ for the parents.

Nursing intervention must deal with the needs of the baby, such

as _____, asepsis, and therapy, as well as helping

the parents to deal with the stress associated with maternal-infant

_____ and the illness of the baby.

crusts;

heat

bacitracin; neomycin;

hexachlorophene

stressor

isolation;

separation

POST-TEST   Indicate whether each statement is true or false by circling the appropriate letter. Then turn to page 507 and see how well you have done.

1. The most common cause of a nonhealth state in the neonate is acrocyanosis.   T   F

2. Infection in the neonate can be intra- or extrauterine in origin.   T   F

3. Often it is difficult to identify symptoms of infection in the newborn.   T   F

4. Parents always understand why their child has been removed from the regular nursery.   T   F

5. The nurse is a casefinder for early diagnosis and treatment of neonatal infection.   T   F

6. A common extension of infection in the newborn is to the meninges.   T   F

7. Thrush is caused by a gonococcus.   T   F

8. Thrush is an infectious, oral neonatal infection.   T   F

9. Thrush always is identified in the nursery and thus treated quickly.   T   F

10. Ophthalmia neonatorum, if untreated, can cause irreversible blindness.   T   F

11. Ophthalmia neonatorum can be prevented entirely by postdelivery care of the neonate's eyes with either silver nitrate or antibiotic ointment.   T   F

12. Congenital syphilis is completely preventable.   T   F

13. The mother with syphilis need not be treated early in pregnancy because the fetus does not develop symptomatology.   T   F

14. Impetigo of the newborn resembles no other rash.   T   F

15. The infant suspected of having impetigo always must be isolated.   T   F

16. The exudate in the blebs is the vehicle for the transmission of impetigo.   T   F

17. Impetigo is particularly dangerous because it is very difficult to treat.   T   F

In the specific areas with which you had difficulty, return to the material and review.

BIBLIOGRAPHY Babson, S. Gorham and Ralph C. Benson: *Management of High-Risk Pregnancy and Intensive Care of the Neonate*, 2d ed., C. V. Mosby Co., St. Louis, Mo., 1971.

Brown, William J., "Acquired Syphilis, Drugs and Blood Tests," *American Journal of Nursing*, Vol. 71, pp. 712–715, April 1971.

Burchall, Dorothy, "Caring for the Infant with Thrush," *American Journal of Nursing*, Vol. 61, pp. 55–56, Jan. 1961.

Infection Control in the Hospital, 2d ed., American Hospital Association, Chicago, 1970.

Klaus, Marshall and John Kennell, "Mothers Separated from Newborn Infants," *Pediatric Clinics of North America*, Vol. 17, pp. 1015–1035, Nov. 1970.

Larsen, Bryan and Rudolph P. Galask, "Protection of the Fetus Against Infection," *Seminars in Perinatology*, Vol. 1, No. 2, pp. 183–193, April 1977.

Standards and Recommendations for Hospital Care of Newborn Infants, 5th ed., American Academy of Pediatrics, Evanston, Ill., 1971.

Vaughan, V. and R. James McKay: *Nelson Textbook of Pediatrics*, 10th ed., W. B. Saunders Co., Philadelphia, 1975.

PRETEST ANSWERS 1. Infection   2. An oral infection caused by *Candida albicans*   3. Vagina   4. White, curdlike patches in the mouth   5. 1 percent gentian violet; mycostatin   6. Delivery, as the infant descends through the birth canal   7. Gonococcus   8. Penicillin I.M. to the neonate   9. Placenta   10. Fourth; antibody and inflammatory response develops   11. Any of these: maculopapular rash on palms of hands, soles of feet, back, and thighs; lesions of mouth and perianal area; snuffles; hepatomegaly; splenomegaly; anemia; pseudoparalysis; osteochondritis; periostitis   12. Penicillin; erythromycin; tetracycline   13. An infectious skin rash   14. Staphylococcus; streptococcus   15. Red papules with a purulent exudate found on opposing moist surfaces   16. The exudate in the blebs   17. Denuding the area; applying heat; applying bacitracin or neomycin ointment   18. Mother-child separation

POST-TEST ANSWERS 1. F   2. T   3. T   4. F   5. T   6. T   7. F   8. T   9. F   10. T   11. T   12. T   13. F   14. F   15. T   16. T   17. F

CHAPTER SEVEN
CONGENITAL INTERRUPTIONS

OBJECTIVES *Define congenital anomaly.*

Define teratogenic agent.

Identify two aberrations of the gastrointestinal system.

Identify three types of congenital heart disease.

Identify three aberrations of the central nervous system.

Identify three aberrations of the urinary system.

Identify one aberration of the musculoskeletal system.

Identify symptoms and medical management of the aberrations.

Identify nursing intervention when caring for a child with a congenital malformation.

GLOSSARY *Anomaly:* A deviation from normal
Coarctation: A narrowing
Teratogenic agent: A nonspecific stressor, such as a drug or an organism, which
causes congenital malformations

PRETEST   In the spaces provided, fill in the word or words that best complete(s) the statements. Then turn to page 518 and check your answers.

1. A congenital anomaly is _____

    _____ .

2. A teratogenic agent is _____

    _____

    _____

    _____ .

3. A cleft lip is _____

    _____ .

4. A cleft palate is _____

    _____ .

5. Two nursing problems in caring for an infant with cleft lip and/or cleft palate

    are _____ and _____ .

6. Two nursing evaluations that may give evidence of imperforate anus are

    _____ and

    _____

    _____ .

7. The greatest cause of death in the first year of life is _____

    _____ .

8. The effect of a spina bifida depends upon the _____

    _____ and the _____

    _____ .

9. Anencephaly is _____

    _____ .

10. Hydrocephalus is a condition in which there is too much

    _____ in the _____ .

11. A nursing observation that would help in the diagnosis of hydrocephalus is

    daily _____

    _____ .

12. The infant with hydrocephalus presents a _____ problem

    and must be protected from _____ .

13. Hypospadius is _____

_____

_____.

14. Congenital dislocation of the hip often can be identified by the nurse during

_____

_____.

15. A nursing measure that must be taught to the mother of an infant with congenital dislocation of the hip is _____

_____.

Developmental interruptions that result in some form of obvious or concealed handicap at birth are called *congenital anomalies*. These accidents can be caused by many and various things. Teratogenic agents, for example, drugs and organisms such as the rubella virus, usually cause damage to the unborn child during the period when the organs and systems are developing, or during the first trimester. Poor maternal nutrition or injury can result in damage to the fetus during any time before birth. Genetic aberrations also can cause congenital anomalies.

The resulting developmental aberration can wreak havoc in the lives of the nuclear and the extended family. As we have previously discussed, parents expect a normal, healthy child no matter what the maternal fantasy has been. They are completely unprepared to have to deal with the emotional and financial strain brought about by the birth of a child who may need long-term care, surgery, or special educational facilities or one who may not survive at all.

The parents are concerned about how the child looks, how he or she will be accepted by friends and family, how they have felt in the past about crippled or retarded children. If there are other children in the family, the parents must explain this handicapped child and be asked questions that, many times, cannot be answered: Why did it happen? Whose fault is it? Will it happen again?

When there are no concrete reasons that can be given for the handicapping condition, parents often will seek an explanation for themselves. They will endeavor to find reasons why this terrible thing happened to them. They will think, "It must be my, his, or her fault." If the baby was unplanned or unwanted initially, it is often looked upon as Divine punishment.

The staff, too, often have many problems in dealing with the child and his parents. The nurse may feel sad—"This poor baby doesn't have a chance"; uneasy; or angry at the parents who, as in the case of drug abusers, may be somewhat responsible for the plight of the child, or who seem to reject the baby. It is essential that the nurse recognize these feelings as stressors that must be dealt with before there can be any positive interaction with the parents.

The parents should be shown the baby and the defect, if obvious, as soon as possible. The situation must be faced in reality rather than allowed to grow in fantasy.

Teratogenic agents can be _____ or _____ that can cause developmental damage during intrauterine life.

drugs; organisms

Developmental aberrations may be _____ at birth or may be concealed, with the _____ of the handicap as the warning that something may be wrong.

obvious;

symptoms

Not only the parents but also the _____ family | entire

will be affected by the birth of a handicapped child.

Often staff also are affected by the _____ of | stress

having to work through their own feelings.

In dealing with their feelings, parents may evidence rejection, withdrawal, grief, or denial. The nurse must carefully identify the defense mechanisms being used by the family, introduce reality after the grief has been worked through, and capitalize on the positive adaptive mechanisms that have been identified.

We will not discuss any of the handicapping conditions in detail but rather will talk of some of the interruptions in the various systems of the neonate caused by genetic or environmental aberrations. Let us first identify some of the obvious interruptions, such as those of the gastrointestinal tract. A *cleft lip* and/or *palate* are seen as soon as the child is born. This malformation is considered to be primarily genetic in origin and is evidenced by a unilateral or bilateral fissure in the upper lip and a fissure in the center of the roof of the mouth which may involve both the hard and soft palates. The infant looks very disfigured and often is frightening to the parents. This anomaly can be corrected very successfully with surgery. The problems in the nursery are mainly ones of feeding and prevention of infection due to aspiration of feedings. An asepto-syringe or Brecht feeder may be used to feed the baby. Some babies feed well with a long, soft nipple. Frequent burping is necessary. The baby must be held in a sitting position while being fed so that aspiration is prevented. As soon as possible, the mother should be introduced to the feeding techniques as well as to the normal care of the neonate.

It is felt that cleft lip and palate are _____ in | genetic

origin.

A cleft lip is a unilateral or bilateral _____ in the | fissure

upper lip.

A cleft palate is a fissure in the _____ of the | roof;

mouth and may include _____ palates. | both

The parents may become _____ by the appearance | frightened

of their baby and also may feel revulsion initially.

You are able to tell these parents that the malformation can be

successfully _____ by surgery. It might be helpful to | repaired

show them before and after pictures when they indicate that they are

ready to discuss the future.

The components of physical care that are important in this condition are concerned with _____ problems and the prevention of respiratory _____.

feeding;

infection

Another aberration in the gastrointestinal system which may occur is *imperforate anus*. This may be caused by a membrane that covers the anal orifice or by atresia of the rectum without any anus. An imperforate anus usually will be identified on the admission evaluation when taking of the temperature of the baby is attempted. It also will be revealed by the lack of passage of meconium. Surgery will correct this aberration. In the absence of an anus, the initial surgery usually is a colostomy, a temporary measure until a complete repair can be done. This type of surgery needs much explanation and allowance of venting of feelings for the parents.

An "imperforate anus" means that there is no patent opening into the baby's _____.

rectum

This aberration may be present because a _____ covers the anal opening from the rectum or there is no _____ at all.

membrane;

anus

This anomaly can be picked up by the nurse when attempting to take the baby's _____ rectally or revealed by the lack of the passage of _____ by the baby.

temperature;

meconium

Surgery must be done to _____ this problem.

correct

Interruptions in the circulatory system seen in various kinds of *congenital heart disease* may or may not show immediate symptoms. Congenital heart disease is responsible for more first-year deaths than is any other anomaly. The symptomatology will depend upon the type of problem the child has. For instance, cyanosis will be present only if there is a right-to-left shunt. Some of the most common defects will become apparent as the communication closes between the two atria and the aorta and pulmonary artery. These defects are: persistence after birth of the opening between the aorta and pulmonary artery (*patent ductus arteriosus*); persistence after birth of the opening between the two atria (*patent foramen ovale*); and *coarctation of the aorta*, which can be suspected when palpation of the femoral arteries fails to reveal pulsation. In any instance, when congenital heart defects are suspected, x-ray examination studies and/or cardiac catheterization are indicated so that a differential diagnosis can be made. Should the nurse observe cyanosis or dyspnea, she should immediately administer oxygen to the baby and notify the physician.

⇩

The symptoms of congenital heart disease _____ or   may;
_____ be immediately apparent.   may not

These anomalies cause more deaths than do any other anomalies
during the _____ of life.   first year

A patent ductus arteriosus means that the opening between the
_____ and _____   aorta; pulmonary artery;
did not close after birth. A patent foramen ovale means that the
opening between the _____ and   right atrium;
the _____ did not close after   left atrium
birth.

Coarctation of the aorta can be suspected when pulsation of the
_____ artery is not felt.   femoral

The nurse should immediately administer oxygen to the neonate
if she observes _____ or _____.   cyanosis; dyspnea

Congenital anomalies of the neurological system create problems
concomitant with their extent and location. *Spina bifidas* are malformations of the bony portion of the spinal canal; through these defects,
the spinal fluid, meninges, and/or nerve roots may protrude. Spina
bifidas vary from the mild, innocuous *spina bifida occulta*, which is
evidenced by a dimple in the lumbar spine and has no effect on the
individual, to a *meningomyelocele*, in which the meninges and the spinal
cord are outside the spinal column. The latter defect results in a protruding sac on the baby's back which must be protected from injury
and infection. This defect may be repaired surgically later, and the
residual neurological damage to extremities and systems will depend
upon the location and extent of the lesion.

Spina bifidas are malformations in the _____   bony;
portion of the spinal canal through which _____ fluid,   spinal;
_____, and/or _____ roots may protrude   meninges; nerve;
in a visible _____.   sac

This sac must be protected from _____ and   infection;
_____.   injury

Anencephaly is an anomaly in which part of the skull and brain
is absent; this condition is incompatible with life.
Hydrocephalus is a condition in which there is interference with
circulation of cerebrospinal fluid. The fluid accumulates in the ventricles

of the brain, causing the head to become large, with tense, bulging fontanels, and often causes mental retardation. One usually treats this anomaly by tapping the fluid to relieve intracranial pressure and by later introducing a catheter into the cerebral ventricle, passing it into the carotid artery or sometimes the peritoneal or pleural cavity, thus feeding the fluid into the circulatory system, where it can be disposed of.

It is important for the nurse to take a careful measurement of the circumference of the baby's head daily in order to make various diagnoses and observe the fontanels for bulging. The child should be held in an upright position for feeding, fed slowly, and prevented from aspiration because vomiting is seen more frequently with increased intracranial pressure. Since the infant's head is very heavy, the nurse must take care to move the head in alignment with the body. The head must be kept dry and protected from infection and pressure areas.

The anomaly in which part of the brain and skull is absent is called _____.

> "anencephaly"

In hydrocephalus, the head grows abnormally _____ because of a collection of _____ fluid.

> large;
> cerebrospinal

Measurement of the circumference of the baby's head is a _____ measure as is care in feeding and protection from _____.

> nursing;
> infection

The most common anomalies of the genitourinary system are *cystic or polycystic kidneys*. However, since the symptoms do not appear during the neonatal period, these conditions do not fall within the scope of this book.

Hypospadius is a condition in which the urinary meatus opens somewhere on the underside of the penis because the urethra does not extend to the end of the penis. The repair usually is done before the child enters school to prevent the trauma of his peers taunting him for being different. It is essential that babies with hypospadius not be circumcised because the foreskin is utilized in making the repair. This fact will have to be explained carefully to parents of the Jewish and Moslem faiths, to whom circumcision is a religious ritual.

Undescended testicles may be identified by the small appearance of one side of the scrotum. Although the testes normally may not be completely descended into the scrotum for several weeks after birth, the parents should be told about the possibility of an undescended testicle so that they will follow through with an examination in a well-baby clinic or at the office of the pediatrician.

The most common malformations of the kidneys are not obvious early in life. These are _____ or _____ kidneys.

cystic; polycystic

"Hypospadius" means that the urethra has not extended to the _____ of the _____ and that it opens on the _____ of the penile shaft. Babies with this condition should not be _____ because the foreskin is necessary for a later repair.

end; penis;

underside;

circumcised

A scrotum that appears to be smaller on one side than on the other may be evidence of an _____ testicle.

undescended

The last system that we will mention is the musculoskeletal system. If you remember the newborn evaluation, you were asked to check the extremities for _____ and to flex the baby's thighs on the abdomen to see if the knees reached the same _____ and _____ easily to a frog position. This was done to rule out the possibility of *congenital dislocation of the hips*. This condition is caused by the head of the femur not fitting properly into the acetabulum. Dislocation of one hip is more common than involvement of both, and it is found more often in girl babies than in boy babies. Early recognition and treatment are essential to prevent permanent damage.

equal movement;

height; abducted

X-ray examination may show evidence of a potential or full dislocation. In a potential dislocation, the head of the femur does not rest securely in the shallow joint. It is important to maintain the joint in abduction by positioning the legs, using a padded diaper placed between the buttocks and the diaper and held in place or using a Frejka splint.

If the head of the femur does not fit properly into the acetabulum, the baby is said to have a congenital _____ of the _____.

dislocation;

hip

If congenital hip dislocation is untreated, when the child attempts to stand and walk, the head of the femur will become more and more displaced and there will be severe malformation of the head and socket of the joint. When the child is older, surgery may be necessary for open reduction and a cast will be used to immobilize the joint position.

POST-TEST Indicate whether each statement is true or false by circling the appropriate letter. Then turn to page 518 and see how well you have done.

1. A congenital anomaly is caused only by teratogenic agents. T F

2. The entire extended family needs help in dealing with the crisis precipitated by the birth of a defective child. T F

3. A cleft lip can be unilateral or bilateral. T F

4. A cleft palate is a fissure only in the soft palate. T F

5. Feeding the child with a cleft lip and/or palate can present difficulties. T F

6. Feeding a child with a cleft lip and/or palate is too difficult for an inexperienced person such as the mother to do it. T F

7. Cleft lip and palate can be repaired surgically. T F

8. An imperforate anus need not be repaired until the child is ready to start school. T F

9. Absent femoral pulses are normal in the neonate. T F

10. A patent foramen ovale is a persistent opening between the aorta and the pulmonary artery. T F

11. The condition in which there is interference with cerebrospinal fluid circulation is called "hydrocephalus." T F

12. Hydrocephalus occurs when the head of the neonate becomes abnormally enlarged. T F

13. Hypospadius is caused by a short urethra. T F

14. Hypospadius is repaired by utilization of the foreskin. T F

15. Congenital dislocation of the hips may be classified as complete or potential. T F

16. The infant with congenital dislocation of the hip should be kept with the legs abducted. T F

In the specific areas with which you had difficulty, return to the material and review.

BIBLIOGRAPHY Kapke, K., "Spina Bifida: Mother-Child Relationships," *Nursing Forum*, Vol. 9, No. 3, pp. 310–320, 1970.

Lewis, C., "Nursing Care of the Neonate Requiring Surgery for Congenital Defects," *Nursing Clinics of North America*, Vol. 5, pp. 389–397, Sept. 1970.

Nadler, Henry L., "Prenatal Diagnosis in Inborn Defects," *Nursing Digest*, pp. 63–67, Fall 1976.

Nitowsky, Harold, "Prenatal Diagnosis of Genetic Abnormality," *American Journal of Nursing*, Vol. 71, pp. 1551–1557, Aug. 1971.

Ross, R. B. and M. C. Johnston: *Cleft Lip and Palate*, Williams and Wilkins Co., Baltimore, 1971.

Vaughan, V. and R. James McKay: *Nelson Textbook of Pediatrics*, 10th ed., W. B. Saunders Co., Philadelphia, 1975.

PRETEST ANSWERS

1. A developmental interruption that occurs in utero   2. A nonspecific stressor, such as a drug or an organism, which causes a congenital anomaly   3. A unilateral or bilateral fissure in the upper lip   4. A fissure in the center of the roof of the mouth   5. Feeding problems; infection   6. Taking rectal temperature; observing lack of passage of meconium   7. Congenital heart disease   8. Location of the lesion; extent of the lesion   9. The absence of part of the skull and brain   10. Cerebrospinal fluid; ventricles   11. Measurement of the circumference of the head   12. Feeding; infection   13. The opening of the urinary uretha on the underside of the penis   14. Nursing evaluation of the newborn   15. To keep the leg abducted

POST-TEST ANSWERS

1. F   2. T   3. T   4. F   5. T   6. F   7. T   8. F   9. F
10. F   11. T   12. T   13. T   14. T   15. T   16. T

CHAPTER EIGHT
DOWN'S SYNDROME

OBJECTIVES *Identify the three types of chromosomal aberrations that can result in a child with Down's syndrome.*

Identify the differences in the heredity patterns of nondysjunction and translocation types of Down's syndrome.

Identify the major problems associated with Down's syndrome.

Identify observable physical characteristics associated with Down's syndrome.

Identify nursing intervention in situations in which a child with Down's syndrome has been born.

PRETEST In the spaces provided, fill in the word or words that best complete(s) the statements. Then turn to page 525 and check your answers.

1. Another name for Down's syndrome is _____.

2. Down's syndrome in a child born to a mother over thirty-five years of age usually is caused by the chromosomal aberration called _____.

3. Down's syndrome in the child of a younger mother is usually caused by the chromosomal aberration called _____.

4. Children with Down's syndrome have some degree of _____ _____.

5. These children may have physical complications such as _____ _____, _____, _____, or _____.

6. Some of the observable physical characteristics of Down's syndrome are _____, _____ _____, _____ _____, _____ _____, or _____ _____.

Many genetic errors can occur as a result of the parents' chromosomal makeup or problems during meiotic division. The resulting interruptions in the development and growth of the child will, of course, depend upon the chromosome affected. We already have discussed genetic makeup and the effects of carrier states, dominant and recessive genes, and abnormal chromosomes on the fetus. As an example of these effects, we will briefly discuss *Down's syndrome*, an autosomal aberration known in lay terms as "Mongolism."

This syndrome is the result of chromosomal aberrations. The most common type of Down's syndrome is trisomy 21 due to nondysjunction. *Nondysjunction* is the abnormal division of the chromosomes so that one cell contains an extra chromosome. When this occurs during meiosis, the ovum ends up with an extra 21 chromosome. Following fertilization, the total chromosomes number 47 instead of the normal 46, and the child will be said to be trisomic for chromosome 21. Trisomy 21 occurs more frequently in children born to women over thirty-five years of age than in children of younger mothers and occurs through chance rather than because the parent is a carrier. There usually is no familial history with this type of chromosomal error; it is felt that it may be due to the age of the ova causing nondysjunction. Investigations are also being carried out to determine if the incidence may be related to diagnostic x-rays of the abdomen, viruses, or high levels of thyroid autoantibodies. However, this type of interruption can occur with mothers of any age.

Other chromosomal aberrations that occur less frequently and cause Down's syndrome are translocation and mosaicism. *Translocation* tends to be familial and occurs frequently because one parent is a carrier, having one of the number 21 chromosomes attached to another chromosome. The parent has the proper chromosomal complement, but at the time of gametogenesis, another number chromosome with the 21 chromosome attached carries this extra genetic material to the offspring so that the child has three 21 chromosomes. The type of translocation that occurs most frequently involves the D group, and the most prevalent chromosomal attachment is with the number 14 chromosome. The number 15 is occasionally involved, but the number 13 rarely is. These D-group translocations show a 50 percent inheritance rate, whereas G-group translocations involving the number 22 chromosome are infrequent but are 100 percent inherited. *Mosaicism* is very rare; at fertilization the embryo has 46 chromosomes, but as the embryo develops, one cell line alters to 47 chromosomes. The child usually does not have the severe characteristics of Down's syndrome.

If there is nondysjunction of a chromosome, it usually will occur during _____.

    meiosis

"Nondysjunction" means that the chromosome pair does

_____ divide in the ovum so the child has _____

chromosomes instead of the usual _____.

     This extra chromosome is number _____ and the condition

gives rise to _____ syndrome.

     Translocation occurs because the parent is _____.

     When translocation occurs, the extra 21 chromosome is

_____.

     When mosaicism occurs, it happens following _____,

and 47 chromosomes are found _____.

not; three;
two (pair)
21;
Down's
a carrier
attached to another chromosome
fertilization;
in one cell line

All children with Down's syndrome have mental retardation, but the degree of retardation varies with the individual child and the children who have mosaicism are only mildly retarded. There are 100 different stigmata associated with Down's syndrome, and each child may exhibit some of these characteristics. At birth, if the child has six or more of the cardinal signs, a diagnosis can be made on clinical observations. Some of these symptoms are a short, thick neck; a flat face when seen in profile; dysplastic ears, small and misshapen; slanted eyes; a simian palmar crease; poor muscle tone; marked depression of the Moro reflex; space between the big toes and the other toes; and a tongue that protrudes because the oral cavity is small. The hands are short and broad, with an incurved fifth finger. Associated with Down's syndrome are many complications, such as cardiac problems, ventricular septal defect, duodenal atresia, leukemia, and visual problems.

     Some of the observable characteristics shown by most of the

children with Down's syndrome are a neck that looks _____

and _____, a nose that seems to have a _____

profile, dysplastic _____, and slanted _____.

The muscles are _____; the

tongue often _____. In addition, the hands are

_____ and have an _____ fifth finger. Additional

problems often associated are _____,

_____, _____

_____. _____, and _____.

short;
thick; flat;
ears; eyes;
atonic (limp);
protrudes;
broad; incurved;
cardiac problems;
visual problems; duodenal
atresia; leukemia

The best time to inform the parents that their child has Down's syndrome is the time of delivery. At this time the parents need much support and assistance in dealing with their feelings of grief and loss that their child is not normal. The staff should be available to answer the parents' questions and to assist the parents in looking at the situation realistically. The family senses the feelings of the staff, and it is important that the nurses be cognizant of their own feelings before interacting with the parents.

Usually a genetic work-up is done to determine the type of Down's syndrome the child has. The nurse must interpret this information to the parents while helping them to handle their feelings, often those of guilt and anger. The parents must determine their ability to bring up this child, and, at times, placement in an institution is the choice.

When the family is taking the child home, it is important to refer them to a community agency for nursing follow-up to help them cope with the many difficult situations that will arise. Parents may be referred also to their local group of parents with retarded children; this type of interaction often is most helpful. Feelings are shared, and the best information on ways of handling the teaching of developmental tasks often comes from other parents who have dealt with a similar situation.

The nurse's role is very broad when working with parents who face a lifetime of daily living with and planning for a handicapped child. Parents can begin to move into a positive family relationship only if the staff, present when the baby is born, help the family to utilize all of their adaptive mechanisms by first allowing them to grieve, talk, cry, and vent their feelings of anger and frustration.

POST-TEST Indicate whether each statement is true or false by circling the appropriate letter. Then turn to page 525 and see how well you have done.

1. Down's syndrome always is an inherited characteristic. T F

2. Children with Down's syndrome are mentally retarded. T F

3. Down's syndrome of the nondysjunction type is most common in children born to women over thirty-five years of age. T F

4. There are physical characteristics common to children with Down's syndrome. T F

5. If the parents seem to adjust well, there is no need to refer them for follow-up services. T F

6. The parents of a child with Down's syndrome should be made aware of genetic counseling services in their areas. T F

7. It is better to keep the parents of handicapped children isolated because they seem to capitalize on their sorrow and grief when they are with other parents in the same circumstances. T F

In the specific areas with which you had difficulty, return to the material and review.

BIBLIOGRAPHY Barnett, Henry L.: *Pediatrics*, 15th ed., Appleton-Century-Crofts, New York, 1972.

Caplan, Gerald, "Emotional Crisis," in Albert Deutch and Helen Fishbein (eds.): *The Encyclopedia of Mental Health*, Vol. 2, Franklin Watts, New York, 1963.

Owens, Charlotte, "Parents' Reaction to Defective Babies," *American Journal of Nursing*, Vol. 64, No. 11, pp. 83–86, 1974.

Stewart, Janet, "Genetic Counseling," in Joy Clausen et al. (eds.): *Maternity Nursing Today*, McGraw-Hill Book Co., New York, 1973, pp. 234–237.

Vaughan, V. and R. James McKay: *Nelson Textbook of Pediatrics*, 10th ed., W. B. Saunders Co., Philadelphia, 1975.

PRETEST ANSWERS 1. Mongolism   2. "Nondysjunction"   3. "Translocation"   4. Mental retardation   5. Cardiac problems; duodenal atresia; leukemia; visual problems   6. Any of these: short, thick neck; broad hands; curved fifth finger; flat face in profile; simian palmar crease; atonia; dysplastic ears; slanted eyes; protruding tongue (due to small buccal cavity); space between the big toe and the other toes; depressed Moro reflex

POST-TEST ANSWERS 1. F   2. T   3. T   4. T   5. F   6. T   7. F

CHAPTER NINE

PREPARATION FOR RETURNING TO THE FAMILY

OBJECTIVES *Identify the special parental tasks that must be accomplished when the parents take home a child with a health interruption.*

Identify the nursing intervention with these families in the community.

PRETEST   In the spaces provided, fill in the word or words that best complete(s) the statements. Then turn to page 531 and check your answers.

1. When the parents have a child with an interruption in health, the parent-child relationship should be initiated _____

    _____ .

2. If the baby is going home and needs special treatments, _____

    _____

    _____ .

3. Before discharge from the hospital, the nurse can help the family plan

    _____ .

4. If the child needs many treatments and medical visits, an important aspect

    is _____ .

5. Parents' groups offer _____ .

6. Parents may not want to go out with the child if _____

    _____ .

7. A nursing responsibility to the community is to _____

    _____

    _____ .

When a child is born with an interruption in health, be it a congenital anomaly, prematurity, or respiratory distress syndrome, a crisis state is produced. The family must mobilize their various resources and adaptive mechanisms to begin to deal with this situation. In this unit, we have discussed the initial responses of the parents to their child and some of the common feelings and concerns that the parents have. Often the hospital stay for the mother is three to four days whereas the infant who has a problem remains in the hospital for a much longer period of time. During the initial contact with their child it is hoped that the parents will have begun to establish the parent-child relationship and begun their parental roles, with the support of the staff, who have provided time and support to the family.

The parental responsibilities outside the hospital will often determine whether the parents can visit and participate in the care of their child. Ideally, the parents will come to the hospital frequently so that their relationship with their child is ongoing and so that they know what normal behavior for their child is. If any special treatments or procedures are necessary, the parents will have learned and practiced them at the hospital.

As the time for the discharge of the baby arrives, it is very helpful for the nurse to sit down with the parents and discuss a day's activities, including all the feedings and the special treatments. It is very helpful to have a public health nurse who will visit the family at home, come to the hospital and meet the parents, and join in with the hospital staff as plans for discharge are made. In this way, the parents are supported in their task of learning child care and they also are aware that they have resource persons available to them.

If the child has a problem, the parents often feel that further difficulties may arise, such as with the premature infant; often the parents are so anxious that the baby gain weight that the infant soon becomes overweight. Instances also occur in which so much attention is directed to the infant that the other siblings are left out and neglected. A visiting nurse often can assess that these difficulties are occurring and help the family to adjust more effectively before this pattern of behavior creates a severe problem.

Often medical expenses are very high for families, especially if treatments and doctor's visits are ongoing and multiple hospitalizations are necessary. Referrals to social and government agencies that make available funds and assistance for special types of equipment are important.

The parents can receive much support from a parents' group, such as the Association for Retarded Children. The members of the group share their experiences and reactions and in this way help the parents to recognize that others have gone through much the same experiences that they are dealing with. Also, the parents thus learn methods of dealing with the children's specific problems and discover ways of doing things or accomplishing goals with more ease. For example, if the child has a feeding problem, the parents in the group will relate ways that have worked for them, such as how the other siblings were involved and shared in the family problems so that there was no neglect. Directions also are given for help with agencies and finances.

One of the major difficulties for the parents of a child with an anomaly is introducing their new child to the members of the extended family and their friends. Often there are comments such as "If you hadn't done this during pregnancy" or "Your family is responsible for this," which can cause much trauma to relationships and to the feelings of the parents as "good parents." If the child has visible anomalies, then comments often are made by strangers or acquaintances. The parents then tend to withdraw and shelter the child and themselves from these abuses. The nurses and parents' groups can provide support and help the parents strengthen their egos so that they can cope more effectively with these difficulties.

Another nursing responsibility is to teach and inform the community about health interruptions and to clarify misconceptions and misinformation. The nurse can be the go-between who provides information to various people—religious advisers, employers, and others. In this way, the parents' resumption of their responsibilities and roles is supported and the various strengths of the families are utilized as they adapt to the new stressors.

There are instances where families take the child home and become increasingly disorganized and disrupted; when this situation occurs, crisis intervention is necessary to assist the members of the family.

POST-TEST Indicate whether each statement is true or false by circling the appropriate letter. Then turn to page 531 and see how well you have done.

1. It does not matter at what time the parent-child relationship is initiated.   T   F

2. The parents do not need to understand about the special treatments for the child.   T   F

3. The nurse can assist the family in realistically organizing the care of the child at home.   T   F

4. A visiting nurse can assess if there are problems arising among the members of the family once the baby goes home.   T   F

5. The family often needs referrals to agencies for assistance.   T   F

6. The extended family always is supportive of the nuclear family.   T   F

7. There is a need for nursing to teach the public about various interruptions in health.   T   F

In the specific areas with which you had difficulty, return to the material and review.

BIBLIOGRAPHY   Korones, Sheldon B.: *High-Risk Newborn Infants*, C. V. Mosby Co., St. Louis, Mo., 1972.

Miller, Mary-Ann and Dorothy A. Brooten: *The Childbearing Family: A Nursing Perspective*, Little, Brown, Boston, 1977.

Vaughan, V. and R. James McKay: *Nelson Textbook of Pediatrics*, 10th ed., W. B. Saunders Co., Philadelphia, 1975.

PRETEST ANSWERS   1. Early in the hospital   2. The parents should learn and practice these in the hospital   3. For daily activities   4. Finances   5. Support and assistance   6. The public makes comments about the child   7. Inform the people of the community about health interruptions

POST-TEST ANSWERS   1. F   2. F   3. T   4. T   5. T   6. F   7. T

Student: _____

THE HIGH-RISK NEONATE

When caring for, observing, or simulating experiences concerned with the high-risk neonate, the student will:

			Satisfactory			Unsatisfactory		
*	1. Identify three infants who may be classified as high-risk because of any of the following: 　　a.　Prematurity							
	b.　SGA or LGA							
	c.　Maternal diabetes							
	d.　Maternal infection							
	e.　Premature rupture of membranes							
	f.　Blood incompatibility							
	g.　Neonatal respiratory problems							
	h.　Congenital defects							
	i.　Low Apgar score							
	j.　Dystocia							
*	2. Select an infant that you consider to be high-risk and determine priorities of care							
B	3. Differentiate between the characteristics of a normal neonate and a premature infant							
*	4. Identify special nursing measures related to a specific high-risk situation other than prematurity							
*	5. Discuss the symptoms of neonatal hypoglycemia							
*	6. Rank-order nursing actions in the event of: 　　a.　Neonatal hypoglycemia							
	b.　Neonatal respiratory distress							
	c.　Neonatal jaundice in the first 24 hours							
*	7. Discuss and/or carry out the care of a newborn in an isolette (Temp., O_2)							
*	8. Prepare or discuss the preparation of an infant for phototherapy							
A	9. Discuss the physiologic reasons for phototherapy							

Instructor Comments:

Student: _____

			Satisfactory						Unsatisfactory				
*	10.	Explain to a specific mother the meaning of jaundice in her baby											
*	11.	Prepare a mother whose infant is being put under the bilirubin lights with appropriate information											
A	12.	Discuss the condition and needs of a premature infant with the mother/father/family											
B	13.	Identify the reasons for and/or include the parents in the care of a high-risk infant											
*	14.	Communicate information to the mother/parents regarding the status of their high-risk infant											
B	15.	Obtain feedback from the mother/parents regarding her/their understanding of the progress and prognosis of the high-risk infant											
A	16.	Identify the sociocultural meaning of the birth of a specific high-risk infant to the mother/family											
*	17.	Identify the stages of grief and grieving in the mother/parents/family of a high-risk infant											
*	18.	Identify ways in which the nurse can support the mother/parents/family in their positive adaptation mechanisms											
*	19.	Discuss and/or carry out the nursing role when an Rh infant is being transfused											
*	20.	Assist the mother/father/family to prepare for discharge without the baby											
*	21.	Discuss the preparation of the home to receive an infant after a prolonged hospital stay											
A	22.	Utilize other health team members to meet specific identified mother/family needs											
*	23.	Report the status of a high-risk infant (as appropriate)											

Instructor Comments:

**UNIT VII
EXAMINATION**
The following multiple-choice examination will test your comprehension of the material covered in the seventh unit of this program. Remember, you are not competing with anyone but yourself. Therefore, do not guess in order to answer the questions; if you are unsure, this means that you have not learned the content. Return to the areas that give you difficulty and review them before going on with the examination.

Circle the letter of the best response to each question. After completing the unit examination, check your answers on page 541 and review those areas of difficulty.

1. The best time to inform the parents that their baby has a disability is:
   a. During the first day postpartum
   b. Only after there has been a thorough work-up of the condition
   c. Only if both parents are together
   d. Following the delivery in the delivery room

2. If you noticed the father and grandparents of a premature infant standing for long periods in front of the premature nursery window looking at the baby, you would:
   a. Stop, smile, and comment on how cute and perfectly formed the baby is
   b. Stop and suggest that they were only increasing their anxiety by being there so much . . . and that the doctor would let them know if the baby became worse
   c. Suggest that they seem concerned and ask if they would like to sit down and talk about it
   d. Suggest that they spend more time with the mother, who is very anxious and really needs them

3. The nutrient that the premature infant needs in greater quantity than the normal full-term baby is:
   a. Proteins
   b. Fats
   c. Carbohydrates
   d. Minerals

4. In caring for a premature infant who is in an incubator, it is important for you to know that the prevention of retrolental fibroplasia depends upon:
   a. Covering the baby's eyes during the administration of oxygen
   b. Administering oxygen at the lowest possible concentration for the shortest possible periods of time
   c. Keeping the humidity in the incubator at a constant high level
   d. Administering an oil-based protective eye drop when oxygen concentrations have to be high

5. You would suspect that the infant is postmature if you observed which of the following signs?
   a. Lethargy and large size—over 8 pounds

      b.   Soft skin and a lot of vernix caseosa
      c.   Dry, parchment-like skin and a small size—under 6 pounds
      d.   Lanugo and little hair on the head

6.   If the infant is postmature, then you would observe the infant for signs of difficulty because, during labor, there is a high incidence of:
      a.   Ruptured membranes
      b.   Fetal distress
      c.   Tetanic contractions
      d.   Prolonged labor

7.   You are working in the high-risk nursery, and an infant is admitted with the probable diagnosis of respiratory distress syndrome. The factor that is deficient, producing poor lung expansion, is:
      a.   Hemoglobin
      b.   Amino acids
      c.   Surfactant
      d.   Factor VIII

8.   You are working in the nursery, and a premature infant is admitted with respiratory distress syndrome. You are aware that there is a deficiency of surfactant, which produces the characteristic finding:
      a.   Cardiomegaly
      b.   Atelectasis
      c.   Hyperbilirubinemia
      d.   Bronchiole occlusion

9.   A clinical sign that often occurs when the infant has RDS is:
      a.   A decreased respiratory rate
      b.   Peripheral vasodilation, producing a flushing of the skin
      c.   A loss of tissue turgor due to fluid loss
      d.   Retractions during respirations

10.   If you observe an infant and see nasal flaring, this is an indication of:
      a.   Tachycardia
      b.   Hypotension
      c.   Respiratory distress
      d.   Fever

11.   In the nursery you may observe that the infant with RDS has an expiratory grunt. This adaptive mechanism serves to:
      a.   Reduce the amount of inspired air
      b.   Increase the residual capacity, thereby increasing the pO_2
      c.   Increase the cardiac output
      d.   Decrease the need for oxygen

12.   One of the first signs that indicates that the infant has respiratory distress syndrome is:
      a.   An increased respiratory rate of over 60 per minute

b. Peripheral vasodilation
c. A loss of body fluid
d. A tense, hyperactive response to stimuli

13. Cephalohematomas indicate that:
    a. The head of the baby has been misshapen temporarily during the process of adapting to the bony pelvis
    b. There is bleeding under the periosteum of the infant's skull bones
    c. There is a soft swelling on the scalp of the newborn
    d. There is intracranial hemorrhage in the neonate

14. When caring for the infant with a subarachnoid hemorrhage, you would:
    a. Provide adequate stimuli for the infant
    b. Keep the head elevated
    c. Keep the infant flat on the side so that he will not aspirate
    d. Provide cool O_2 so that the metabolic rate is slowed

15. During delivery, the infant sustained injury and developed Erbs-Duchenne paralysis. The prognosis is good following the treatment, which is:
    a. Traction applied to the affected arm
    b. Immobilization of the arm in abduction
    c. Application of a splint to the arm
    d. No intervention and a return of function within four weeks

16. Thrush in the newborn is caused by contact with which infection in the mother's vagina during the birth process?
    a. A gonococcal infection
    b. A trichomonas infection
    c. A spirochete infection
    d. A *Candida albicans* infection

17. Clinical signs of congenital syphilis include:
    a. Poor feeding and high-pitched cry
    b. A coppery rash on the hands and feet and snuffles
    c. Anemia and poor kidney function
    d. A purulent discharge from the eyes

18. If an infant in the nursery develops impetigo contagiosa, it is important to:
    a. Isolate the infant
    b. Structure the feeding schedule
    c. Cover the area with bandages
    d. Apply alcohol to the blebs

19. If the infant develops impetigo contagiosa, the infection can be spread because organisms are present:
    a. In the nasopharynx
    b. In the blebs
    c. In the urine
    d. In the feces

20. Hydrocephalus occurs when:
    a. There is trauma to the head during the birth process
    b. Circulation of the cerebrospinal fluid is interrupted
    c. The infant is delivered by forceps
    d. Delivery is by cesarean section

21. Signs of hydrocephalus in the infant include:
    a. Depression of the fontanels
    b. Premature closure of the sutures
    c. Increasing head circumference
    d. Increased size of the tongue

22. Spina bifida occulta was noted in a newborn. You are aware that this interruption of the spinal column will lead to:
    a. Severe neurological deficit
    b. A mild neurological problem found in the lower extremities
    c. No consequence unless another problem is complicating this
    d. A problem that needs immediate surgery

23. When an infant has a meningomyelocele, this means that:
    a. There is only an incomplete closure of the vertebrae
    b. There is an incomplete closure of the vertebrae, and the dura protrudes through this opening
    c. There is an incomplete closure of the vertebrae, and the spinal cord, nerve roots, and dura protrude through
    d. There is an absence of vertebrae, and the spinal cord stops at the thorax area

24. When an infant with a disability is separated from the parents, the parents have difficulty in:
    a. Establishing a relationship with the infant
    b. Wanting to visit the infant
    c. Maintaining an interest in the child
    d. Relating to the staff who are caring for the infant

ANSWERS TO UNIT EXAMINATIONS

Unit I: 1. b   2. c   3. d   4. a   5. c   6. d   7. c   8. b
9. d   10. b   11. a   12. b   13. a   14. b   15. d   16. b
17. c   18. d   19. d

Unit II: 1. b   2. a   3. c   4. c   5. d   6. b   7. a   8. b
9. c   10. c   11. b   12. d   13. b   14. c   15. d   16. c
17. c

Unit III: 1. c   2. c   3. d   4. c   5. c   6. a   7. b   8. c
9. c   10. a   11. c   12. d   13. a   14. a   15. b   16. b
17. c   18. a   19. c   20. b   21. c   22. a   23. c   24. c
25. c   26. b

Unit IV: 1. a   2. d   3. b   4. d   5. c   6. b   7. d   8. c
9. d   10. c   11. d   12. a   13. a   14. b   15. d   16. b
17. d   18. b   19. b   20. a   21. b   22. d   23. c   24. d
25. a   26. b   27. c   28. b   29. a

Unit V: 1. c   2. c   3. d   4. c   5. b   6. b   7. b   8. b
9. b   10. a   11. a   12. d   13. a   14. a   15. b   16. c
17. b   18. d   19. d   20. b   21. c   22. c   23. b   24. d
25. c   26. b

Unit VI: 1. a   2. b   3. c   4. b   5. d   6. a   7. c   8. c
9. b   10. c   11. a   12. d   13. b   14. c   15. c   16. c
17. d

Unit VII: 1. d   2. c   3. a   4. b   5. c   6. b   7. c   8. b
9. d   10. c   11. b   12. a   13. b   14. b   15. b   16. d
17. b   18. a   19. b   20. b   21. c   22. c   23. c   24. a

INDEX